Go, and Do Thou Likewise

A HISTORY OF
CORNELL UNIVERSITY-NEW YORK HOSPITAL
SCHOOL OF NURSING
1877–1979

Shirley H. Fondiller, EdD, RN, FAAN

All photos courtesy of Medical Center Archives of NewYork-Presbyterian/Weill Cornell except the following:

Lillian Wald's Henry Street "family"
Public health nurse home visit

ISBN 13: 978-0-615-14173-2

Contents

Acknowledgments

The preparation of a serious historical work involves a long period of investigation that at best becomes a solitary pursuit. At the same time, the success of such an effort depends not only on the acquisition and interpretation of authoritative sources, but also on the observations of key people who have been parties to the School's history. The recollections of many individuals are invaluable because they build on the available archival data and generate fresh insights.

To begin with, I extend my appreciation to the Alumni Association, which granted me the privilege of researching the history of one of the most prestigious schools in the nation. I am particularly grateful to the many nurses—alumni and others—that graciously shared with me their experiences as students, faculty, and staff. I value the support of Mary Millar, chair of the History Committee. She generously gave her time and suggestions that helped to identify sources, sustain the momentum, and fuel the investigator's enthusiasm. Another outstanding resource was Louise Hazeltine, who authenticated much of the data, including the chapters that covered the years of her tenure at the school. As a reviewer of the entire manuscript, nurse historian Dr. Eleanor Krohn Herrmann superbly carried out the task of a providing a substantive and constructive evaluation. My gratitude also goes to Arlene Shaner, reference librarian at the New York Academy of Medicine, and Professor Emeritus Jerome Ziegler of Cornell University, who provided information that illuminated the study.

Indispensable to the research were the transcripts of in-depth interviews conducted mainly in the early 1970s by the late Doris

Schwartz. Her searching questions of the nursing leadership of the school, after it was integrated into the Cornell system, produced some compelling information. Other transcripts of Dr. Judith Allen's later interviews with former faculty and deans added greatly to the data cited in official records. A special thank you goes to Dr. Alma Woolley and Mary Millar for their skillful editing of several audiotapes, which involved a scrupulous and tedious process.

Cheryl Wurzbacher is recognized for her role in getting the book into print. Her skill and experience in book design and production were essential throughout the final steps of the publication process.

Finally, I acknowledge James Gehrlich, head of archives at the New York Weill Cornell Medical Center Archives, and his assistant Elizabeth Shepard, to whom I will be forever indebted for the courtesy, cooperation, and assistance rendered to me throughout the research process. Jim's genuine interest in the project and his extensive knowledge of nursing and medical history became a strong motivator as I pursued the work. Furthermore, his review of the documentation and his expertise in formatting the completed work helped me prepare it in its final form.

Shirley H. Fondiller,
EdD, RN, FAAN

Preface

In 1991, the Board of Directors of the Cornell University-New York Hospital School of Nursing Alumni Association began to consider the possibility of the dissolution of the organization. Membership was declining as a consequence of the School's closure in 1979. Without the addition of alumni from successive graduating classes, financial support was declining. The future of the association was in jeopardy.

The Board issued a call to alumni for ideas about how to dispose of any remaining organization funds in the event of dissolution. Alma Schelle Woolley '54 repeated a proposal that she first put forth in 1984 for the creation of a lasting legacy. She proposed that the Alumni Association support a project to "collect, preserve, and disseminate the history and collected wisdom of the School of Nursing during its existence." In her proposal to the Board, Dr. Woolley elaborated as follows:

> There is much to be learned from the history of the New York Hospital School of Nursing. Its rise, its development, and its fall are closely related to many societal factors, and its influence on the profession was considerable at the time. Although we all have strong emotional ties to the School, there are many cogent reasons for preserving the history in scholarly form, among them the accurate documentation of its existence for future scholars of nursing and history.

Two histories had already been written, with the first presented on the occasion of the School's 75th Anniversary in 1952. Written by Helene Jamieson Jordan, the special assistant in public relations for nursing, it was published as a small volume by the Society of The New

York Hospital. The work described the School from its inception in 1877 until 1952. In 1982, Dr. Judith Cormack Allen, a 1960 graduate, completed her doctoral dissertation on the history of the School when it operated as a collegiate program affiliated with Cornell University from 1942 to 1979.

Between 1994 and 1998, the Board laid the groundwork for preparing a comprehensive history of the School by determining the nature and condition of the School's documents and memorabilia housed at the New York Weill Cornell Medical Center Archives. The Board also took steps to restore and preserve photographs.

In 1999, under the leadership of President Pam Bennett-Santoro '77, the Board established a history committee to ensure that the archival material was catalogued and preserved in a safe and accessible place. Further, the Board directed the committee to provide a detailed scholarly record of the School that included its beginnings, evolution, and accomplishments in the nursing profession and health care. Strong support for attaining these objectives continued when Linda Vecchiotti '71 became president in 2004.

The search for a qualified individual interested in writing a history of the School began in 2001, and the following year resulted in the selection of Shirley H. Fondiller, EdD, RN, FAAN, a seasoned writer and nurse historian. Her scholarship, diligence, and enthusiasm were essential throughout the intense process of research, analysis, writing, and revision.

We are indebted to Dr. Fondiller for helping us realize our goal of creating an accurate, scholarly, and readable record of the illustrious contributions of the Cornell University-New York Hospital School of Nursing to nursing practice and education in service to society.

Mary L. Millar, MA, RN
Class of 1954
Chair, History Committee

Foreword

The history of nursing education is an important lacuna in general histories of nursing in the United States. Although numerous articles, monographs, and other historical works have been written about individuals, events, and concerns of the times, the complete story has yet to be told of how the nursing profession entered the mainstream of American education. The 100-year history of the Cornell University-New York Hospital School of Nursing was undertaken and supported by its Alumni Association, not only to preserve the history of this remarkable school, but also to add an important piece to the history of nursing education as a whole.

Nursing was a latecomer to academia. Although universities and faculties were established in traditional disciplines by the 12th and 13th centuries, nursing education did not begin to become integrated into the system until the early 20th century, and our long struggle for recognition in the academic community continues today.

As part of public history in the United States, nursing education can cite many accomplishments in the realm of health care policy. Nurses have used the political system to support their education, improve working conditions, and advance the profession. Subsets of nursing education also have lent themselves to historical inquiry in the public domain in such areas as federal aid for nursing education, nursing practice acts, and state licensure and education laws.

Biographies of prominent people frequently reveal significant information about economic conditions, social and political environments, and the prevailing thought patterns of the past. Scholarly studies of schools of nursing are important because they reflect the profession's social history, particularly in relation to education, the struggle of women for autonomy, and, of course, public health and the health care system.

Nurse scholars offer a compelling case for the development of nursing through an historical lens. Faculty members who value nursing history convey their appreciation to students as opportunities arise in both classroom and clinical teaching. Historical inquiry is included in most research courses, but aspiring investigators soon discover the dearth of available funding to support their projects. Other problem areas include the lack of mentors and advisors with dissertation expertise and the difficulty encountered in accessing the required source material.

Schools of nursing present a special case since relatively few have attempted to document their history. Most programs that have closed have retained or warehoused their records, but sorting through reams of data is a challenging task for the researcher. Some schools have published hastily compiled histories at the time of their demise, while others have written brief histories for anniversaries and fundraising campaigns. Although necessarily celebratory, focusing on the accomplishments of the schools and their illustrious alumnae, these histories may be of dubious scholarly quality.

Each year it becomes more important that the history of nursing education be written and that records be carefully collected and preserved in archives. In an age of electronic communication, it is crucial for our profession to place a high priority on the preservation and storage of records. Computerization has tended to obliterate the kind of carefully written documentation of thought processes, discussions, decisions, and events formerly preserved by nursing leaders. As a consequence, source materials are becoming increasingly scarce. Nursing's present history will not be supported by the kind of papers and correspondence that have helped to chronicle our past.

More than two decades ago, noted nurse historian Dr. Eleanor Krohn Herrmann shared her thoughts in the following commentary on the importance of studying nursing history:

> Our profession and our practice continue to evolve. Our students will participate in this process of evolution, but they will perceive it as evolution only if they look behind and beyond the

present. It is my belief that the uncertainties of the future and the tribulations of the present can be borne with better grace, more stamina, and a clearer vision by those who understand the past.

Alma S. Woolley, EdD, RN
Class of 1954
Professor Emerita
Georgetown University, Washington, DC

The above foreword was written by Dr. Woolley for the present work, a few months before her untimely death on December 17, 2005. Her devotion to nursing education and history will remain an inspiration to future scholars.

Introduction

"Whatever withdraws us from the power of our senses; whatever makes the past, the distant or the future, predominate over the present, advances us in the dignity of our thinking beings."

—Samuel Johnson, in
A Journey to the Western Islands of Scotland

In its broadest sense, the history of the Cornell University-New York Hospital School of Nursing parallels the development of the nursing profession, while responding to the health concerns of the day in a climate of discovery at a progressive teaching hospital. Covering a span of 100 years, the work identifies the major players in the School's remarkable evolution as well as events in American life that transformed it into a compelling social force. Most revealing are the values and attitudes of the times as shown in the relationships of the nurses with the hospital and medical hierarchy, particularly in the early Victorian period, and later with University officials when the School became part of the Cornell system. As the story unfolds, the indomitable spirit of the pioneers in the nursing and medical community is illuminated as they valiantly cope with disease, epidemics, wars, and other crises.

Decades before the training school for nurses came into its own in 1877, The New York Hospital claimed an impressive record of service as the second hospital in the nation and the first and only general care facility in New York City. On June 13, 1771, George III, King of England, granted a charter of corporation entitled, "The Society of the Hospital in the City of New York in America" (later changed to The

Society of The New York Hospital). At the time, scarcely 20,000 inhabitants were concentrated in the lower tip of Manhattan.

Operated by a Board of Governors elected by the Society's members, the Hospital opened in 1791. In the ensuing years, the patient population consisted of poor people, while private physicians saw those who could afford medical treatment at home. From 1792 to 1856, The New York Hospital received grants from the State of New York ranging from $5,000 to $22,500. Some reimbursement to the institution came from the U.S. Treasury Department for the care of indigent seamen certified by the U.S. Customs Office.

Described as a handsome structure among shaded lawns and majestic elms, the Hospital was situated on five acres of land on lower Broadway not too distant from the original site of the city's almshouses. Among the 87,465 patients treated between 1792 and 1849, half were first-born Americans while the other half had emigrated from several European countries. After the Hospital began admitting patients, it organized clinical lectures for young men interested in a career in medicine. Dr. Valentine Seaman, a prominent surgeon who gave instruction on maternity care and practice on the wards, introduced the first systematic courses for the training of nurses, midwives, and attendants in 1798. Prior to the advent of modern nursing, women employed to care for the sick were untrained, often incompetent, and classified as servants.

The 19th century ushered in an age of activism, with medical progress and humanitarian reforms dominating American society. Scientific medicine expanded, generating the transformation of medical theory and practice. Along with the decline in the number of indigent patients, The New York Hospital modified its mission to one of emphasizing cure rather than merely providing a place to house the sick. In 1870, it suspended operations, and seven years later the second New York Hospital, located between 15th and 16th Streets West of Fifth Avenue, opened its doors with a 250-bed capacity. As part of the complex, nurses' quarters became the home of a small group of pupil nurses entering the training school for the first time.

The present research scrutinizes the early recruits, who became pupil nurses drawn into a world of service and sacrifice markedly different from the lifestyle enjoyed in previous years. What motivated the privileged young women to enter nursing, and how did they survive the rigors and deprivations of the training period? Also, what was the role of the heads of the Training School and the nature of their leadership in administering the program while coping with the discipline and controls exerted by the institution's power elite? When a principal did not capitulate to the wishes of the governing or medical boards, which usually meant a lowering of standards, the individual was asked to leave or "gracefully" resign.

A significant part of the School's history is recorded in the achievements of the pioneering graduates, who recognized many of the burgeoning health and social concerns in the larger society and bonded together in alumni associations and national organizations. To protect nurses and the public, they were committed to improving health care by strengthening educational programs and promoting legislative initiatives to regulate practice. A number of those extraordinary women journeyed to lands, near and far, to establish training schools which had begun to proliferate in the nation by the end of the 19th century. The public health nursing movement took off, headed by the incomparable Lillian Wald and her "family" of Henry Street nurses, along with Mary Beard, in a position of great influence with the Rockefeller Foundation, and Annie Goodrich, who became the foremost educator of her time and an international leader. The contributions of such illustrious graduates gave a structure to nursing and to the School, whose fine reputation endured for decades to come.

The compelling wartime experiences of the graduates come alive through graphic descriptions in their memoirs, letters, and logs. A childhood acquaintance with Clara Barton, the Civil War heroine and a family friend, inspired Anne Williamson to volunteer as a Red Cross nurse in the Spanish American War. The reader accompanies the young nurse on her assignments as she responds to the harrowing conditions in the army camps, and tries to soothe her patients suffering from the typhoid fever sweeping through the wards.

Another distinguished graduate, Julia Stimson, rose to the position of chief nurse of the American Red Cross Nursing Services in France during World War I, which merited her the American Distinguished Service Medal bestowed by General John Pershing. The copious letters to her family not only provide insight into the travesty of war, but also show the courage, humor, and humanity of the nursing volunteers. Stimson continued to serve the profession with numerous accomplishments, which included a major role in World War II when a fresh crop of graduates of the School of Nursing responded to the call to military service.

The study chronicles the series of events leading to the establishment of The New York Hospital-Cornell Medical Center Association in 1927. Created by a joint agreement between the Society and the University, their partnership held great promise for the advancement of patient care, education, and research. Five years later, construction of an expansive Medical Center was completed and the Society's third Hospital, an imposing structure towering over East 68th Street, was ready to admit patients. The historic occasion brought great joy to the nursing community with the opening of a splendid-looking, 16-story nurses residence located adjacent to the Hospital and the Medical College.

A salient feature of the history involves the long struggle of the School to acquire university status during the Great Depression. The efforts of Anna Wolf, the visionary nursing director, are recounted in her relationships with officials of the two parent organizations, which determined policy and the conduct of the School when it became a reality in 1942. In the succeeding years, the work shows the gradual but steady development of the Medical Center in establishing modern methods of research and greater knowledge of preventive medicine and social service. A growing contingent of highly qualified nurse faculty began initiating innovative programs, joining those whose nursing service projects employed the latest medical and surgical procedures.

Critical to understanding the history of the School is the exploration of the role and relationships of the three nursing deans since 1946, and the outcomes generated by their respective leadership styles. What were their strengths and weaknesses? How did they interface with influential officials in the Medical Center and the University? How did they relate to faculty, students, and alumni? Credible conclusions can be drawn from a compendium of rich information found in class records, documents, correspondence, writings, and other memorabilia.

As the story of the Cornell University-New York Hospital School of Nursing approached journey's end, the fateful decision to terminate its programs in 1979 might have seemed inevitable in light of the failure to secure an endowment. To lessen or end speculation, an in-depth analysis of the contributing factors, internal and external, that hindered the goal, may put the matter to rest or at least produce some interesting observations. Thus, the question as to whether the demise of one of the oldest and most prestigious schools of nursing in the United States could have been prevented continues to be an intriguing proposition.

CHAPTER 1

A Training School for Nurses: Its Time Had Come

The founding of The New York Hospital Training School for Nurses in 1877 turned out to be an auspicious event, following closely on the establishment of the training school at Bellevue Hospital, the first in the nation functioning on the principles espoused by Florence Nightingale. Each school operated in New York City and revealed commonalities as well as dissimilarities created by the governance of one nursing program in a public institution and the other in a voluntary hospital (1). Both schools of nursing made their entry into society in an era characterized by Mark Twain as the "Gilded Age," which highlighted the nation's poverty and riches, political corruption, reform movements, and changing roles of women.

The most compelling reasons for establishing the training schools were the rise of scientific medicine and the beginning movement toward the emancipation of women, accelerated by the Crimean War in England and the Civil War in the United States. In the medical world, theory, training, and practice underwent transformation with Lister's principles of asepsis in surgery, an outgrowth of Pasteur's germ theory. The dramatic demonstration of sulfuric ether as an anesthetic, performed at Massachusetts General Hospital on October 16, 1846, by Dr. William T. G. Morton, a dental surgeon, hastened the momentum toward the professionalization of medicine. After the event, The New York Hospital successfully introduced the anesthetic the following month and later contributed $500 to a fund established for Morton (2).

With great strides underway in medical and scientific exploration, the public perception of nurses could not have been more unfavorable, with nursing viewed primarily as menial work and unacceptable employment for well-bred ladies. No one fit that stereotypic model more aptly than the disreputable and fictional Sairey Gamp, whom Charles Dickens immortalized in *Martin Chuzzlewit* (3). During the 1850s, physicians at The New York Hospital lamented the abuse and neglect inflicted upon patients, while criticizing the class of people employed as nurses (4).

Not until the 1860s, when Florence Nightingale proposed sweeping reforms that led to the emergence of modern nursing, did the process of changing the image of nursing assume some significance. Proper training seemed essential to enable nurses to organize and provide instruction to others, as well as improve patient care. An integral part of Nightingale's model was the training of the district nurse, the forerunner of public health nursing (5). She viewed nursing as one of the highest callings of women—second only to motherhood—and believed that nurses should control their teaching and practice (6).

Responding to the burgeoning scientific discoveries of the 1800s, the Board of Governors of The Society of The New York Hospital collaborated with the Board of Health in efforts to control epidemics of cholera, yellow fever, typhus, and other life-threatening diseases (7). They recommended that iron beds be installed and that clean white sheets be used for the patients (8). In addition, they urged construction of a sewage system to improve sanitation (9).

Eager to offer safer obstetrical care, the Governors took an important step in 1801 to become associated with the Lying-in Hospital (10). Concerned also about the care of the mentally ill, they recommended that a building be constructed separate from the Hospital; and, in 1821, Bloomingdale Asylum opened on Morningside Heights where the Low Library of Columbia University now stands (11). Flourishing over the years with a patient population comprised of the upper and upper middle classes, and the addition of several more buildings, the asylum relocated in 1894 to White Plains, New York, where the name was eventually changed to Bloomingdale Hospital (12).

Following the move, the Governors instituted a school of instruction in White Plains to train male and female attendants. In 1912, a complete reorganization established a nursing school that was registered with the State Department of Education, and affiliations were arranged with The New York Hospital (13). The program was terminated in 1936, the year the Board of Governors renamed Bloomingdale Hospital The New York Hospital-Westchester Division (14).

Prior to building Bloomingdale Asylum, the Hospital had maintained a department to house psychiatric patients. It was one of the first institutions in the United States to recognize mental illness as a disease—at a time when most people regarded those afflicted as animals or degenerates. Some years later, a feisty retired New England schoolteacher became one of the early pioneers in mental health reform, and began a crusade meriting national and international recognition. Incensed by the inhuman conditions at the Middlesex House of Corrections in East Cambridge, Massachusetts, Dorothea Lynde Dix launched an 18-month survey in 1841 of every jail and almshouse in the state (15). Following a visit to Bloomingdale Asylum in New York, she reported her observations to the Board of Governors, who acknowledged the "inadequate arrangements for bathing, heating, and ventilating in the Loges . . . and that funds should be raised immediately to improve and enlarge the buildings" (16).

In one respect, Dix's role as a spokesperson for the mentally ill illustrated how the functions of women working out of social benevolence—referred to as the "charitable impulse"—played in the national political system (17). During this period, rumblings of liberation from women relegated to domestic activities that were supported by a male-dominated society began to echo throughout the nation. Women of all classes responded to the ideal of egalitarianism, although they could not yet vote.

In 1848, at a historic women's rights convention at Seneca Falls, New York, convened by Elizabeth Cady Stanton and Lucretia Mott, an enthusiastic assembly issued its Declaration of Sentiments. Based upon the Declaration of Independence, the document enunciated several demands of these early activists. Under the remarkable leadership of Stanton and her partner Susan B. Anthony, who joined the cause in 1851, the campaign for Women's Suffrage began its long struggle. Although both women devoted 50 years to further their mission, they did not live to see the passage of the 19th Amendment in 1920 giving women the right to vote.

The advent of the Civil War profoundly affected the status of women in American life. Imbued with a national consciousness, many women launched fund-raising efforts to support the U.S. Sanitary

Commission and armies in the field. Florence Nightingale played a major role as an expert and consultant in the care of the sick and wounded. From her solitary boudoir in Victorian England, nursing's *grande dame* gave continuous advice to the Commission and the women who took charge of relief work (18).

At the outset of the war, Dix was appointed superintendent of Union Army nurses. Helping to set up and staff infirmaries in the Washington, D.C. area to care for the soldiers, she received strong support from the Women's Central Association of Relief (WCAR), which became New York City's agency for coordinating the contributions of women to nursing (19). WCAR established a bureau for the registration of candidates eligible for medical instruction as nurses. A committee was formed that arranged with The New York Hospital and Bellevue Hospital to train 91 nurses (20).

The concept of volunteerism dominated 19th-century American life, and nowhere was this trend more evident than in the formation of Ladies Aid Societies that demonstrated the response of women to the national calamity (21). Many volunteers from the North and South offered their services, furnishing the soldiers with food, clothing, and shelter; while those with nursing experience provided care and comfort to the men and established schools of nursing after the war (22). Among the women involved in the war effort, perhaps no one has been portrayed more heroically than Clara Barton, the daughter of a farmer from North Oxford, Massachusetts, and the lone lady in black silk who became known as the "Angel of the Battlefield" (23). She independently operated a large relief operation arranging for supplies for the army and established the first national cemetery at Andersonville in Georgia. Recuperating from nervous prostration after the war, Barton spent a few years in Europe learning about the International Red Cross, and then spearheaded the founding of the American Red Cross on her return to the States (24).

An accomplished writer, Louisa May Alcott served briefly as a nurse in the Civil War; she was assigned in December 1862 to the Union Hotel Hospital in Washington, D.C.'s Georgetown section. Her reading of Nightingale's *Notes on Nursing* hardly prepared the sensitive young woman for the appalling conditions—sagging beds for the suffering men and the long corridor "haunted with evil smell" (25). Later, while convalescing at the family home in Concord, Massachusetts, Alcott wrote *Hospital Sketches*, based on her recollections and letters to relatives, which graphically described her wartime experience through the eyes of "Nurse Periwinkle" (26).

During the war, several gentlewomen served as voluntary nurses at The New York Hospital. In an arrangement with the military authorities in New York State and Washington, D.C., the institution received and treated soldiers en route to the battlefield and those wounded on returning home. One of the buildings was set aside to provide free treatment to more than 3,000 men over a four-year period (27).

The Civil War represented a culmination of events that gave impetus to a movement already brewing in the country, one created by social and political conditions. Volunteerism was a crucial phenomenon because it expanded and demonstrated the competence of women and, for the first time, resulted in the acceptance of those who worked outside the home. The stage was now set for the evolving modern service professions such as nursing and for the entry of the training school into American life.

A time of reconstruction followed the Civil War when the nation underwent a process of reunification. Striking developments ensued with financial prosperity, rapid population growth, urbanization, and industrial, technologic, and scientific advancement. The expanding capitalism dramatically transformed the economy and led to changes in the workplace, creating opportunities for women in their drive toward independence. As people from rural areas and immigrants from Europe poured into American cities, crowded urban slums began to spring up accompanied by a host of social and health problems.

Fortified with a newly acquired freedom that gave them respite from the restrictions of domestic life, women became socially active, organizing a variety of clubs ranging from sewing and dramatics to the arts and sciences. Many sought jobs as typists, secretaries, and factory workers, while others took the education route. Coeducational acceptance at state public universities and the establishment of liberal arts women's colleges such as Smith, Mount Holyoke, Wellesley, Radcliffe, Barnard, and Goucher drew young women eager to prepare for professional careers (28).

A policy of admitting female students existed from Cornell University's beginnings when Ezra Cornell, a Quaker of great vision, founded his university in 1868 in the scenic village of Ithaca, New

York, a thriving settlement of about 8,000 people (29). Designated as coeducational, the school, however, did not provide dormitory facilities for women until 1873, five years after admitting the first students. A man of strong ideals, Cornell believed he had created an institution in which any person could find instruction in any study (30). In his founder's address, he poignantly shared his dream:

> I hope we have laid the foundation of an institution that will combine practical work with liberal education, which shall fit the youth of our country for the professions, the farms, the mines, the manufactories for the investigations of science, and for mastering all the practical questions of life with success and honor (31).

Ezra Cornell had great confidence in his experiment in coeducation, although Andrew Dickson White, the University's first president, and the Board of Trustees were not too eager to contest the sex-sectarianism of that period (32). Cornell, however, remained firm in his intentions to include both sexes, as did his wife Mary Ann and their daughters, who had attended Vassar. When Jennie Spencer "hoisted up her skirts (to her ankles) and plodded her way up the hill to the Cornell campus," she became the first woman to matriculate to the University in 1870 (33).

Changing attitudes, as well as the policies of colleges and universities, generated movement toward the equality of women in the post-Civil War years. Other important developments evolved nationwide with improvements in the care of hospitalized patients. The marked influx of wealthy people residing in elegant mansions along New York's Fifth Avenue, plus the latest clinical information and treatments, attracted many physicians to the city (34). Specialization had begun to flourish in a competitive environment, and those who followed the trend dominated institutional positions (35).

At The New York Hospital, demographic changes became evident with the declining number of indigent patients and shifts in ethnic populations. For example, the number of patients of Irish descent decreased from 31.8% to 20.6%. Concerns plaguing the Board of Governors and the Medical Board deepened when the annual mortality rate continued at 10% (36). The high incidence of virulent infections, previously not experienced, prompted the Governors to appoint a committee to explore the problem. In their report, they concluded that atmospheric conditions caused the spread of disease and that the Hospital's buildings located in lower Manhattan were no longer suitable or adequate (37). They pointed out that scientific advances of the past two decades called for "a different type of structure as most conducive to the recovery of the sick" and a change of location seemed desirable (38). Furthermore, there would have to be some rethinking about the mission of the institution if the buildings were to become "places of cure rather than receptacles for sickness" (39).

A new locale may have seemed to resolve the problem, but public protest favoring the existing site delayed any action (40). While debate continued, an investigating committee of the Board of Governors reported a decrease in the Hospital's census, with the wards only half full due to insufficient funds of the poor. They believed that a relocation of quarters would provide accommodations to the poor at a rate of compensation to be determined by the financial resources of each applicant for relief (41).

On February 19, 1870, The New York Hospital closed, and construction started on a modern new building between 15th and 16th Streets west of Fifth Avenue. Conscious of their responsibility to maintain emergency care in their former location, the Governors established a small facility at a vacant police station in 1875, which was called the Chambers Street House of Relief (42). Designed to provide medical care to accident victims, provisions were also made for its first ambulance and a dispensary to handle minor and surgical cases. Several years after the House of Relief opened, it moved to new quarters on Jay and Hudson Streets (43).

During the early 1870s, a group of reform-minded society women, including former WCAR members, organized volunteer visiting committees. Impressed by Florence Nightingale's model for educating nurses, they charged the committees, consisting of men and women, to inspect public hospitals, almshouses, poor houses, and insane asylums in New York's 60 counties (44). In April 1872, the visiting committee formed at Bellevue Hospital observed that "little more could be done with the present system of nursing" (45).

With approval from Bellevue's Medical Board, the first training school in the nation was organized in the spring of 1873, and instruction began for the entering class of young women (46). The new training school committee estimated that $20,000 would be needed to finance the program's first year. Responding to a request for contributions, the Board of Governors of The New York Hospital authorized a donation of $500 along with furniture from the old hospital (47).

The Bellevue Training School operated under the direction of a committee of women known as Lady Managers who advised the Medical Board and worked closely with the superintendent of nurses (48). Early on, the Managers won the confidence of the Board and their relationship strengthened over the years. In 1877, the Medical Board passed a resolution stating that "the training school for nurses proved of incalculable benefit to Bellevue Hospital, by securing intelligent, skilled, and faithful nursing" (49).

Pupil nurses learned their craft diligently by "doing," functioning on a rigorous schedule of 12 hours daily on the wards six days a week, plus instruction and off-duty homework. Discipline, order, and cleanliness became the work ethic of the program and elevated the image of nursing by the example of the pupil nurses (50). The patients they attended were primarily charity cases consisting mostly of first-born Americans and English and German immigrants.

Bellevue's nursing program had been progressing well for four years when a committee appointed by the Governors of The New York Hospital completed arrangements for occupying their new buildings. Staffing would include physicians and surgeons committed to maintaining their lofty standards, which enhanced the Hospital's reputation as a leader in medical and surgical practice. Reporting to the Governors, the Building Committee boasted with pride that the facility would be "as safe as in the most luxurious home" (51). At the inauguration ceremony on March 16, 1877, architect George B. Post received high praise for endowing New York City with a structure that captured the public's imagination. A writer for *Harper's New Monthly Magazine* glowingly described the Hospital, particularly the solarium where "huge and beautiful fish filled the aquarium" (52).

What struck the eye immediately was the stunning exterior of red brick and consisting of a Mansard roof, as well as "wrought iron balconies and railing of lightening rods along the ridge pole . . . its ornamental ventilating towers looking like Flemish dovecotes, its stained glass and its Romanesque main door and the pillars rising beside its tall windows" (53). Designed to house about 250 patients, the seven-story building was equipped with two elevators running from the basement to the top floor. Among the latest furnishings and appliances rarely found in other hospitals, speaking tubes added to the convenience of patients who required the attention of the nurse occupied at the far end of a ward (54). In addition to the standard wards, private rooms with one or two beds were available for strangers "of a respectable class" who took ill while visiting New York City (55).

In his remarks at the opening ceremony, Dr. William H. Van Buren sparked a growing interest in launching a training school for nurses at The New York Hospital where he was a consulting surgeon. Observing that the preservation of life was the aim of surgery and medicine, he stated that good nursing must be recognized as necessary for recovery. Van Buren, who was also a professor of surgery at Bellevue, as well as a member of the Bellevue Medical Board, had visited hospitals in England and stressed "the advantage of having thoroughly trained nurses" (56).

Shortly after the new Hospital began operating, expectations for a training school for nurses moved toward realization when the Governors acted in 1877 to establish provisional rules in preparation for the event. Their intent was to recruit young women of high caliber who desired to devote themselves to a specialty with education provided therein (57). Grateful for the Society's earlier financial contribution to Bellevue's training program, the Lady Managers offered to lend their graduates to set up the proposed school and to suggest the first nursing superintendent (58). The Governors declined, however, having decided to make their own choice. In July 1878, they adopted the first bylaws of The New York Hospital Training School for Nurses, which clearly revealed an approach to governance different from the Bellevue pattern (See Appendix A) (59).

Accountable to the Board of Governors, the superintendent of the Hospital served as the chief administrative officer, overseeing its daily operations and enforcing regulations (60). Charged to perform general supervision throughout the institution, the Society's Visiting Committee recommended that a Conference Committee, consisting of three Governors and two members of the Medical Board, be appointed to address concerns affecting the School and the Medical Department (61).

In the summer of 1877, the Board of Governors engaged Juliet E. Marchant to be the first principal of the new School of Nursing for a term of one year. Shortly after she started, friction arose between this strong-minded woman and the Governors and the Medical Board. The School had barely opened when she submitted her resignation to the Visiting Committee, stating that "as circumstances now exist, it would be a waste of time to continue . . . there being no recognition of the School as such by the professional department nor of my position as its teacher" (62).

Marchant agreed to stay on until April 1878 when Jane A. Sangster, a Bellevue graduate, accepted the position after the Lady Managers recommended her to the Board of Governors. After four months, she presented a progress report and commented on the marked improvement in the students' system of work that had been lacking at the beginning of her administration. To elevate standards, Sangster instituted many lessons on practical instruction learned at Bellevue. What greatly disturbed her, however, were the crowded, unpleasant living conditions of the pupil nurses, which she considered a drawback to recruiting women of superior character, education, and refinement (63).

At the time of admission, the pupil nurses were required to sign an agreement obligating each one to stay the full 18 months and an additional six months if their services were needed (64). After a successful probationary period, they were guaranteed the sum of $10 a month for clothing and personal expenses. Throughout the program, the students were divided into three classes for three terms, spending the first six months as junior assistants, the next six months as senior assistants, and the third six months as head nurses.

In September 1878, the Conference Committee approved the design for the School's diplomas and ordered 100 engraved copies (65). The following January when the students passed their examinations conducted by the Conference Committee, the diplomas were awarded for the first time. That same month, another Bellevue graduate, Eliza W. Brown, replaced Sangster as the School's third principal.

At the outset of her term, Brown was distressed to discover that a substantial number of students were sick, largely due to the menial work of washing and cleaning in the Hospital (66). One of the Governors, David Coden Murray, reported to the Visiting Committee that the "duties of the nurses on the wards are so onerous they are breaking down in health" (67). Realizing that these tasks were necessary but interfered with proper training, Brown set out to improve the situation. When she approached the Governors about employing a maid for each ward, they acceded to her request and authorized the hiring of permanent workers to carry out the housekeeping duties (68).

During the summer of 1879, a subcommittee assumed the responsibility for planning a systematic course of instruction. One of its first recommendations was to shift the beginning terms of the Training School from January and July to April and October, to correspond with the Hospital's staffing schedule and provide more convenient arrangements for the course of lectures (69). For the autumn session, the subcommittee planned 40 lectures to be given by physicians at a rate of $15 compensation per lecture on the teaching of anatomy, physiology, sick room nursing and hygiene, medical and surgical emergencies, and surgical dressings (70).

In the early 1880s, the curriculum was modified to reduce the number of lectures to 28 by combining some of the subjects and including new ones. Obstetrical training was acquired at the State Emergency Hospital on Ward's Island and the New York Infirmary. One of the most popular courses enjoyed by the pupil nurses included the cooking lessons taught by Miss Pavla, a dietetic specialist (71).

Following Eliza Brown's resignation, the Governors selected Zilpha E. Whitaker, one of their own graduates, on October 2, 1882 (72). Within a few months, Whitaker related her concern to the Conference Committee about the dearth of candidates who could meet the required standards for admission. Citing the School's lack of visibility to the public, she prepared a historical sketch to be printed and distributed widely (73). Whitaker also approached the Conference Committee about selecting a suitable badge to be presented to each member of the graduating class. The badge would identify the nurse when working and serve as protection against the growing trend of young women falsely passing themselves off as graduate nurses (74).

At the June 1883 graduation exercises, the new regulation badge was awarded for the first time along with the diploma. It was not the initial emblem of the School, however. Some years earlier, the nurses had been issued a round gold medal that hung from a bar that displayed a bas-relief of The New York Hospital and the inscription

"Training School for Nurses, 1877." On the reverse side, the name of the student and date of graduation appeared (75).

When the Conference Committee issued its five-year report on the School, it singled out the improved appearance of the wards and the discipline and quiet of the surroundings (76). In 1883, the Conference Committee announced a total of 74 graduates since the program's inception, with nine pupil nurses abandoning the profession (77). That spring, the Governors furnished a library with a collection of literary works for the students (78).

Despite the favorable evaluation of the Training School, an underlying discord between Whitaker and the Board of Governors began to surface in 1885. Six months earlier, a registry had been instituted for the graduates seeking employment, mainly in private nursing. A procedure was developed that entitled the nurse to place her name on the register, which functioned under the direction of the principal (79). The issue involved an undermining of Whitaker's authority when the Governors transferred the registry for nurses, located in the School, to the office of Superintendent George Ludlam (80).

When the new policy went into effect, placing Ludlam in charge of the Bureau of Registered Nurses of the Training School, the Governors hailed it as a protection to both nurse and employer (81). Whitaker's position was further weakened by the Conference Committee's recommendation that the Training School operate as a department under the direct supervision of the Hospital. Even more disconcerting to her was the Committee's proposal that in lieu of the position of principal, a "supervising nurse" be employed to instruct the students and assign them to duty on the wards (82).

The changes to be incorporated into the 1886 bylaws prompted Whitaker to resign and accept a position as superintendent of nurses at a hospital in Worcester, Massachusetts. Shortly after arriving at her new quarters, she wrote to the Conference Committee of the Training School questioning the circumstances regarding her former post:

> When I requested to sever my connection with your Committee, I received no explanation, nor have I ever had any reason given to me for the action taken. I feel it my duty to know why my services were not acceptable to you (83).

A response from the Conference Committee contradicted Whitaker's perception of her leaving and indicated that she had resigned voluntarily (84). The facts of the matter remained unclear, even though in the Conference Committee's annual report the Governors had lauded her faithful, untiring devotion (85). For the first time, the report carried information emphasizing the authority of the Hospital superintendent to exercise supervision and control over the School (86).

When the Conference Committee interviewed Irene H. Sutliffe as a candidate for the position of supervising nurse, she expressed a willingness to head the program, but with a different title. The Conference Committee capitulated and recommended her as directress of nursing (87). A much-admired graduate of the class of 1880, Sutliffe embarked on her new adventure with great gusto and a creative spirit. In time, she would emerge as an important figure in American nursing. During her 16-year reign, she received recognition not only for her superb leadership in the Training School and devotion to The New York Hospital, but as a pioneer in a young profession.

CHAPTER 2

The Formative Years: The Way They Were

In the summer of 1877, a small group of spirited young women first passed through the tall, wrought iron gates along curved pathways leading to the high-arched entrance of The New York Hospital. A striking façade indeed for beginning nursing students, most of them from privileged backgrounds, who chose to leave behind the comforts of a secure home for a markedly different lifestyle. How many would brave the challenges of this early exposure to the hospital world and survive the rigors of training? The records from that early period revealed that of the seven pupil nurses listed in the first class, two remained one year, four graduated after 18 months, and one more graduated after two years (1).

A high attrition rate in the beginning was not unusual for aspiring neophytes, who in some cases dropped out in less than a day or after a few months and even weeks before completing the program. Many had entered the training program with false and romantic notions and when faced with the reality of the hard work abandoned the course. Others left because of ill health, family problems, unsuitability, or performance below standards (2). As time went on, however, the majority of pupil nurses persevered, with several of the graduates becoming national and international nursing leaders.

From the inception of the School, the Governors had set an age limit of not younger than 25 years for the entering class. In view of their desire to attract more mature applicants, it was not surprising that a large number of students had already pursued education beyond high school in seminaries, academies, liberal arts colleges, and normal schools (3). Several had some college preparation, while a few earned academic degrees from well-known colleges and universities. Before admission to the Training School, most had sought employment as a schoolteacher, governess, office worker, or companion (4). Those who did not work outside the home ran family households, raised siblings, or took care of infirm parents. Ninety-five percent of the applicants were unmarried, and the rest either widowed or divorced (5).

A small number of the pupil nurses were daughters of farmers or craftsmen, but the majority came from families of means, whose fathers were professionals or businessmen (6). When Annie Warburton Goodrich entered the nursing program in 1890, she had an impressive background that included private schooling in France and England following a childhood under the tutelage of a governess. Her training at The New York Hospital marked the beginning of a long friendship with Lillian Wald, a senior student who introduced Goodrich to her first work experience on the ward (7). In addition to being attractive, slender, energetic, and of the same height, both women shared mutual goals and values (8).

Some of the students claimed ancestry as far back as the American Revolution, even predating it as in the case of Mary Brewster, a descendent of the renowned Pilgrim Reverend William Brewster. Jane Hitchcock, the daughter of a physician who was also a professor at Amherst College, could trace her forebears to Peregine White, the baby born on the *Mayflower* (9). Another student, Julia Stimson, class of 1908, had family roots going back to the Thirteen Colonies (10). When admitted to the Training School, she had already earned a bachelor of arts degree from Vassar College and completed graduate studies in biology at Columbia University. As a member of the distinguished Stimson family of New York City, she enjoyed the privileges of the social elite. Some years later, when interviewed by a reporter from the *New York Sun* about her desire to pursue nursing, Stimson confessed that she wanted a career in medicine until her uncle, a surgeon at The New York Hospital, persuaded her to wait (11). She changed her mind, however, and became a student of Goodrich, who directed the School at the time and greatly influenced Stimson's professional life.

Lillian Wald exemplified the 19th- and early 20th-century woman who sought a career for self-fulfillment. In her 1889 letter of application, she indicated that the life of a young lady did not suit her because she longed for "serious definite work, a need perhaps more apparent since the desire to become a professional nurse has both" (12). Jennie Richie and Alice Bird expressed similar zeal, in revealing their intentions to combine nursing with missionary work (13).

Another inspirational story came from Anne Williamson's recollections of Clara Barton, a close friend of her mother, who visited the family home in Massachusetts in the early 1880s. An impressionable 12-year old, young Anne sat quietly on a footstool near her mother in the parlor while listening to a spirited discussion about the American Red Cross. Mesmerized by their guest, she could not resist blurting out how she wanted to be like Barton and do things for people (14). Undoubtedly, the seeds of Williamson's beginning interest in nursing must have been planted then.

The drive toward economic independence was a strong motive among some of the young women, such as Josephine Hill, a Southerner whose family suffered financial reverses in the Civil War. A letter from Georginia Spratt and her twin sister Margaret noted that they were compelled to seek employment because of financial troubles. When Sara Neff applied to the School, she wrote that her father had lost most of his fortune to unwise investments (15).

Whatever reasons spurred these women to prepare for nursing in the early period, they all began as probationers during a month of brief but fresh discovery. Prior to admission, there were certain prerequisites to be met, such as vaccinations within two years, correcting teeth needing attention, providing evidence of good health, and studying anatomy, physiology, and the metric system in a prescribed text (16). Among some of the clothing and other items required were three washable dresses in a color of choice, a dozen white aprons, a pair of blunt-pointed scissors, and a watch with a second hand.

Williamson vividly remembered her first evening as a "probie" when Irene Sutliffe, then the directress, gathered all the newcomers in a classroom to explain hospital ethics and the rules of seniority. In those days, certain protocols were established that would become traditional practices for decades in hospital schools. Sutliffe informed the new recruits of what they were expected to know about standing or sitting in the presence of doctors and seniors, with the admonishment of never preceding anyone of higher rank into an elevator. As for relationships between doctors and nurses, social contact off duty was forbidden, and any infringement of the rules could lead to dismissal (17).

The probationary period may have had its vicissitudes, but most students survived and became full-fledged pupil nurses. When officially accepted into the School, they received an organdy cap with a ruffle trim, a regulation long-sleeved blue plaid uniform extending a few inches from the floor, and a full white apron. In the months that followed, the young women became acclimated to the conditions imposed upon them in their new status. Recalling her training at The New York Hospital, Wald commented on the grimy scrub work, washing dishes, polishing brass, and simple cooking. "It was a strenuous time," she noted, "but a wonderful human experience for an undisciplined, untrained girl" (18).

Mary Beard, a 1903 graduate, characterized her nurse training as "the era of the 12-hour day and the 12-hour night. If time could be spared from the ward, the pupil was granted a day off" (19). One of the best-known nurses of her time, Beard declared that on top of the rigorous work schedule, she had to attend classes in the evening.

At the beginning of the 1890s, the Board of Governors at Sutliffe's urging agreed to extend the length of the program to two years in light of the growing interest expressed in the School and the added months of student affiliation at Sloane Maternity Hospital, which had been initiated by the directress (20). In 1895, a third year was added, and the admissions age requirement was reduced from 25–35 years to 23–33 years. With the increasing enrollment, the graduates of the Training School were becoming a visible force in a profession on the move.

For several years, the Conference Committee of The New York Hospital had enjoyed a harmonious relationship with the Training School, but in the mid-1890s, the committee members bristled over a resolution submitted to the Board of Governors. The Visiting Committee had indicated its desire to assume authority over the School, thus shifting the responsibility away from the Conference Committee (21). The action evoked some dismay and ignited a written response signed by 59 of the graduates:

We the undersigned wish to express our entire satisfaction with the past and present government of the School and to thank the gentlemen of the Conference Committee for their kind and watchful care over its best interests . . . .We feel that the school is in prosperous condition and should regret any changes that would place the government of it in any other and less experienced hands (22).

The question of governance affecting the conduct of the School came to a head in May 1886 when the Conference Committee was discontinued and its powers to direct and manage the program were transferred to the Executive Committee of the Board of Governors (23). Created by a bylaws change, the new policy occurred a few months after Sutliffe assumed her post as the fifth head of the School.

Sutliffe's adaptability to work well with colleagues and without antagonism toward subordinates became evident from the beginning of her appointment. She brought something fresh to her role, generating productivity and a high morale among the pupil nurses and staff nurses working on the wards or "pavilions," as they came to be known. The fact that she herself was an outstanding graduate of the School may have been a factor in her ability to establish cooperative relationships with the hospital hierarchy from the outset, but more likely it was her keen understanding of human nature and superb interpersonal skills.

Among the pupil nurses enrolled in the program, she left an indelible impression on many as they moved along in their career. Some years later, Wald recalled her initial interview with Sutliffe, which she claimed had intensified a beginning interest in nursing (24). Another graduate of that period, Anne Williamson, described her initial exposure to Sutliffe. Expecting to find a foreboding, unapproachable person, the anxious new recruit was stunned to find herself warmly shaking hands with a "blue-eyed, golden-haired young woman barely five feet tall" (25).

Sutliffe's administrative ability must have been recognized early as a student, having been approached almost immediately after graduation to establish a training school in Pennsylvania. Following a few years as superintendent of nurses, she left to develop the Long Island College Hospital School of Nursing in Brooklyn, New York, where harrowing conditions awaited her. She would never forget "the beds full of vermin, insufficient supplies, inadequate facilities for scrubbing patients, and the servants and orderlies discharged for drunkenness" (26).

After returning to The New York Hospital to administer the Training School, she strengthened the curriculum offerings and provided affiliation opportunities at other facilities. One of her earliest challenges occurred on December 15, 1886, while attending a meeting of the Board of Governors' Executive Committee. Dr. William Turnbull, the chairman, reported on a special subcommittee to explore the best methods of instruction and management of the Training School (27). For some years, the question of too much theoretical content had been a sensitive issue created by the interference of physicians eager to increase the practical experience of the pupil nurses.

The previous month, Dr. William Hoppin, chairman of the subcommittee, had sent a communication to the Medical Board describing the results of an investigation of 10 prominent training schools. He noted that several similarities existed among the schools, but the program at The New York Hospital was not carried out as systematically and elaborately as it should be (28). A prickly response followed at the December meeting when Dr. Thomas M. Markoe, president of the Medical Board, and Dr. George C. Peabody, an attending physician, indicated that the chief source of dissatisfaction was "not that our system is not carried out as it should be but at present is too *elaborate*" (29).

Pinpointing the crux of the disagreement, they added that the school gave too much attention to the scientific training of the nurse and not enough to the commonplace daily routine of her work (30). Peabody went so far as to state that experience showed the futility of giving nurses any useful instruction on anatomy and physiology as well as putting books in the hands of students. It was ironic that two years earlier, Clara Weeks, a classmate of Sutliffe, had written the first nursing textbook by a nurse that became a classic in the profession (31).

Peabody offered a simplistic alternative when he prescribed the use of manuals dealing solely with principles of nursing (32). Although mindful of the Medical Board's protestations, the subcommittee held a different view and pointed out the danger of mechanically carrying out instructions consisting of arbitrary rules. They cautioned that the quality of the School would be compromised and good nursing would deteriorate (33). The controversy seemed to be settled, at least for the time being, when the medical staff agreed to continue with the scientific lectures because they wanted the Training School to rank high among others in the nation (34).

Sutliffe took great pride in her students, determined to sustain their motivation and provide them with a satisfying and productive learning environment and a positive self-image. Dissatisfied with the regulation uniform, a plain washable dress covered by an apron, she designed a new look after selecting attractive blue plaid fabric made in Scotland exclusively for the pupil nurses (35). Throughout the years, hundreds of students proudly donned their distinctive uniform until World War II. Because the war disrupted commercial shipping, the class entering in 1942 wore a uniform made of blue-checked fabric. The class entering in 1949 resumed wearing a blue plaid uniform from fabric manufactured in the United States which differed slightly from the pre-war fabric.

Like her predecessors, Sutliffe had deep concerns about the living conditions of the pupil nurses, particularly with illness persisting in large numbers. With the 10th anniversary of the School approaching in another year, changes appeared to be overdue. Before the dissolution of the Conference Committee, Hoppin had referred to the manner of accommodating the students as rest deprivation and lack of proper ventilation (36). In addition to being subjected to cramped, low-ceilinged rooms that were originally designed for the general help, two or three pupil nurses not only shared quarters, but also had access to only one bathroom and two water closets (37).

At an Executive Committee meeting in February 1888, Sutliffe delineated the most pressing needs of the Training School and echoed many of the observations in an earlier report of the Visiting Committee to George Ludlam, the Hospital's superintendent (38). During the discussion, Ludlam pointed out that other hospitals in the city, such as Bellevue and St. Luke's, had erected special buildings for their training schools and "our hospital, which from its position and influence should be the lead in all these matters is far behind" (39). He also noted that the present roster of 40 students was inadequate, noting that one-third of the probationers were not equipped for ward work requiring certain skills, and four pupils rotated on affiliation at Sloane

Maternity Hospital (40). Furthermore, three more pupils were expected to take a leave of absence or become ill, leaving only the remaining 20 as an effective work force in the Hospital (41).

Ludlam suggested that consideration be given to demolishing the site at the northeast corner of the property and erecting a large fireproof building to meet the requirements of the Training School (42). Subsequently, the Governors agreed to a temporary measure of renting quarters in the neighborhood until a permanent building would be ready for occupancy. They recommended that as soon as the accommodations were available, the limit of the School should be fixed at 60 pupil nurses (43).

It was a festive occasion in 1891 when No. 6 West 16th Street became the site of the first real home of the students enrolled in The New York Hospital Training School for Nurses. The imposing eight-story structure that had cost $223,567 was modern and well furnished, displaying a pathological cabinet or museum on the first floor to preserve "specimens of morbid anatomy" (44). The library was located on the second floor, while the Training School occupied the remaining six stories.

Living arrangements consisted of six suites on each floor to accommodate the desired number of 60 students, with two students sharing a suite of two bedrooms separated by a sitting room. Provision had been made in a tower for an isolation ward for seriously ill students. Also available was a rooftop area that became the favorite spot for lounging during the summer months (45). The year following the opening, the installation of wiring for electric lighting proved a welcome addition (46).

A pronounced contrast to the meager surroundings endured by pupil nurses over the previous years, the new Nurses Home represented more than merely a handsome building. It connoted a symbol of recognition by the Hospital of what the Training School had accomplished and its future potential through the nursing leadership and the quality of the graduates. It conferred an identity on the present students and became a haven of fulfillment to many nurses in the decades ahead.

Class records of 1,022 graduate nurses of The New York Hospital Training School from 1878 to 1920 provide a compendium of demographic information, revealing that they represented a total of 30 states as pupil nurses. The majority (61.4%) came from New England and the Middle Atlantic states, with 43.1% from New York State and 15.7% consisting of New York City residents. Also represented were Canada, particularly the Province of Ontario, the United Kingdom, and Scandinavia (47). In 1896, Helen Fraser, a Bellevue graduate and superintendent of a training school in Japan, recommended a young Japanese woman for study at The New York Hospital rather than at her own school. She explained her reasons in the following letter:

> The moral influence of Bellevue is such that I would not like to take the responsibility of sending an inexperienced Japanese there, who is not accustomed to American life. I feel she would be safer with you (48).

Although the Training School had a non-sectarian admission policy, the vast majority of the graduates were Protestant (Episcopalians comprised the largest group at 32. 8%) and only 5.9% were Catholic. There was only a small number of Jewish women; others may have been drawn to the nearby school of Mount Sinai Hospital, which opened in 1887 and conducted an active recruitment program (49).

Records of the marital status and careers of the graduates surveyed over 40 years revealed that 548 remained single and 474 married (50). Only a small proportion of the single group was unable to practice because of health problems, family obligations, or retirement. The majority of married nurses discontinued their careers, a trend that persisted for several years. A large number married professional men, especially physicians (51).

In his address to the 1911 graduating class, Peabody commented on the "matrimonial proclivities" of the nurses (52). One of the earlier graduates, Caroline Hampton, relocated to Baltimore where she worked as the surgical nurse of Dr. William Halsted, surgeon-in-chief at the new Johns Hopkins Hospital. A romance between them flourished, which may have resulted from an unusual surgical innovation. When Hampton complained of the harsh effects of an antiseptic on her hands, Halsted approached the Goodyear Rubber Company to make her a special pair of thin rubber surgical gloves (53). The event had a greater significance because it led to the nationwide introduction of rubber gloves to protect the hands from corrosive substances and later from blood-borne infections (54). In 1890, Hampton married her supervisor!

Most of the Training School graduates began their practice in private nursing, both in the Hospital and home. They were notified of their engagements through the registry, which permitted flexibility in assignments. Some nurses expressed a reluctance to take patients with scarlet fever, diphtheria, measles, and venereal disease as well as alcoholics and the mentally ill. Fewer than 5% refused to take care of black patients with tuberculosis (55).

The families who requested private nurses listed in the registry generally belonged to the upper middle and upper classes. Not all cases, however, involved seriously ill patients, and it was not unusual for a nurse to accompany a patient with a chronic condition on an overseas trip, or to be employed in the home for an extended period (56). An attractive feature of private practice was the independent nature of the work and the opportunity to be in complete charge of the patient except during the physician's visits.

When an occasional impropriety was discovered or reported that involved a graduate of the School, the nurse was required to return her diploma and badge while under investigation. If the guilty party was a private-duty nurse, she also had to withdraw her name from the registry. When and if cleared, the nurse's credentials would be returned and her name replaced on the registry with the understanding that she had to inform the Hospital's Executive Committee of the name and address of the physician on the case (57).

During the 1880s, private nurses in New York hospitals earned $20 to $25 a week, with a gradual increase in the fee to $25 to $30, plus an additional $6 a day for 12-hour duty and $7 a day for 24-hour duty. In the early 20th century, their annual wages ranged from $500 to $1,500, averaging $950, a slight increase over the income of head nurses and operating room nurses, who additionally received room and board. Occupying the most prestigious position, the head of the Training School could earn up to a yearly $1,200 in the 1880s; this salary rose to as much as $3,000 during the first two decades of the next century (58).

Among the early graduates of The New York Hospital Training School for Nurses, private nursing remained the most popular as well as viable choice, but by 1913 it showed a decline, from 68.4% in 1893 to 49.3% for nurses practicing in New York City. Conversely, it continued to be on the rise in other cities, from 5.8% to 14%, while institutional nursing climbed from 16.4% to 24.1% (59). Some nurses chose district nursing (2.0%), medicine (2.7%), army nursing (2.9%), public health (0.2%), and non-nursing work (1.1%) (60).

During its nascent period, The New York Hospital Training School for Nurses showed great potential in responding to a desperate and important public need for competent nursing care by preparing qualified practitioners. The developing career patterns of the graduates opened new frontiers that captured the imagination of young women seeking purpose and utility in their lives. Many of these women became pathfinders, establishing some of the best schools in the United States and other countries. With amazing productivity, they wrote textbooks, served on state boards of nurse examiners, held high office in national nursing and health organizations, organized the Army School of Nursing, and instituted new models of patient care delivery. These adventurous nurses spread their message throughout the world and helped provide a foundation for an evolving profession.

CHAPTER 3

The 1890s: A Fateful Decade

The late 19th and early 20th centuries ushered in a number of reform movements which captured the interest of nursing leaders, who knew they were not alone in their struggle to improve the health care of the public. Philanthropic groups abounded, promoting social betterment as well as changes needed in overcrowded tenements, food inspection, and communicating information to people about healthy living (1). The supply of pupil nurses increased as medicine and technology advanced, the nation's population grew, and more health services became available. Admissions to The New York Hospital for 1891 rose in all services, with 61% of the inpatients receiving free care while the outpatient department was thriving (2). Responding to over 3,000 calls, a busy ambulance service transferred a third of the people to other facilities (3).

On the wards, pupil nurses were expected to spend 12 hours a day or night in practical experience with minimal attention given to theoretical instruction although the medical staff, the directress of the School, and senior nurses on the wards continued to provide some lectures to the students. This pattern, which existed in nursing schools throughout the nation, nurtured a system of education that deeply troubled the superintendents of leading programs, particularly with the marked proliferation of training schools.

At the beginning of the 1890s, 35 schools reported a student enrollment of 1,552; 10 years later the figures rose to 432 schools and 11,164 pupil nurses (4). Recognizing the need for self-government and curriculum standardization, nursing's pioneers knew their goals would have to undergo severe testing before being realized. The greatest opposition came from members of the medical community who viewed nurses as becoming too independent and threatening to the position of physicians (5). Equally disturbing was the profit motive of the governing boards of most hospitals. They found the training schools to be extremely lucrative by relying on pupil nurses to provide a pool of essential labor. The schools became an important asset to the institution's management, and the preparation of nurses an economic expedient (6).

Because nursing education assumed a secondary role, the superintendents of training schools were forced to offer nursing preparation in a system with little regard for women's education, roles, or professions. Their observations generated a strong call for collective action in a united front designed to upgrade nursing's professional status. The determination of these women marked the beginning of a new movement that characterized the period from 1890 to 1900 as the fateful decade in American nursing (7).

In June 1893, a group of superintendents of training schools came together during the World's Fair in Chicago to explore the pressing issues in the field. As a visible spokesperson at the event, Irene Sutliffe presented a paper urging the profession to organize in order to maintain high ideals and standards (8). A historic outcome of the gathering was the adoption of a resolution to form the American Society of Superintendents of Training Schools for Nurses (ASSTSN), the first national nursing organization, which changed its name to the National League of Nursing Education (NLNE) in 1912 (9). From its inception, the association enunciated its objectives of establishing and maintaining a universal standard of training, promoting fellowship among members, and furthering the best interests of the nursing profession (10).

Sutliffe's outside professional activities in no way lessened her loyalty to the School and the Hospital, but rather gave stature to her position. Through supportive relationships with colleagues from other schools, they bonded in a common cause to advance nursing education. She believed that the ASSTSN would become the vehicle to strengthen all training school programs and develop nursing as a profession.

During the years of Sutliffe's administration, the Governors seemed highly satisfied with her performance, which had placed the nursing program at The New York Hospital among the top-ranking training schools. Her record of accomplishment had not escaped them as the number of desirable pupil nurses increased along with improvements in the quality of patient care. She extended the length of the course, helped settle the students in their new Nurses Home, arranged affiliations with other institutions, and created the first diet kitchen in the United States, which demonstrated the significance of nutrition in both health and sickness (11). In addition, she initiated a postgraduate refresher course at the School for nurses who wanted to strengthen their skills in the Hospital (12).

In 1892, the Governors granted Sutliffe a six-week leave of absence to study training schools in other countries. They agreed with the Special Committee on Examination of Nurses that the trip would be "beneficial not only to Miss Sutliffe but her observations will be of great benefit to the School" (13).

Sutliffe had many qualities that endeared her to colleagues and students, but perhaps it was her humanity that made her so unique. Nothing illustrates this quality in her nature more poignantly than the story of Laura York, the baby who captured everyone's heart. Laura York Sutliffe's story in Sutliffe's own words follows on page 30.

After the founding of the ASSTSN, Sutliffe actively participated in the work of the organization while maintaining a rigorous schedule at the Hospital. The Governors gave her permission to attend the organization's annual conventions held in major cities in the nation and Toronto. Between 1894 and 1899, more than 200 nursing superintendents represented schools at these events where prominent nurses addressed the assembly. In 1897, Agnes Brennan, superintendent of the Bellevue Training School, presented a paper dealing with the timely issue of the value of theory versus practice and observed the following:

> An uneducated woman may become a good nurse but never an intelligent one; she can obey orders continuously and understand a sick person's need, but should an emergency arise, where is she? She works through her feelings and therefore lacks judgment (15).

No reports of the involvement of black nurses appeared in the organization's work (16). This was not surprising since a quota system

OUR HOSPITAL BABY*

Very early one bitter cold morning, March 10, 1889, two policemen were standing on the corner of Tenth Avenue and Eighteenth Street; one to relieve the other when they heard a peculiar wail. One of them said, "That is a cat". The other replied, "No, it is a new born baby". Following the Sound in the darkness they, descending about ten feet in an excavation, found a tiny baby girl wrapped only in part of a New York Herald. A rag tied about the neck had evidently been placed over her mouth to stifle her. One of them, putting her under his coat, ran to the nearest police station. The other summoned an ambulance. The little one was soon receiving every attention at the New York Hospital. It was many days before we thought she would survive the terrible experience. She was wrapped in cotton, put in a small basket and placed on a radiator. She was baptized, Laura York Sutliffe, after two of the nurses and the Hospital. 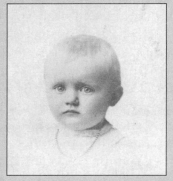 Her recovery was, however, not satisfactory until a wet nurse was procured, and later she with this nurse and the nurse's own baby, were sent to the seashore for the summer. When the wet nurse left us she said "she loved our baby as well as her own". I think she told the truth. They returned in October and our baby was taken to the apartment of the Directress of the School for Nursing, and finally adopted by her. It seemed a miracle that the puny, wrinkled baby, looking like an old woman, should return to us a most beautiful child, a perfect blonde with wonderful dark blue eyes and rosy cheeks.

Everyone connected with the Hospital was interested and most of them loved her. She was certainly very lovable and loving. Many of us still remember her on Christmas Eve when our tree was revolving, and our dear baby, looking like a little fairy danced around it, calling, "Come down and see the tree go wound". She received more attention than the tree. She said once, "I love all the nurses but I just love more the night nurses". They would stop on their way to their rooms and after searching for her would find her hiding behind a door or chair. Then a dance and such shouts of laughter. She was an anxious child but a very happy one, always obedient and most affectionate.

On January 13, 1892, she died after three days illness. Her memory will always be cherished by those who loved her.

I.H. Sutliffe.

*This first-person recollection is transcribed verbatim as it appeared in the Historical Scrapbook, Alumnae Association, 1893–1932.

had restricted the admission of black students ever since the first nursing schools were established. The New York Hospital Training School for Nurses was no exception. Admission requirements specified in recruitment material that "applications of colored candidates will not be considered" (17). To deal with this discrimination, 19 all-black schools with diploma programs existed in the nation between 1896 and 1900, and before long the number proliferated (18).

During its first decade, the ASSTSN reported considerable progress in working toward its goals. The members were an elite group within the profession who recognized the importance of an organization dedicated to the needs of practicing nurses. In February 1897, their efforts led to the founding of the Nurses Associated Alumnae of the United States and Canada, renamed the American Nurses Association in 1911. The new organization aimed to "strengthen the union of existing nursing organizations, to elevate nursing education, and to establish and maintain a code of ethics" (19). Among the 40 local groups represented, the Alumnae Association of The New York Hospital Training School for Nurses became one of the nine charter members (20).

In September 1893, when 47 nurses met at The New York Hospital to launch the School's Alumnae Association, they announced that the organization's purpose was to initiate a sick fund for nurses and a registry for graduates engaged in private nursing (21). The next month they expanded some of their activities to include lectures by doctors to inform the alumnae of medical and surgical progress. Another topic of growing interest concerned legal regulation of the profession for the graduates of the School (22).

At the annual meeting of the Alumnae Association in March 1894, dues were determined and voting was held; Sutliffe was elected president, Maria Greene vice president, Ada Stewart secretary, and Sutliffe's sister Frank treasurer (23). The following year, 131 members of the Alumnae Association expressed interest in attending a series of lectures at Columbia College under the auspices of the St. Barnabas Guild (24). By 1896, the organization claimed a membership of 150 nurses.

For some time, the Alumnae Association had hopes of finding a home in New York City for nurses who had no other choice than to live in boarding houses (25). In February 1898, the Nurses Club House opened at 54 East 49th Street as a residence primarily for unmarried women who had graduated from the Training School, but it eventually welcomed other nurses, librarians, teachers, and students (26). Undaunted by the trains of the New York Central Railroad running along the rear of the building, the residents seemed satisfied with their accommodations until faced with landlord problems. When the Nurses Club House relocated to a new and larger home on West 92nd Street, the Alumnae Association expressed its gratitude to the Board of Governors for their donation of $2,325 to the house fund (27). Eventually, Sutliffe established residence there after her retirement.

The Nurses Club House served another purpose when the Alumnae Association decided to launch its own Nurses Registry at the same site as a convenience for the residents. Under Sutliffe's guidance, the facility operated as a business with a salaried registrar and fees from the members (28). During its first year of operation, over 400 calls were received and the number nearly doubled the following year. In 1905, the Governors discontinued the Hospital Registry, which had not been too successful, and referred all inquiries to the Nurses Club House.

Three years after the alumnae organization was established, the first copy of its newsletter appeared as a single sheet with the title "Officers of the Alumnae Association of the New York Hospital Training School for Nurses" (29). The publication aimed to keep the graduates in close touch with one another and to share information about programs and events. In 1907, it became officially known as *The Alumnae News*, adopting a new look as a quarterly, with Mary Young as the editor.

Among the influential members of the Alumnae Association were Lillian Wald and Mary Brewster, who had actively supported its founding. Only two years out of the Training School, these dedicated young women introduced their seminal work at the Henry Street Settlement and pioneered their experiment during a period when the country was experiencing a burgeoning settlement movement. In the fall of 1898, Jane Addams, the dynamic leader of the famous settlement in Chicago, visited Wald at Henry Street for the first time. That meeting marked the beginning of a warm friendship and enduring professional relationship (30).

In the interval between her nursing school graduation and involvement at Henry Street, Wald entered the Women's Medical

College of the New York Infirmary for Women and Children in 1892. During the program, she taught home nursing to women living on the Lower East Side. While on a brief journey through the streets of densely packed neighborhoods, Wald was devastated when she saw the poverty, squalor, and poor health conditions. This initial exposure prompted Wald to forsake her medical studies and begin a mission that would become her life work (31).

From the outset, she and Brewster decided to live among the tenement dwellers and bring nursing services directly into the homes of the immigrant families. During the first year of their work at the Settlement, the small corps of nurses they recruited made 3,600 visits and treated 5,032 patients (32). They climbed up and down hundreds of flights of stairs and scrambled over connecting rooftops to reach their patients. Over the years as the services expanded and the number of staff increased, these women demonstrated a uniqueness, not only in their bedside care but in their interest and involvement in the social, cultural, and environmental factors of the community (33). Required to live in the neighborhoods where they worked, the nurses were unmarried and mostly in their thirties and forties. They were viewed as Wald's family and generally referred to her as "The Lady" (34).

In nursing circles, Wald was characterized as one of the great triumvirate that included Mary Adelaide Nutting of Teachers College, Columbia University, and Annie Warburton Goodrich, an 1892 graduate of the Training School, who succeeded Sutliffe as superintendent and later became the director of the Henry Street Settlement Nursing Service. Another prominent alumna and one of the first four nurses at the Settlement was Jane Hitchcock, a former classmate of Wald, who devoted her career to the development of public health nursing and to the improvement of the basic preparation of nurses for public health work (35).

During the early 20th century, the Henry Street nurses participated with the New York City Board of Health in anti-tuberculosis campaigns, instructing families on personal hygiene. In May 1907, The New York Hospital followed their lead and employed a visiting nurse in the outpatient department to educate patients with tuberculosis about their care and nutritional needs. The patients were supplied with eggs and milk. By the end of seven months, the Hospital had dispensed 960 dozen eggs and 4,158 quarts of milk (36). The visiting program gradually expanded to include the home care of patients discharged from the wards, and in time a second visiting nurse was assigned to the outpatient department along with services provided to children hospitalized on the wards (37).

Through the work of the Henry Street nurses under the leadership of graduates of The New York Hospital Training School for Nurses, district nursing among the poor evolved into public health and social service nursing. In 1909, Sutliffe volunteered her services as a social worker in the Hospital, which became the impetus for establishing a social service department (38). During this period, the successful implementation of the visiting program in the outpatient department prompted The New York Hospital to combine the tuberculosis service with social service work. This action created a new department titled "Convalescent Relief" that operated under the direction of a nurse (39). In 1912, the Executive Committee approved a proposal to organize a Ladies Auxiliary Committee to volunteer for social service activity in the Hospital. Composed of at least 10 women, the group was expected to meet monthly with the Executive Committee to discuss the cases in progress with the director Hannah Josephi, a 1901 graduate of the Training School (40). The Auxiliary contributed a valuable service in raising funds that helped to maintain long-term support for the department.

On her return from an extended leave of absence in the mid-1890s, Sutliffe found a disturbing situation concerning the affiliation at Sloane Maternity Hospital. Pupil nurses complained of harassment from the supervising nurse at the institution. Mostly affected were the students on night duty, whose sleep during the day was repeatedly interrupted by the supervisor. They were told to arise, get dressed in full uniform, and return to the ward to correct a trifling error or attend to an unimportant detail (41).

After exploring the matter, the Visiting Committee of the Board of Governors met with the hospital director at Sloane and was reassured that the annoyance would cease. In a communication to the Executive Committee in April 1897, Superintendent George Ludlam explained that "the complaint is not based upon the fact of being compelled to attend to these details but upon the manner in which the rebuke is declared to be arbitrary, unreasonable and unjust" (42).

When the problem showed no improvement, Sutliffe terminated the arrangement with Sloane and transferred the affiliation in obstetrics to Lying-In Hospital, then located at 17th Street and Second Avenue. Known for its high standards, Lying-In accepted only pupil nurses who had been at the School for more than a year. Two nurses at a time would enter the three-month experience at four- or six-week intervals (43). In this way, the number of entering students was kept low, assuring more in-depth learning and more careful supervision.

While changes were underway in the obstetrical affiliation, the Board of Governors made an important decision concerning the disposition of books and related materials in the Hospital library. For some time, a number of physicians complained that because of the limited and dated holdings they had to do their research at the New York Academy of Medicine (44). A special committee charged to investigate the difficulty concluded that a substantial appropriation would be needed to refurbish the library. Selecting another option, the Governors determined that it would be more feasible to close the facility and donate a certain portion of the books, amounting to 23,000 volumes, to the Academy with the stipulation that an area be designated as the Alcove of the Library of The New York Hospital (45).

Toward the end of the 19th century, two major events occurred that profoundly affected the Hospital and the Training School for Nurses. The year 1898 saw the founding of the Cornell University Medical College and a proposal to establish a course on hospital economics for graduate nurses at Teachers College, Columbia University. On September 1, 1898, the Sunday edition of the *New York Herald* carried a front page headline: *FINEST MEDICAL COLLEGE IN THE COUNTRY WILL BE IN NEW YORK* (46). This historic undertaking resulted from the generosity of Colonel Oliver Hazard Payne, who donated $1,500,000 to endow the Cornell University Medical College. The action had been made official the previous April by the University's Board of Trustees, thus beginning the alliance between Cornell and The New York Hospital (47).

Born into an affluent family in Cleveland, Payne was the son of a Standard Oil founder. He became interested in supporting medical education through his friendship with Dr. Lewis A. Stimson, a Yale classmate, and his physician, Dr. H. P. Loomis, who were both associated with University Medical College, an autonomous department of New York University (48). In describing the proposed structure for the Medical College, which was to be located at First Avenue between 27th and 28th Streets, Stanford White, the famous New York architect, noted that the building would be five stories high and "designed in a severe style of Renaissance architecture and be built of Joliet and Indiana limestone and red brick" (49).

When the Medical College's new building opened in the fall of 1900 much pomp and ceremony accompanied the event with addresses by Theodore Roosevelt, then Governor of New York, President Seth Low of Columbia University, President Jacob Gould Schurman of Cornell University, and Dr. Lewis A. Stimson representing the faculty (50). For the next 20 years, Stimson, who was professor of surgery, and Dr. William M. Polk, dean of the Medical College and professor of gynecology and obstetrics, would become key figures in the development of the Medical College.

During the first year, a total of 278 students, including 26 women, registered at the College (51). The four-year course had an unusual feature in that the first two years could be taken either in New York City or on Cornell's Ithaca campus before transferring to New York. Women students, however, who comprised about 15% of each class, were required to spend the first two years in Ithaca (52). In adopting coeducation in medicine, Cornell followed the example of Johns Hopkins (53). Eventually, the upstate program closed and all classes were held at the Medical College in New York City.

In 1908, a new admissions policy stipulated that all entering students be required to have a bachelor's degree before acceptance to the school (54). Four years later, an event of some note occurred when a gift of $250,000 formalized an affiliation between Cornell University Medical College and The New York Hospital (55). The benefactor was George F. Baker, a prominent banker and a member of the Board of Governors, whose donation aimed toward promoting medical research, aiding the care of patients, and furthering the education of medical students (56).

During the formative period of the Medical College, discussions about a uniform curriculum in training schools for nurses dominated the annual conventions of the ASSTSN. Concern was also expressed about the qualifications of the superintendents and the faculty. At the Fifth Annual Convention in 1898, the organization's newly formed Education Committee wrote to Dean James Earl Russell of Teachers College, Columbia University, to explore the possibility of introducing a course of studies to be titled "hospital economics," designed expressly for superintendents and teachers in hospital schools of nursing (57). When this proposal became a reality in October 1899, it was the first nursing course in the United States located in a university (58).

Enthusiastic about the program, Sutliffe brought it to the attention of the Board of Governors and proposed that a scholarship be provided for the graduates of the Training School. She pointed out the potential of the course for attracting nurses to positions in the Hospital as well as an incentive to new students. The Board concurred and voted to underwrite the sum of $460 to be given annually to a nurse from the graduating class, who would be eligible to attend the course. All fees, books, board, and incidentals would be included for 12 weeks in addition to lodging for 35 weeks (59).

When the program on hospital economics was launched, the nurses enrolled for one year and received a certificate upon completion. Faculty in such disciplines as psychology, science, household economics, and biology offered courses to a limited number of students. In 1905, the program was extended to two years with a diploma awarded when completed. Two years later, Mary Adelaide Nutting resigned from her position as the principal of the training school for nurses at Johns Hopkins Hospital, and assumed the administrative reins at Teachers College; she became the first professor of nursing education in the world (60). She invited well-known nurses to give lectures on various topics that included training school administration, history of nursing, and hospital administration. In one of her lectures, Annie Goodrich spoke on working essentials and hospital construction (61).

Determined to strengthen the hospital economics course, Nutting recruited leading physicians in New York to give a series of lectures on hospital organization. Among the group was Dr. Thomas Howell, who became superintendent of The New York Hospital in 1909 (62). The hospital economics course flourished under her leadership and in 1910 a gift of $150,270.32 from Helen Hartley Jenkins endowed a Department of Nursing and Health at Teachers College (63). The inspiration for such a sizeable donation came from Lillian Wald, whom Jenkins greatly admired. The new department offered courses in public health nursing to graduate nurses for the first time, and as a lecturer, Wald tied academic studies to practical experience at the Henry Street Settlement (64). The introduction of public health nursing in the curriculum at Teachers College signified the beginning of a pattern that would continue for several years.

As America moved toward the close of the century, it became embroiled in a war—albeit a short one—in which nurses prepared in training schools served for the first time. In April 1898, President William McKinley declared war on Spain two months after the sinking of the U.S. battleship the *Maine* in the harbor at Havana, Cuba, resulting in the loss of 260 men (65). The New York Hospital responded to the call for medical and nursing volunteers; 41 graduates of the Training School offered their services in Cuba, Puerto Rico, and the Philippines (66).

George M. Sternberg, surgeon general of the United States, believed that the military should not employ women and that army camps were no place for a decent woman (67). When letters of protest poured into his office, the Red Cross came to the rescue and offered to arrange all details involving recruitment. The one exception was that each nurse had to be vouched for by the Daughters of the American Revolution (DAR) before being accepted (68).

Under the guidance of Dr. Anita Newcomb McGee, assistant surgeon general, the DAR selected the nurses to be assigned to the camps and military hospitals. When McGee resigned after the war, Dita Hopkins Kinney replaced her and became the first superintendent of the Army Nurse Corps (ANC) in 1901 (69). An 1892 graduate of the Massachusetts General Hospital Training School, Kinney had joined the army as a contract nurse during the Spanish-American War and assisted the surgeon general. Throughout her eight years with the ANC, she organized the system and improved the working conditions of army nurses nationwide. She also accorded them a distinctive identity with a green enamel badge (70).

When war became imminent, The New York Hospital mobilized its forces and enlisted the participation of volunteer graduate nurses.

Irene Sutliffe took a brief leave from her position at the School to direct the nursing service at Camp Black in Hempstead, Long Island. One of her former students, Canadian-born Isabelle Jean Walton, who graduated in 1895, signed up with the military and was stationed at Fort Hamilton on Governor's Island as the chief nurse. After the war, Walton returned to The New York Hospital, where for the next 26 years she headed the outpatient department. On her retirement in 1928, the Board of Governors honored her with the following tribute: "…she created an atmosphere of interest and kindliness which forever will be a happy memory to the patients and an inspiration to the nurses, and to all the staff of the Hospital" (71).

From the beginning of the Spanish-American War (which lasted only eight months), local organizations of the Red Cross known as auxiliaries were formed, with each group assuming responsibility for a certain branch of war work (72). Anne Williamson became one of the first nurses to report to Red Cross Auxiliary Number 3, whose chief task was to supply graduate nurses. At the orientation, the nurses had their credentials examined and were informed of the regulations to be followed, such as restriction on wearing white uniforms in the field hospitals (73). The Red Cross agreed to pay $25 a month to any nurse who had a dependent (74).

Before volunteering for military duty, Williamson could still hear the words of Clara Barton echoing in her mind as she recalled the visit of the Civil War heroine to her home several years earlier. "God forbid that we have another war," Barton had declared, "but remember as you grow old, there are many ways you can be useful to the Red Cross in serving humanity" (75). That opportunity had arrived, and Anne Williamson unhesitatingly began her first assignment which took her to Charleston, South Carolina and from there to Sternberg Hospital at Camp Chicamauga in Tennessee.

Williamson was exposed to a raging epidemic of typhoid fever sweeping through the wards (76). "The wards reminded me of the picture of Dante's Inferno," Williamson later recalled. "If I ever thanked God for my training, it was that night when the ward in perfect chaos was turned over to me and I realized that thirty seven soldiers were looking to me for their comfort and even their being" (77).

When the war ended, representatives of Spain and the United States signed a Peace Treaty in Paris on December 20, 1898. Spain had lost control over the rest of its empire, including Cuba, Puerto Rico,

Guam, the Philippines, and other islands. The loss in lives would never be known, but it was estimated that the number of civilians who died from famine, disease, and related causes ranged from 200,000 to 600,000 (78). Over 1,000 army nurses had contributed their services in the country and abroad, while on the home front, The New York Hospital and the House of Relief provided care to the wounded soldiers (79).

An important outcome of the Spanish-American War was that it gave legitimacy to the trained nurse in contrast to the untrained volunteer. Another positive result was the establishment of the Red Cross Nursing Service (80). Eighteen days after the Peace Treaty, the executive committee of the Nurses Associated Alumnae (NAA) met in the Nurses Home of The New York Hospital to explore the possibility of proposing legislation that would place army nursing under the control of trained nurses (81). When a special committee of the organization formulated a bill that died in Congressional committee, delegates to the NAA convention in 1900 reaffirmed their support of an army nursing service to be directed by a qualified nurse (82).

In 1901, the year of President McKinley's assassination, the Army Reorganization Act was enacted, which established the Army Nurse Corps; seven years later, the Navy Nurse Corps was formed (83). These actions proved to be significant in a developing profession striving to advance and to achieve a modicum of autonomy. The legislation specified a standard of competency and provided for the supervision of nurses *by* nurses.

CHAPTER 4

A New Century: Action in Adversity

A long with the expanding industrialization and urbanization, the first decade of the 20th century spawned a series of extraordinary events that produced phenomenal changes in American society. The creative spirit and technology gave birth to a host of remarkable inventions, such as the escalator, air conditioner, polygraph machine, and the subway system in New York City. Other "firsts" capturing the public's attention included the Wright Brothers' historic flight at Kitty Hawk, the silent movie, *The Great Train Robbery*, and Thomas Edison's talking picture. The teddy bear made its appearance in 1902 and soon erupted into a national craze. In the world of science and medicine, Albert Einstein proposed his theory of relativity, while Sigmund Freud published his theory of sexuality (1).

Nurses in public health and social work emerged as a mobilizing force in the drive to increase public interest in humanitarian reforms. Fifty-six hospitals in the nation extended their training programs to three years, five institutions to two years, and five more to two years and several months (2). Some reduced the hours of pupil service to 10 and in a few cases to eight, such as the schools of Johns Hopkins Hospital in Baltimore and the Harper Hospital in Detroit (3).

Toward the end of the 19th century, The New York Hospital Training School for Nurses claimed an impressive number of graduates, with 504 engaged in active practice. They spread their talents in different directions, including 182 working in private nursing, with 157 practicing in New York and 25 outside the city. Fifty-eight nurses chose institutional nursing, and 22 performed settlement work, district, school, and army nursing. While 10 of the graduates earned degrees in medicine, others established training schools in the United States and service abroad (4).

In the fall of 1900, the Hospital planned to erect a new building for private patients to open by the end of the year. Located at 10 West 16th Street, the 10-story building provided accommodations for 60 patients as well as for house and resident staff, and a large dining room for pupil nurses (5). The anticipated increase in the admission of patients prompted the Governors to authorize the hiring of graduate nurses to lessen the extra workload that would be required of the students (6).

Another change occurred with the placing of a permanent nurse in charge of the operating theatre and the new sterilizing room (7). At the time, there was a stirring of excitement when the Hospital acquired an electric ambulance, which eventually eliminated the need for the traditional horse-drawn vehicle (8). It would not be long before Henry Ford's Model T appeared on the market after its dramatic introduction in 1908.

The New York Hospital continued to expand its property and demolish existing sites to erect new buildings. In 1901, the administration building underwent a complete reconstruction as a two-story structure consisting of an outpatient department and a suite for the Board of Governors, the treasurer, and the records room (9). Long connecting corridors provided convenient access to the other buildings situated within the complex.

When Irene Sutliffe retired in 1902 for health reasons, the Governors appointed Annie Warburton Goodrich to head the Training School. Over the years, she would become one of the most charismatic figures in the annals of American nursing. Before beginning her career, Goodrich was well known for her strong will, delightful sense of humor, and driving need for independence—the same characteristics demonstrated throughout her four-year tenure at The New York Hospital (10).

Prior to her appointment, she claimed a record of accomplishment as superintendent of nurses at two training schools in New York City. During her seven years at Post Graduate Hospital, she initiated the requirement of a high school diploma for the admission of students, introduced a probationary period, and strongly advocated state regulation and licensure for nursing (11). At St Luke's Hospital, she implemented the first graduation ceremony, among other innovations for pupil nurses (12). Throughout her professional life, it would be Goodrich's pattern to institute changes far ahead of the time that they eventually became standard procedure.

Before accepting the position at The New York Hospital, she established certain ground rules with the Board of Governors. Goodrich had a passionate desire to place the School on a more educationally sound basis and to give increased administrative authority to graduate nurses (13). She proposed the title of superintendent instead of directress, which would lend more prestige to the Training School, and requested that the general supervision and control of the program fall within her jurisdiction (14). In addition, she expected that certain responsibilities of the Hospital's superintendent would be transferred to her, such as: (1) correspondence with applicants to the School, (2) selection of probationers, and (3) the appointment and dismissal of ward maids and orderlies (15).

In March 1904, at a special meeting of the Training School Committee, formed two years earlier, the members approved Goodrich's recommendation to extend the probationary period to six months. She believed that the change from two months would eliminate a number of undesirable applicants and attract more young women of superior education and culture. Another recommendation was to shift evening classes to the daytime and pay competent instructors to teach the students (16). Goodrich suggested that five scholarships a year be made available to pupil nurses who could not complete the course because of financial difficulty (17). She informed the committee that other training schools had successfully adopted the system she proposed (18).

One of Goodrich's concerns related to the practice of providing an allowance to the pupil nurses. Beginning with the class of 1908, she urged a change in policy, in which payment would be discontinued, but students would be provided uniforms, caps, textbooks, and other necessities connected with their work (19). She pointed out that Presbyterian Hospital had distributed circulars announcing its nonpayment plan, and Bellevue and St. Luke's Hospital were in the process of exploring the matter (20).

In the spring of 1905, the Governors concurred with Goodrich's desire to resume the affiliation with Sloane Maternity Hospital and reduce the number of pupil nurses at Lying-In Hospital (21). The following January, she explained to the Training School Committee the changes underway in the distribution of graduate nurses, who would be responsible for instructing pupils and probationers on the wards. In the private patients building, senior students would be placed in charge of three floors under the supervision of graduate nurses (22). At the end of the year, 26 new pupil nurses were enrolled in the School, joining 28 seniors, 25 intermediates, 23 juniors, and an additional 12 probationers (23).

The following March, some subtle changes surfaced that undermined Goodrich's authority. The Medical Board began to assert greater control over staffing in the operating theater by appointing a committee to oversee personnel and equipment as well as supervision of all engaged in the department (24). The committee recommended that the nursing staff include two paid graduate nurses, four pupil nurses, two orderlies, and one general utility man. When Goodrich learned of the action while on a summer holiday in Nova Scotia, it distressed her, particularly the inadequate complement of anticipated staff in light of the tasks involved. In a letter to Dr. William Hoppin, chairman of the Training School Committee, she expressed her concern:

> I understand the entire control of graduate nurses and pupil nurses would be in the hands of the surgeons. That this should be so I do not dispute but believe me when I say that the dignity, loyalty, and proper discipline of the school can only be maintained when the authority is used through the woman who has been placed in charge of the school (25).

In November 1906, when Goodrich submitted her resignation to the Board of Governors, she indicated that Mrs. William Church Osborne, president of the Board of Bellevue and Allied Hospitals, had offered her the position of general superintendent of the Training School (26). She pointed out that they might view her new position as a compliment because Bellevue selected one of The New York Hospital's graduates to direct the reorganization of "The Great City School" (27). The Governors lauded her intelligent administration of the department, her loyalty to the Hospital, and the high standard of excellence (28).

A month after Goodrich resigned, the Medical Board wasted no time in abolishing many of her reforms and accelerated its control over the School. The majority of physicians concurred on a proposal to reduce the length of the program to two years, which would limit the amount of theoretical instruction. They noted that the "knowledge obtained is necessarily of the most superficial and fragmentary character, and if it had any influence at all, the nurse's conduct is apt to make her less rather than more useful in the sickroom" (29). On February 4, 1907, the Training School Committee also decreased the probationary term from six to two months (30). These actions generated considerable protest from the School's Nurses Alumnae Association, which declared that it was a practical impossibility in two years time to move a large body of pupil nurses through all the wards of a large hospital (31).

Some years later, Mary Beard reflected on the reversal of The New York Hospital's policies regarding the School. She believed that Goodrich's decision to leave did not occur on the spur of the moment, but rather because she had a sense of the Medical Board's increasing control. A 1903 graduate, Beard had fond recollections of the personal interest Goodrich took in the pupil nurses, especially when they were ill. "The students could feel the stimulus of her personality from the moment they arrived. Even when many of the reforms were discontinued, more still remained as a nucleus which could not be killed. Miss Goodrich made it a school!" (32).

In the early 1900s, the anxieties of nursing leaders were heightened by the proliferation of training schools, as well as the uneven entry requirements and controls imposed by external forces. Various patterns of course work existed in nursing programs that ranged from six months to three years, with each school setting its own standards. Furthermore, the service demands of the hospitals took priority over the educational needs of the pupil nurses. In the existing system, a graduate of any school could call herself a "trained" nurse, and the public was unable to differentiate the safe from the unsafe practitioner (33). Before 1910, only 10.2% of women who worked as nurses were trained (34).

Between 1898 and 1902, registration as a mechanism for eliminating unqualified and incompetent nurses was gaining momentum with the formation of state nurses associations. At the first meeting of the International Council of Nurses (ICN), held in Buffalo, New York, in September 1901, Ethel Manson Fenwick described the need for a system of registration to be regulated by nursing to guarantee the qualifications of the nurses (35). Founder of the ICN and Great Britain's most fervent advocate for registration, Fenwick furthered her cause through the pages of the *Nursing Record* (later changed to the *British Journal of Nursing*), which she acquired in the early 1890s (36).

In 1903, the first bills requiring registration for nurses were enacted in North Carolina, New York, New Jersey, and Virginia (37). When the profession proposed the legislation, it was patterned after the laws establishing state boards of medical examiners (38). However, unlike the medical licensure laws, which were originally established to eliminate quackery, comparable legislation for nurses was not intended to correct abuses of independent practice, but rather to protect the nurse and the public from unqualified and unethical workers (39).

When the Board of Governors authorized Annie Goodrich to register the Training School with the Regents of the University of the State of New York, the action was necessary to comply with the new nurse practice act, which stipulated that before a school admitted students to examination for licensure, it had to undergo inspection (40). In the ensuing years, members of the New York State Nurses Association (NYSNA) and the Alumnae Association of The New York Hospital, as well as other institutions, worked tirelessly to strengthen the law. Their efforts to achieve legislative recognition and propose reforms were vehemently resisted by physicians and hospital administrators.

At a conference of the American Hospital Association in 1913, representatives of The New York Hospital's governing body opposed a bill proposed by the state nurses association, claiming it would give too much power to the Board of Nurse Examiners (41). Unquestionably, any changes suggested in the nurse practice act intimidated the Governors, who believed that the state nursing group tended to "pay little attention to any interest other than their own" (42). Superintendent Howell pointed out that the Regents had the authority to make rules and regulations "prejudicial to the hospitals" (43).

In May of the same year, Dr. Howard Townsend, vice president of the Board of Governors, sent an urgent letter to the Reverend A. S. Kaufman, chairman of the executive committee of the Hospital Conference of New York City. He urged a united front of all hospital members to protest a bill sponsored by the NYSNA proposing that only a registered nurse should practice nursing (44). Townsend contended that any such legislation would interfere with hospital management. He informed the chairman that a special committee of the state association consisting only of nurses was advising the Regents on matters affecting hospitals (45). The committee, he noted, should also include two nurses, two physicians, and two hospital trustees.

The attempts of hospital and medical boards to regulate the practice of nursing, as demonstrated by the profession's struggle to achieve state registration, continued to be a serious issue facing nurses. Nevertheless, by 1913, 20 states had passed licensing laws and in time the rest followed. For some years, the laws controlled practitioners and titles but not the practice itself, and thus they were called *nurse* practice acts rather than *nursing* practice acts, the name by which they later came to be known (46).

During the critical years when state nurses associations and alumnae groups participated in the registration movement, Adeline Henderson, successor to Annie Goodrich, served as the superintendent of the Training School of The New York Hospital. Soon after beginning her position in March 1906, she appointed Anna Reutinger, a graduate of the program, as assistant superintendent. When Henderson shared with students the news about reducing the length of the program, she encountered some resentment, particularly among the junior class (47). At the time, the course had shown a steady increase in the number of pupil nurses enrolled.

At the outset of her administration, Henderson was eager to return to the former system of giving the students an allowance of $10 a month instead of furnishing them with uniforms, books, stationery, and other items. The Governors supported her recommendation to reverse the policy and suggested including the probationers. She explained her reasons as follows:

> The majority of applicants now come from the class of those who regard the training as a means of social elevation. No self-

respecting woman cares to have her clothes furnished. Every
woman prefers to purchase her wearing apparel and always takes
better care of what has cost her time and money (48).

On February 24, 1909, the proposed student affiliation with
Sloane Maternity Hospital was approved, and after it began operating,
Henderson submitted monthly reports to the Training School
Committee. She noted that the pupil nurses on affiliation there had
performed excellent work, receiving high marks and showing "exceptional punctuality" (49). That same year, she introduced a course
designed specifically for graduate nurses who expressed interest in
institutional management (50).

Adapting the models offered at the Massachusetts General
Hospital in Boston and Detroit's Grace Hospital, the six-month program was launched in October with two 1896 graduates of the School
who were employed at the Hospital (51). It included course work and
exposure to several departments of the institution; upon completion,
the participants received a certificate. A year after the postgraduate
course had proceeded well, Henderson considered decreasing the
length to four months, believing it would be more beneficial to nurses
as well as attracting a larger number (52).

By 1910, the Training School had achieved national recognition,
as evidenced by the competence and leadership skills of the graduates.
Requests from other schools to affiliate at the Hospital increased
markedly, with formal agreements made with the French Hospital,
White Plains Hospital, and Watertown Hospital. The courses and practical training proved to be invaluable to the students because they
could observe first hand the advances in diagnosis and treatment performed at The New York Hospital. Heralded by the Medical Board as
the "Spirit of Modern Medicine," the era of specialization had arrived
(53).

During this period, the Hospital began to limit the number of
patients receiving free care and shifted its focus to serving a more affluent population (54). New procedures and experimentation were continually underway, such as the policy regarding the discharge of
patients. In his annual report to the Executive Committee in March
1915, Superintendent Howell indicated that with fewer infections
occurring postoperatively and when a wound had completely healed,
the surgeons were justified in sending patients home earlier than pre-

viously. Howell pointed out that whereas The New York Hospital kept patients undergoing hernia surgery in bed from 12 to 14 days, Johns Hopkins discharged their hernia patients after 8 days. "It is our duty to pass patients through their beds as rapidly as is consistent with good work and their welfare," he asserted, adding that the Mayos in Minnesota claimed it was "dangerous for a patient to remain long in bed after an operation" (55).

Unlike the more progressive hospitals or medical schools, not all institutions had responded to the changes resulting from scientific advances. Concerned groups raised questions about the educational status of medical schools as well as their relationship to the general program of medical education. In 1908, Henry S. Pritchett, President of the Carnegie Foundation, asked Abraham Flexner, an educator and not a physician, to undertake an extensive investigation of American medical education (56). Two years later when the Flexner Report appeared, it yielded some shocking findings. Flexner provided detailed accounts of the existing medical schools in the nation, revealing that (1) 22 schools required two or more years of college, (2) 50 schools required only a high school education, and (3) 80 schools lacked a clearly defined standard for the admission of students (57).

Flexner recommended closing 120 of the existing medical schools, while maintaining about 30 schools with 300 students each located in different regions of the country (58). The Report earned the support of the American Medical Association and its Council on Medical Education, which forced the medical profession to initiate significant reforms in medical education (59). The study had a profound effect on nursing leaders such as Sutliffe and Goodrich, who had worked zealously with their national organizations and alumnae associations to strengthen nursing practice acts and raise standards in the training schools, which had soared to over a 1,000 by 1910. They recognized the need for a similar investigation of nursing education, but it would be more than a decade before such a hope could be realized.

In the same year that the Flexner Report was published, another epochal event occurred when the University of Minnesota opened a school of nursing with Bertha Erdman, a Teachers College graduate as director (60). Although a positive step toward moving nursing into higher education, the program differed little from the three-year pattern of the hospital school leading to a diploma. In time, the university substituted a five-year program, offering a bachelor's degree and including two years of academic study (61).

The ASSTSN welcomed this development because of a long-standing goal advocating university affiliation. At the time, however, its membership realized that the majority of training schools were controlled and administered by hospitals, and because of the lack of standardization, the programs were difficult to assess. In 1914, a Curriculum Committee of the newly titled National League of Nursing Education began developing a guide with appropriate criteria for basic nursing preparation (62). Three years later when the *Standard Curriculum for Schools of Nursing* was published, it had a marked impact on the training schools but was not well received by all groups, particularly the hospital and medical community, which found the standards too high (63).

By this time, interest in public health nursing had grown markedly, and graduates of the Training School joined Lillian Wald and her family of nurses at the Henry Street Settlement. In November 1912, the new National Organization for Public Health Nursing (NOPHN) rented headquarters in New York City at $75 a month, in the drawing room of an old private home on East 34th Street (64). As the organization's founder and first president, Wald keynoted the first convention and emphasized that public health nursing was not a service for the poor but for all people (65).

In 1914, Adeline Henderson reported that the number of students in the program had increased to 100 (66). This was good news for The New York Hospital, particularly when sobering events loomed on the horizon in the world at large. War clouds threatening Europe prompted the American government to begin gearing up for the war effort. At the Hospital, the Board of Governors announced that five of the surgical staff and 14 nurses "have already gone on this errand of mercy" (67).

According to Henderson, graduates of the School responded generously to the call for nurses in war-stricken countries. Anna Reutinger and other nurses were sent abroad under the auspices of the Red Cross (68). Wasting no time, the Alumnae Association met on October 5, 1914, to form plans and appoint a committee to begin the task of supplying clothing and materials for the relief of the people of Belgium who had endured hardships (69). When Henderson died in 1915 after a long illness, the Governors recruited Minnie Jordan from the French Hospital, with a return to the title of directress. From the outset, she succeeded in convincing the Governors to reinstate the length of the course to three years, which would include three months of affiliation at both Bloomingdale Hospital for mental illness and Willard Packer Hospital for contagious diseases (70).

In the winter of 1916, Colonel J. R. Kean, director general of military relief of the American Red Cross, requested The New York Hospital, Bellevue Hospital, and Presbyterian Hospital to collaborate in organizing and enrolling personnel for three base hospital units of 500 beds each (71). In the opinion of the Governors, only a limited number of professional and administrative staff would be needed to enroll in the base hospital unit. They decided to choose the recruits from the oldest and youngest surgeons, leaving the associates to staff the Hospital (72). The officers and enlisted men were sent to Governor's Island, while the nurses and civilian employees went to Ellis Island for indoctrination and training (73).

These were unsettling times for the Hospital, with war preparations in progress while an epidemic of infantile paralysis ravaged New York City. The Board of Governors offered to equip the old vacated Orthopaedic Hospital on East 59th Street, which had been at the disposal of the Board of Health (74). By August 1916, the facility was operating again, with the ever-dependable Irene Sutliffe volunteering her services as superintendent until a number of patients were discharged and the building and equipment turned over to Bellevue Hospital (75). During that summer, a marked depletion of the nursing staff occurred at The New York Hospital, but Jordan remedied the situation by replacing most of the nurses with younger graduates (76). The greatest loss, she explained, appeared to be in private nursing, with 215 nurses enrolling in the Red Cross and 7 in the Army Nurse Corps (77).

On April 6, 1917, the United States entered the war, and four months later 23 medical officers, 60 nurses, a chaplain, and enlisted personnel from The New York Hospital sailed on the *S.S. Finland* (78). The majority of nurses on board were graduates from the classes of 1908 through 1917 (79). The Alumnae Association seemed particularly pleased that Mary Vroom had been appointed chief nurse of Base Hospital Unit No. 9, and indicated as much in their newsletter to the members: "We feel fortunate in securing a woman of Miss Vroom's capabilities, personality, and high ideals, and also that the high standards of our graduates will be maintained in their service to the country" (80).

At The New York Hospital, the war was undoubtedly on the minds of the graduating class of 1917 as they listened to the inspiring words of Virginia Gildersleeve, dean of Barnard College, who spoke in the Governors' Room of the administration building. "The demand for nurses who have in addition to their technical training a good background of general education is, I am told, very large," she declared. "Buckle your armor and move forward with courage into the many fields of opportunity before you" (81).

It was not long before one of the new graduates volunteered and joined the other nurses on the voyage to France. Throughout the trip, the chaplain, Padre Raymond Brown, maintained a detailed record and commented on the frivolity that took place, with people laughing at the hardships and discomfort. "The nurses at Base Hospital No. 9 burlesqued their life on the *Finland*," he wrote in his log, "which caused so much merriment and applause that the captain had to call out from the bridge 'less noise!'" (82).

After spending a day in St. Nazaire where the ship landed, the nurses, doctors, and other personnel left for Savenay, a quiet Brittany town where they were joined by the staff of Base Hospital Unit No. 8, also from New York City (83). In September 1917, they moved to the small village of Bitray, which became their permanent location. The unit established a hospital in 32 one- and two-story buildings constructed of stone and stucco (84). A former mental facility, the hospital expanded from 700 to 2,000 beds within a year. The chief surgeon designated the institution, which began as a general hospital, as the Orthopedic Center of the American Expeditionary Forces (85).

Although Base Hospital Unit No. 9 had its own contingent of nurses from The New York Hospital, many graduates of the Training School had signed up with other hospital units. On May 15, 1917, Julia Stimson, class of 1908, set sail for Europe as chief nurse of Base Hospital Unit No. 21 of St. Louis, which served with the British Expeditionary Forces in France (86). In 1911, she had been recruited to

St. Louis, Missouri from New York to develop the hospital's social service department at Washington University (87). For the next six years, she held the simultaneous post of superintendent of nurses at Barnes Hospital and worked closely there with Dr. G. Canby Robinson, chief of the medical clinic of the outpatient department. Some years later, Robinson would become an important figure in the establishment of The New York Hospital-Cornell Medical Center. In his autobiography, he recalled Stimson's leadership qualities and how their association "awakened in me an interest in medical social work that has never abated" (88).

Stimson's daily correspondence with her family during the war years graphically described her experiences after landing on foreign soil. Writing to her mother on July 25, 1917 from Rouen, France where the base hospital unit was stationed, she expressed her feelings in this way: "There are so many pitiful people over here it keeps one's heart torn up. It is before your eyes every waking moment and in your ears even when you sleep." (89). In a September 11 letter, she informed her mother that her younger brother Philip, a medical officer, had been wounded and was hospitalized in Flanders. "I'm going to raise the roof today and see why the boy can't be brought here!" (90).

Her determination paid off and before long she was on her way, accompanied by an officer to the Chicago Base Hospital that housed her brother. "We had a beautiful trip. Both Captain Veeder and I sat in the front seat with the driver. The car was a great big ambulance that can be used to carry four stretcher cases" (91). After her reunion with Philip, she returned with him to Rouen where the doctor dressed his wound caused by a jagged piece of shrapnel shell that pierced his shoulder and tore the muscles down his back (92). While he convalesced and eventually recovered, Stimson returned to her other duties.

In an entry dated April 6, 1918, Stimson mentioned her appointment as chief nurse of the American Red Cross, which would relocate her to Paris. She wrote that the city was "not a sweet little health resort at present as it has been. But bombs and long distance guns are nothing to me" (93). Recorded in her last entry sent from Paris on May 17, 1918, Stimson expressed her thoughts about the people she worked with. "I was so homesick and lonesome for my children [the nurses], that when some of the officers blew into my office and said they were going back [to Rouen], I decided to go with them" (94).

Six months later, when the signing of the Armistice on November 11 signaled the end of the war, Stimson had the monumental task of overseeing the return of nurses to the United States. The recognition accorded her leadership was given high visibility in a report of the Alumnae Association of the Training School. It highlighted the honors she received from England, France, and the United States, including the American Distinguished Service Award bestowed upon her by General John J. Pershing (95).

The Great War had ended, but it would take some time before the base unit hospital disbanded and released many of the staff eager to return to civilian life. Although rigid mail censorship had been imposed from the beginning of the war, letters poured into The New York Hospital from graduates of the Training School sharing as much as they could. Irene Sutliffe heard from several young women stationed in Europe, who apparently were kept informed of happenings on the home front. Anna Reutinger's letter of November 10, 1918, revealed her awareness of the influenza epidemic in the States. "We hear the flu is raging," she wrote. "I hope dear Miss Sutliffe that you will consider your health – doubtless there will be great demands on nurses" (96).

The epidemic, which struck the nation in the fall of that year and lasted until the following August, became one of catastrophic proportions affecting people of all classes. Strict quarantine measures were instituted along with the closing of churches, public gatherings, and schools. At The New York Hospital, the Governors reported that 560 cases had been treated and discharged from September to December (97). Among the patient population of 322 males and 238 females, the largest number ranged in age from 50 to 74 years followed by those in the 17 to 27 age group (98). Minnie Jordan noted an absence of 55 nurses, while adding that "on the whole and compared with other hospitals, we were very fortunate, as many of the pupil nurses made a very good and complete recovery" (99).

In early 1918 before the disease became rampant, the Governors responded favorably to a request from Dr. A. Lung, medical director of the U.S. Naval Hospital Base. Lung had been authorized by the Navy Department through the Bureau of Medicine and Surgery in Washington, D.C., to explore with officials of The New York Hospital the possibility of using the House of Relief to accommodate 50 or more patients, both officers and enlisted men (100). The Governors agreed with the proposal and in March the facility closed as a civilian hospital to be used solely for the care of sick and wounded sailors in active service (101).

A year later when the arrangement proved successful, the U.S. Government expressed interest in purchasing the property as a permanent institution of the public health service. On February 3, 1920, the Society of The New York Hospital sold the House of Relief for the amount of $225,000 (102). The event was significant because it represented the end of 40 years of emergency service in the lower part of New York City.

During this period, the times were changing with the ending of World War I and the arrival of a new decade offering promises of prosperity and optimism. Annie Goodrich, president of the American Nurses Association, expressed the sentiment that nursing had reached an extraordinary period in the history of the world and that "all consecrate ourselves to the service of humanity through our profession" (103). The challenges that lay ahead in the 1920s not only became a stimulus for energizing The New York Hospital, the Training School for Nurses, and the Medical College, but also led to a dramatic and visionary development: strengthening the bond with Cornell University.

CHAPTER 5

Fulfilling the Dream:
An Evolving Medical Center

Earning the popular sobriquet "The Roaring Twenties," postwar America entered the decade on the brink of a cultural revolution. The era conjured up vivid images of a new generation and introduced prohibition, jazz, and flappers to a nation also mesmerized by the first transatlantic flight and the silent film. People reveled in the availability of modern conveniences, aided by the expansion in consumer credit facilities. Many Americans drove their own automobiles, purchased homes, and enjoyed more leisure time. After years of struggle, women won the right to vote and began to achieve a modicum of economic independence as they flocked to the workplace, becoming a visible force as job opportunities flourished. Some represented the immigrant population that arrived in the "Second Wave" from Southern or Eastern Europe, differing from the "First Wave" that came from Britain, France, and Germany (1).

In the nursing profession, the decade generated a variety of pioneering efforts, most notably those of such remarkable nurses as Mary Breckinridge and Margaret Sanger. Breckinridge, a woman of deep passion committed to reducing the high infant and maternal mortality rates plaguing the mountaineers in rural Kentucky, introduced the first nurse-midwives into the United States (2). She and her gallant corps of nurse-midwives traveled year-round on horseback over rocky terrain and overcame treacherous conditions to reach lonely log cabins and shacks often miles away from neighbors and without electricity. In 1928, Breckinridge founded the Frontier Nursing Service and 11 years later the Frontier Graduate School of Midwifery, the first of its kind in the nation, which helped to establish the role of the educated nurse-midwife (3).

A contemporary of Breckinridge, Sanger was engaged in her mission to promote birth control by establishing classes, writing extensively, lecturing around the world, and working to change restrictive legislation (4). She was instrumental in planning the first National Birth Control Conference and in establishing the American Birth Control League, which evolved into the Planned Parenthood Federation of America in 1942. Through Sanger's influence, funding became available in the early 1950s for the research conducted by Dr. Gregory Pincus that produced the birth control pill (5).

During the 1920s, the opening up of occupations and white-collar positions attracted an increasing number of young women from the middle classes, a trend with a marked impact on schools of nursing. As a consequence, Minnie Jordan noted that the Training School tended to attract more applications from the working class population (6). Nursing leaders complained that most women with the "right character," an attribute stressed by Florence Nightingale, were no longer applying to nursing programs (7). In her annual report to the Governors in 1921, Jordan cited the rigidity of the schools as one of the factors creating the decline of desirable applicants. She noted that nursing programs with the largest number of the best candidates were the ones that maintained the highest educational standards and provided the most desirable living quarters (8). The recent policy of the Board of Governors, instituting an eight-hour working day or night for the pupil nurses, may have been a step in the right direction, but numerous controls continued to be applied in the learning environment (9).

Aware of the problem in many schools, hospital directors and nursing superintendents attempted to seek some resolution by focusing more on transforming the individual's character rather than altering the work process and unfair social hierarchy (10). To retain staff nurses in the working environment, administrators applied the common strategy of appealing to their loyalty by stressing the concept of "our hospital" (11). The tactic often worked because many nurses and other employees experienced a sense of pride about their hospital as well as a commitment to caring for patients and sharing responsibilities.

In 1920, Jordan reported soberly on the drop in enrollment to 95 students from 117 four years earlier. To fill the necessary complement of staff for floor duty, she employed graduate nurses for the Private Patients Pavilion, while less seasoned pupil nurses worked on the wards (12). Although the more experienced students were on affiliation, their absence was counterbalanced by affiliations from several other schools. As part of their four three-month affiliations, senior students had the option of selecting two elective courses, which included the Henry Street Settlement and social service work in the Hospital (13). Most of the arrangements with other institutions worked out well, with the latest affiliations occurring at the Manhattan Maternity and Dispensary and the Maternity Center Association. Another positive experience had occurred with the group of incoming pupil nurses from the Army School of Nursing, sent by Julia Stimson, who had replaced Annie Goodrich as the second dean. Jordan found them to be "bright, alert, and intelligent" (14).

During this period, Jordan began to perceive changing behavior characteristics in the nature of the student body. Unlike the compliant pupil nurses of former years, she claimed that the present crop was restless and "too progressive to settle down, and are on the alert for professional and financial advancement, and rightly so" (15). Another change was the rapid turnover of staff in the Hospital, due largely to the number of other employment opportunities springing up. Jordan pointed out that these developments greatly complicated management of the department.

While superintendents of training programs were trying to deal with the pervasive problem of recruiting suitable students, the profession desperately needed capable nurses to lead, direct, teach, and supervise in hospitals, schools, and public health agencies. In 1923, the findings of a major study sponsored by the Rockefeller Foundation appeared in a publication known as the "Goldmark Report" (16). The significant conclusion reached in the report was that most training schools bore no resemblance to educational institutions, and that they needed to be recognized as well as supported as separate entities consisting of both a training program and a liberal education (17). Nurses serving on the original study committee included Annie Goodrich, M. Adelaide Nutting, and Lillian Wald, and when it expanded, President Livingston Farrand of Cornell University joined the group (18).

The Goldmark Report became a classic in the field, but it did not have the impact on nursing education comparable to that of the Flexner Report on medical education. An important outcome, however, was the establishment in 1923 of the first undergraduate nursing program at Yale University, which operated as a separate department with Annie Goodrich as the dean (19). A bachelor of nursing degree was awarded to the nursing graduates, signifying another "first" for Yale in awarding this credential to women (20). The school began as a five-year experiment with $150,000 funded by the Rockefeller Foundation, which renewed its pledge with a $1 million endowment after the program proved successful (21). In 1924, Mary Beard began her long association with Rockefeller, and through her influence $4,000,000 was donated to the nursing profession, which included funds to help schools implement the Goldmark Report (22).

Although the Report provided fresh insights into nursing education, it represented only a brief survey. Subsequently, the NLNE appointed a Committee on the Grading of Nursing Schools to conduct a series of studies to obtain specific information on the status of nursing schools (23). One of the studies, published as *Nursing Schools Today and Tomorrow* (1934), focused on the supply of nurses and other nursing functionaries. The work reported the existence of 2,000 hospital schools in the nation as compared with 79 medical schools (24). The growth of these schools was phenomenal as well as unchecked, allowing shockingly low standards and unqualified students to graduate. As a result of the findings, the committee considered it crucial to develop "...nursing schools which are directed with a primary educational aim and animated by professional ideals" (25).

While the profession was assessing conditions in hospital schools, university nursing programs were also being explored. In 1924, the NLNE formed a Committee on University Relations to study collegiate programs with the expectation of establishing uniform standards for this type of nursing education (26). By 1928, 38 schools in the United States claimed some connection with a college or university (27).

As head of the Training School for Nurses, Minnie Jordan had kept up with the beginning movement toward collegiate education and the involvement of the NLNE in monitoring this development. She faithfully attended the conventions of the national nursing organizations, where colleagues gathered to discuss pressing issues in the field and to seek ways to advance nursing. In the late 1920s, while members of the Alumnae Association were preparing for the 50th Anniversary of the School, another dramatic event was imminent, which would have marked implications for the future of the nursing program. Planning for the reorganization of the Society of The New York Hospital that had been in progress for some time was concluded, and an important new alliance was formed with Cornell University.

In 1927, nursing alumnae representing every class except two since 1878 congregated in New York City, from May 9–13 to celebrate the 50th Anniversary of the Training School (28). The occasion generated an aura of excitement, nostalgia, and pride as Irene Sutliffe and the anniversary committee greeted classmates, students, hospital officials, and a host of other guests. Not even a stormy night could dampen the spirits of the participants at the formal opening that took place in the Cathedral of St. John the Divine. Irene Sutliffe, Annie Goodrich, and Lydia Anderson led the procession of white-robed, white-capped women marching down the aisle, followed by the graduates and Minnie Jordan with staff close behind (29).

During the week, some of the people visited Bloomingdale Hospital in White Plains and the Henry Street Settlement on the Lower East Side of New York, where Lillian Wald gave an informal talk and served tea from two authentic Russian samovars (30). A highlight of the celebration of particular interest to the alumnae was a tour of the Hospital, which Jane Hitchcock recorded glowingly. "They reminisced, peeped into old beloved corners, or looked with awe upon the new methods and the enlarged equipment" (31).

At the dinner held the last evening in the Hotel Astor, several distinguished graduates of the School's earlier years gave stimulating addresses. The speakers included Mary Beard, associate director, International Health Division, Rockefeller Foundation; Florence Johnson, director of the New York Chapter of the American Red Cross; Major Julia Stimson, dean of the Army School of Nursing; and Lillian Wald, director of the Henry Street Settlement. Also among the group was Annie Goodrich, who spoke passionately about education and nursing and closed her talk with the following comments:

The life of a nurse is filled with meaning . . . .We are but a segment of the great social force whose candles were lighted
through the hard school of practical experience; we have held
high torches and even more light [will] be given to those who
follow (32).

Summing up the week's activities, Minnie Jordan described the
joyful reunion of classmates and old friends. "It was a wonderful inspiration to the staff and student body to meet in this assemblage of pioneers in our profession . . .who carry the message of health and healing to the home, the community, and the world at large" (33).

A month after the School's anniversary, an event of some magni-
tude took place on June 14 with the signing of an historic agreement
establishing The New York Hospital-Cornell Medical College
Association (34). The genesis of this landmark development could be
traced to the early 1920s when the Board of Governors began to consider the future of the Society in relation to medical and surgical education and the general management of the Hospital (35). Their deliberations became more focused when Payne Whitney, vice president of
the Board, donated $100,000 in 1923 to erect and furnish new build-
ings in the Bloomingdale complex (36).

In September of that year, Edward Sheldon, president of The
New York Hospital, reported that Cornell University had reopened
negotiations regarding a permanent arrangement between the two
institutions. He explained that Whitney had been involved in a number of conferences during the summer with representatives of his foundation and the University (37). In May 1924, Sheldon announced that
Whitney had donated a munificent gift of $2,800,000 to The New York
Hospital for the explicit purpose of acquiring a new site (38).

With contracts underway and six plots of land purchased by
Whitney, the Society resolved to carry out in full the terms entered into
between George H. Storm Lumber Company and the Treat Realty
Company. At the time, architectural studies had been initiated and preliminary plans drawn up for a hospital in the block between 68th and
69th Streets, extending from Avenue A (later named York Avenue) to
the East River. In the spring of 1927, the second block was acquired,
which included the area from 69th to 70th Streets as well as the east end
of 69th Street (39).

A major philanthropist, Whitney was the son of a lawyer, financier, and Secretary of the Navy during President Grover Cleveland's administration. As the heir to the estate of his uncle, Oliver Hazard Payne, he received a bequest that made him one of the wealthiest men in America. In December 1926, Sheldon reported that Whitney's gifts, specifically earmarked for the new hospital, totaled more than $4,100,000 (40). Tragically, Whitney did not live to see the results of his generosity, having suffered a heart attack while playing tennis on May 25, 1927, three weeks before Sheldon and Livingston Farrand, president of Cornell University, signed the agreement, thereby creating a stronger relationship between their respective institutions (41). In his will, Whitney left over $40,000,000 in trust to the Hospital to be executed by Sheldon (42). On November 1, 1927, his only son, 23-year-old John (Jock) Hay Whitney was elected to the Board of Governors (43).

The formal agreement solidified the association of the Society of the New York Hospital and Cornell University while preserving their respective rights and obligations. In the preamble, the document stated that the Hospital would participate fully in the educational program and the faculty and staff would be organized on a true university plan encompassing both clinical and laboratory departments (44). Education became a primary concern along with the other functions of patient care and research.

The agreement further stated that a new general hospital would be erected to include all the necessary facilities, laboratories, and equipment as well as accommodations for teaching medical students. Responsibility for building, maintaining, and conducting the new medical college rested with the University, which would confer the doctor of medicine degree. The therapeutic and educational work of the entire enterprise was to be conducted under The New York Hospital-Cornell Medical Association directed by a Joint Administrative Board (JAB) (45).

In her 1927 annual report to the Governors, Jordan noted that according to the joint agreement the Hospital would maintain a training school in New York City for the education of registered nurses, and would erect a building for the school and a nurses' residence (46). For some time, she had been troubled by the limitations imposed on the students and graduate nurses who lived in the same building constructed in 1891, which no longer provided sufficient classrooms and adequate facilities for extracurricular activities. "It is essential that some plan be adopted that will enable us to compete with other schools during the intervening years," she told the Governors, realizing it would take a few years before new housing became available. Although she looked forward to the prospect of larger quarters, the directress had a more immediate goal that she expressed as follows: "The thought of spacious and more comfortable halls is a lesser joy when compared with the anticipation of developing a bigger and broader educational program for the School to enable it to keep pace with the other units of the Association" (47).

The following year, the Board of Governors announced an agreement with the Lying-In Hospital to relocate from its present site to the Maternity Building in the new complex when completed. As a result of sizeable gifts donated from the Laura Spelman Rockefeller Memorial, as well as from J. Pierpont Morgan and George F. Baker, a new building would be constructed for the Lying-In Hospital (48).

At the graduation exercises of the Training School on March 7, 1928, the address of Dr. Walter L. Niles, dean of Cornell Medical College, sounded a positive note on the future of nursing education at The New York Hospital, excerpted below:

> I think the time has come to make a very urgent plea for the adequate endowment on the educational side of the Training School for nurses . . . I should like to see the needs of nursing presented side by side with the needs of medical education, and it is my belief that the day is not too distant when that will be (49).

The activities of the JAB came under the direction of Dr. George Canby Robinson, who was approached in 1926 by Sheldon, Farrand, and Whitney to head the project (50). Robinson had an impressive background that included his most recent position as dean and professor of medicine at Vanderbilt University where he had been the architect of a major reorganization of the medical school and hospital (51). At The New York Hospital, he not only began to institute a system similar to that of Vanderbilt and Johns Hopkins, but also sought Hopkins men for top positions at the new medical center (52). He also had worked closely with Henry R. Shepley of the same Boston architectural firm, which had been engaged for the proposed New York Hospital-Cornell Medical Center (53).

The year after his arrival, Robinson and the Governors were caught up in one of the most devastating events facing the nation when the stock market crashed in October 1929. In its aftermath, the Society of The New York Hospital was forced to liquidate $15,000,000 of its investments (54). As the 1930s approached, there were signs of a pending Depression, but the JAB decided to forge ahead with its work already in progress.

From the beginning of the project, it was understood that the Hospital and the Medical College would be organized and conducted on a university basis. Each division of the Hospital would operate under the direction of a chief of service, who held the title of professor and head of the respective department. The chief physician was salaried and expected to contribute his services full time without financial dependence on private patients (55).

Although the JAB was not incorporated and had no funds in its own name, the authority delegated to it came from the two incorporated bodies, Cornell University and The New York Hospital (56). The members consisted of three Governors of the Hospital, three trustees of the University, and a seventh member to be elected by the other six appointees. The original group from the Hospital included President Sheldon; William Woodward, a banker and horseman; and Frank L. Polk, a lawyer and son of Cornell University Medical College's first dean. Among the University representatives were President Farrand; J. DuPratt White, a lawyer and trustee; and Dean Walter L. Niles. J. Pierpont Morgan became the seventh person to serve on the Board (57).

As executive officer of the New York Hospital-Cornell Medical Association, Robinson was charged to represent the educational and research interests of the Hospital (58). While he assembled the staff and implemented plans to build the Medical Center, the JAB began to consider the problems of nursing, including the education of the pupil nurses. At their April 2, 1929 meeting, the Governors suggested that a special study be initiated on the subject (59). The Committee on Nursing Organization was formed with Chairman Mary Beard, president of the Alumnae Association, assisted by Lydia Anderson and Anna Reutinger, and Annie Goodrich and Minnie Jordan as advisors (60).

To conduct the studies, the committee engaged Ethel Johns in September 1929 (61). She was a well-known nurse researcher from Canada, who had spent the last four years in Paris on the staff of the Rockefeller Foundation. During the next two years, she conferred often with Robinson and the committee, whose main concerns related to the improvement of nursing education, formulation of the hospital nursing service, and financial requirements to meet the needs of the program being advocated (62). Committee members decided to approach the National Organization for Public Health Nursing (NOPHN) to undertake a study that would determine the best methods of teaching health and the prevention of disease in the curriculum (63).

The year before the committee issued its final report, the cornerstone of the new Medical Center was laid on June 3, 1930 (64). According to the Governors, construction would begin soon, and the hospital would be ready for occupancy by the fall of 1932 (65). High on the list of recommendations submitted by the Committee on Nursing Organization was the establishment of a school of nursing in conjunction with Cornell University offering an educational program leading to a bachelor's degree (66).

The committee had estimated that the School would require an endowment of $2,000,000 if it were to continue on a sound educational basis, but the Governors pointed out that no funds could be secured at that time and therefore the proposed relationship with Cornell could not yet be consummated. Nevertheless, they supported the recommendations in principle as well as those of the NOPHN, and suggested carrying out the program as far as existing conditions permitted (67). The JAB would serve as a conduit through which the School related to the University; the director of the nursing program would hold the dual position of director of nursing service; and qualified nurses appointed to higher positions on the staff would participate in the educational program.

The recommendations of the Committee on Nursing Organization and the NOPHN provided a foundation for the policies governing the proposed School and the nursing service of the Hospital. (See Appendix B.) Their implementation, however, did not come easily in light of resistance from the medical community and the uncertainties arising from a full-blown depression. Several years would pass, but with the strong support of Robinson, Farrand, and Sheldon, and their collaboration with a visionary nursing administrator, the dream of establishing a university school of nursing would eventually become a reality.

On June 2, 1931, Mary Beard informed the Board of Governors that the committee had selected Anna Dryden Wolf for the position of director of the School and director of nursing service (68). Beard had approached her in Chicago, where for the past five years she was the director of nursing at the University of Chicago Clinic, and associate professor of nursing at the university (69). As old friends, they shared a close colleagueship with Annie Goodrich and Lillian Wald, which may have been a factor in Wolf's decision to accept the post at The New York Hospital.

Wolf's appointment coincided with the beginning of the Great Depression, which created serious problems for the nursing profession. Throughout the nation, conditions changed rapidly as clinics and public health agencies were overwhelmed with requests from a needy population. In voluntary hospitals, nurse unemployment soared as private-duty nurses found themselves no longer in demand (70).

The daughter of American missionaries, Wolf acquired a world perspective early in life that gave her a tolerance for all people and a commitment to service (71). While assistant superintendent of nurses at Johns Hopkins Hospital School of Nursing, the Rockefeller Foundation had invited her in 1919 to reorganize the school of nursing at Peking Union Medical College Hospital in China. For the next six years, she served as the dean of the first school in that country to prepare women students to care for male patients (72).

During her tenure at the University of Chicago, Wolf learned of the work undertaken by the Committee on Nursing Organization at The New York Hospital, and spoke highly of Ethel Johns, who conducted the studies. "I knew of her as most imaginative and would bring a clear vision of what could be done. She did a stunning job for the committee" (73).

In August 1931, a month after the announcement of Wolf's appointment, Minnie Jordan resigned and informed the Governors that she expected to begin a new position with the Metropolitan Life Insurance Company. At the farewell reception, they expressed appreciation for her 16 years with the Hospital and presented her with an engraved silver tea service, the traditional gift given on occasion to an individual retiring or resigning from the School (74).

During the winter of 1932, the Society decided to expand the scope and size of the Medical Center, and on February 2 the Board of Governors completed arrangements involving a reorganization of Memorial Hospital, which specialized in the treatment of cancer and allied diseases (75). The agreement between the two institutions stipulated that Memorial Hospital would operate on a university basis, with the members of its professional staff eligible for positions on the faculty of Cornell Medical College (76). Prior to February 1, 1937, Memorial Hospital would be expected to find a satisfactory site in the immediate neighborhood of the Medical Center and secure a plan for acquiring an endowment. Memorial Hospital followed through and by 1938 relocated to a new building west of York Avenue opposite the Rockefeller Institute (77).

When Wolf assumed her duties at the School, her vision of how nursing would fit within the changing system included a new curriculum pattern and more well-qualified faculty. As a well-known figure in the profession, she had contacts throughout the world, but before recruiting outside staff she sought Jordan's advice about the present group of nurses working at the School, and requested a list of the names of alumnae (78). Among the senior staff nurses, she retained Sarah Moore as her administrative assistant and later described her as "a wonderful little person who knows every alumna!" (79).

Among the graduates invited to join the faculty was Margery Trieber Overholzer, who retained fond memories of Wolf that she expressed freely after retiring almost 30 years later. "Miss Wolf knew how to appoint appropriate people as the head of a department. She recruited an exceptionally fine group of nurses who served in various capacities and on the school's faculty. Under her leadership we became the first school to put a full time public health nurse on the faculty" (80).

Wolf conveyed her expectations early on to the Governors and the JAB. "I didn't want the nursing school to be under the medical school, and President Farrand and Canby Robinson supported me," she later recalled (81). Throughout her association with Robinson, they had excellent rapport that began soon after she arrived when he introduced her to the Governors, the medical faculty, and others whom Wolf considered sympathetic to the idea of a nursing school operating within the university system. She also enjoyed a close relationship with the Governors, particularly those who came to her office to talk over problems. "You don't see that in many places," she declared (82).

Among the people she greatly admired, Wolf cited President Farrand of Cornell University as her premier counselor. "Livingston Farrand was the greatest man I ever worked with. When you spoke of academic affairs and getting people prepared for their life work, he knew what you meant" (83).

During Wolf's first year at the School, she wrote to G. Howard Wise, secretary of the Board of Governors, expressing her appreciation for the recent action on forming a Council of the School of Nursing (84). In her view, the new Council could play a significant role in shaping present and future policies of the nursing program. Its main purpose was to strengthen the School's relationship with the executive and clinical staff in interpreting nursing education policies and furthering understanding of the expectations of nursing service. Another aim was to establish closer links with the University in Ithaca, inform the public about the School's goals, and gain support for higher standards, as well as attract qualified young women into the profession (85).

Membership on the Council of the School of Nursing consisted of President Edward Sheldon and Governors Wilson Powell and John R. Howard; President Livingston Farrand, Cornell University; Dr. Eugene Dubois, physician-in-chief and professor of medicine, Cornell University Medical College; Dr. G. Canby Robinson, executive director of the New York Hospital-Cornell Medical College Association; and a representative of the College of Home Economics, Cornell University. The nurses included Mary Beard, associate director, International Health Division of the American Red Cross, Mary M. Roberts, editor of *The American Journal of Nursing*, and Anna Wolf (86).

In July 1932, the old Hospital closed, and a month later the Executive Committee held its first meeting in the imposing building towering over East 68th Street at No. 525 (87). When The New York Hospital-Cornell Medical Center opened on September 1 to receive patients, Robinson commented that it was "the most specialized building project ever erected at one time" (88). At the morning convocation of the School of Nursing held in the amphitheater of the Medical

College, Wolf described the event as one to remain in memories: "It must have been difficult for The New York Hospital graduates and students to believe they were among their own, to feel at home in such a mammoth place after the intimacy of the old hospital" (89).

At the School of Nursing graduation exercises, Sheldon announced that Irene Sutliffe, then 82 years young, had been accorded the title of directress emeritus and was honored by the Society with an invitation to membership (90). In addition, she was assigned a permanent apartment in the new nurses residence (91). After Wolf became director of the School, she requested that a handsome oil portrait of Sutliffe, painted by Ernest L. Ipsen, be moved from the Governors' Room in the Hospital to the quarters of the Alumnae Association (92).

In the fall of 1932 when alumnae members met in the new nurses residence for the first time, Sheldon was invited as the guest of honor (93). A splendid looking building of 16 stories, the residence was located adjacent to the Hospital and the Medical College at 1320 York Avenue between 70th and 71st Streets. The first floor was reserved for social rooms filled with elegant and comfortable furnishings, while the entire second floor housed the School of Nursing offices of the director and faculty and the classrooms (94).

Since the building was designed primarily as a home for students and staff, one of its most attractive features was the living quarters area, which included furnished single bedrooms with shared sitting room, kitchenette, and baths on each floor. Also available were two complete apartments and five suites (95). On the ninth floor, the School maintained a health service and a 15-bed infirmary for students who were ill but did not require admission to the general hospital (96). When *The Architectural Forum* highlighted the Medical Center in its February 1933 issue, it described the dining room in the nurses residence: "The walls are of hand-finished plaster painted ice green, with columns and the acoustic plaster ceiling painted white. The floor is of red and light pinkish-gray rubber tile, laid in three-foot squares"(97).

A genuine caring about the living conditions and welfare of the students became apparent early in Wolf's administration. Her respect for them was reflected in the development of the Student Organization, which operated through an honor system and involved the faculty in maintaining student discipline (98). To encourage foreign students, the School registered with the Federal Department of

Labor (99). Wolf lauded the student organization in publishing its first *Handbook*, which she indicated would serve an important need in promoting the best interests of student life. An inspiring welcome to new students that appeared in the publication clearly spelled out her hopes for them:

> For most of you, school life of this kind will be a new experience. Many new fields of endeavor will be open to you and new opportunities will present themselves. If you will but recognize the possibilities around you, you can not fail to find the best that the school has to offer (100).

At the outset, Wolf had set in motion her plans for initiating change and a new direction for the School and nursing service. In reorganizing the curriculum, she was committed to developing a university course of study that would include public health nursing as an integral part, and hired Harriet Frost, a qualified instructor in the discipline (101). The graduate service also needed to be stabilized along with submitting a realistic budget. By October 1, 1932, 26 students were admitted in the first-year class, and two months later, the School increased the matriculation requirements to two years of college work (102). The following year, all 22 of the new students had at least two years of preclinical preparation (103).

A policy was instituted for students with college background to be eligible for a bachelor's degree from the school in which they had previously attended, to be awarded after completing the nursing course (104). Wolf informed the Governors that such an arrangement had been worked out with Temple University, and in another agreement, Cornell University indicated that it would be willing to admit nursing students to the College of Home Economics in Ithaca for further study toward an undergraduate degree (105).

The School's interest in university education was timely because nurse leaders such as Wolf, Annie Goodrich, and Effie Taylor recognized the need to move nursing into the system of higher education. In 1933, supported by representatives of over 20 colleges and universities with nursing programs, they were instrumental in forming a new national organization titled the Association of Collegiate Schools of Nursing (ACSN), with Goodrich elected the first president (106). Its purpose was to develop standards and policies and encourage experimentation in university education for nursing (107). As the ACSN began its formidable task of accrediting or approving collegiate nursing programs, the National League of Nursing Education invited Wolf to serve as chairman of its new Standing Committee on Accreditation. (108). Addressing a conference held at Teachers College, Columbia University, Taylor pointed out that the ACSN and the NLNE should complement and support each other (109).

At The New York Hospital, Wolf turned her attention to strengthening the patient care setting and formed a Committee on Nursing Service to coordinate the activities of all departments in the institution (110). This action aimed to provide support to the medical care organized for the Medical Center. The Hospital consisted of two divisions that included a ward service and an outpatient department to treat patients generally not requiring bed occupancy (111). The inpatient occupancy of 862 beds and 131 bassinets reached a capacity of 85% in the pavilions and 59% in the private service (112).

In October 1934, the Executive Committee discussed a communication from the United Hospital Fund concerning the establishment of the Associated Hospital Services (AHS) (113). The organization came into existence as a result of the Great Depression and the desperation of hospitals for revenue. In time, it would become a significant development in the future of American health care. Several institutions throughout the nation expressed enthusiasm about adopting an experimental plan that focused on hospital employees buying insurance (114). The New York Hospital joined the AHS in 1935, and a number of private and semi-private patients participated in the plan (115).

During the early 1930s, the economic pressures resulting from the Great Depression began to have a dispiriting effect on the progress accomplished by Wolf in raising the standards of the School. At the January 31, 1934, meeting of the Council, the members deliberated over the impracticality of maintaining the admission prerequisite of two years of college preparation, and recommended reducing the requirement to graduation from an accredited high school. They also recommended decreasing the class hours in the curriculum, as well as the length of the clinical experience (116).

In order to give more nursing hours to the Hospital, Wolf pointed out that the clinical practice periods would require a change in the sequential course plan and a decrease in public health and psychiatry (117). Adding a positive tone to the discussion, President Farrand noted that the difficulties involving matriculation requirements might not be insurmountable. He explained to the Council that in making decisions about the present situation "we do so because we believe them to be wise, right and necessary" (118).

Another consequence of the Great Depression was its effect, to a large extent, on Robinson's position as director of the JAB. He came to New York with great expectations of building what Morris Bishop characterized as his "Temple of Medicine" and succeeded brilliantly (119). As the architect of this monumental undertaking, Robinson made up his mind from the outset to bring in the most prominent physicians he had known and did so mostly with Hopkins graduates. He also dispensed with certain traditional privileges that had been previously granted to the faculty of the Medical College (120).

These factors, compounded by financial constraints, created a problem and altered his circumstances. Cuts in salary and the reduced departmental budgets intensified a sense of insecurity. When a change occurred in the chairmanship of the JAB, with Sheldon leaving because of illness, Wilson M. Powell, the Society's new president, assumed the reins. In his autobiography, Robinson claimed that unlike his supportive relationship with Sheldon, Powell made radical changes without consulting him, which he believed weakened his position (121). He also observed that the more aggressive leaders of the faculty had selfish objectives and disregarded what was best for the Medical College. "Their state of mind and feelings were, I thought, unfavorable for the creation of an environment in which medical students should develop" (122).

When Robinson resigned and left the Medical Center, it must have been disappointing to Wolf because of their productive relationship and his support for the School of Nursing. Thirteen years would pass before another director would fill the post at the JAB. In the meantime and throughout the rest of the decade, Wolf would work valiantly during difficult times to carry on her goal of building a foundation for what was to become a long-anticipated university school of nursing.

CHAPTER 6

Mission Achieved:
University Affiliation

During the 1930s, the economic depression subsided as the nation underwent a period of relief, recovery, and reform. Congressional enactment of the Social Security Bill in 1935 illustrated the government's recognition of its role in the health and welfare of the American public (1). The legislation established a system that provided unemployment insurance, old age pensions to workers, and survivor benefits for victims of industrial accidents. Grants-in-aid became available to dependent mothers and children, the blind, and the physically ill, as well as to nurses for training in public health (2).

Federal action initiated by President Franklin D. Roosevelt's administration produced desperately needed work programs and projects (3). Financial assistance to students harked back to the days of Ezra Cornell and his efforts to provide jobs—a policy that could be viewed as the forerunner of modern work-study programs in universities. On the Ithaca campus, the leadership of Livingston Farrand resulted in notable achievements despite economic problems with student enrollment rising to 6,341 by 1937 and a growing general endowment from $12,200,000 to $19,800,000 (4). Cornell Medical College also flourished, drawing increasing numbers of students that helped to sustain financial solvency (5). In 1938, New York City became its permanent site when the Ithaca Division was discontinued. That year, Edmund Ezra Day, a well-known educator from the field of social science, succeeded Farrand as president of Cornell University (6)

75

A noticeable trend by the end of the decade was the decline in hospital diploma programs while enrollments soared in the remaining schools of nursing. Within 10 years, the number of nursing students in the nation reached 94,133, and 380,000 women were practicing as graduate nurses (7). During the late 1930s, nursing leaders had recognized the need to develop a mechanism for evaluating the schools. Subsequently, the National League of Nursing Education (NLNE) charged its Committee on Standards to study various accrediting systems and submit the findings to the board of directors of the NLNE, the American Nurses Association (ANA), and the National Organization for Public Health Nursing (NOPHN) (8).

Another important NLNE initiative related to the concerns of nursing educators about the different curriculum patterns implemented in hospital schools. The NLNE's Curriculum Committee (formerly the Committee on Education) began a thorough revision of the 1917 *Curriculum Guide*, which had been modified only slightly in 1927. The committee aimed to examine critically not only the basic curriculum and instructional methods, but also the goals of nursing and its educational system (9).

This effort was significant because for the first time an in-depth analysis would be undertaken that described the philosophy of nursing education, goals and values to be maintained, and services that nurses should be prepared to render. Also to be determined were the kinds of nursing students to be selected, as well as the appropriate preparation required for the practice of nursing (10). The Curriculum Committee performed its task well, and in 1937 the NLNE released *A Curriculum Guide for Schools of Nursing* (11).

In April of the following year, the Council of The New York Hospital School of Nursing discussed the document and agreed to incorporate many of the suggestions in course titles, such as changing "bacteriology and pathology" to "microbiology"; "nursing principles and practice" to "introduction to nursing arts"; and "materia medica" to "pharmacology and therapeutics" (12).

An indirect by-product of the revised guide was the attention it focused on evaluating the nursing student objectively. Nellie Hawkinson, NLNE president, pointed out that one of the curriculum's weakest links was the "measurement of student achievement" (13). In

1939, the Committee on Nursing Tests was launched with Isabel Stewart, director of the Teachers College Department of Nursing Education, appointed as chairman and R. Louise McManus as secretary. The committee's work resulted in the development of a battery of tests—the Pre-Nursing and Guidance Test Battery—for use by state-approved schools of nursing as an aid in the selection and placement of students (14).

Another group expressing interest in standardized tests were the State Boards of Nurse Examiners, which cited studies that revealed the lack of validity of practical examinations of large numbers of graduates for licensure. During the early 1940s, the State Boards submitted to the League's Committee on Nursing Tests a list of activities applicable to the competent nurse. Their collaboration produced a new test based on objectives contained in the *Curriculum Guide* and eventually led to the establishment of the State Board Test Pool Service and the NLNE Testing Service (15).

Anna Wolf joined other leaders in organizational efforts to raise standards in the profession, while diligently pursuing her goal of placing The New York Hospital School of Nursing on a stronger educational basis. She began by forming faculty committees to help the members interpret the School's aims to the public, and to encourage an open interchange of disparate views on various issues (16). Wolf inspired her faculty to grow professionally by publishing books and articles, presenting papers at conferences, participating in workshops, and seeking continuing education. Among the faculty and staff nurses, 87% held membership in the ANA and 64% in the NLNE (17).

In her 1935 annual report to the Governors, Wolf indicated her desire to establish a closer relationship with Cornell University in order to recruit more mature students with advanced preparation (18). On one occasion, she visited the Ithaca campus where President Farrand had arranged a meeting with faculty members, who she hoped might be interested in teaching nursing students. When nothing later developed, she admitted that her visit might have been "a bit premature" (19).

In her efforts to give visibility to the School and promote its mission among many groups in the public arena, Wolf was delighted when invited to be a guest on a program of the Columbia Broadcasting

System entitled "So You Want to Be a Registered Professional Nurse." As was her style, she spoke eloquently at the broadcast, sharing her knowledge, vision, and concern for the patient and the nursing profession (20).

Wolf continually explored new ways to improve the image of the School of Nursing and succeeded in having the word "training" eliminated from its name. In her view, the old title connoted an apprentice-type preparation rather than one with an educational focus (21). She advised the faculty on curriculum development and increased the complement of instructors for the anatomy and combined chemistry-physiology courses. In addition, she secured the services of Fannie Bradshaw, a well-known voice teacher, to give lessons to the students in diction, voice control, and reading. Wolf believed that the effect of voice on patients was important and "may improve a limitation we experience in many of our students and graduates. It will prove effective in patient care and other contacts," she explained to Council members at their November 1937 meeting (22).

Also offered in the program were personality studies conducted on first-year students by a psychiatrist to provide consultation and help them adjust to the work, as well as determine their fitness for the profession (23). In the fall of 1937, the School admitted 57 students, ranging in age from 18 to 30 years, including nine college graduates, 17 with three years of college preparation, and 30 high school graduates. The majority were New York State residents. By the end of the year, there were 117 students enrolled in the School of Nursing, plus 38 from affiliating institutions, and 41 graduate students (24).

The New York Hospital educational facilities were increasingly used by a number of outside agencies interested in nursing, nutrition, clinical medicine, and the fundamental sciences (25). A spirit of teaching permeated the Department of Medicine with carefully planned instruction given to nursing students, nurses, and house staff. Dr. Henricus Stander, president of the Medical Board, noted that facilities for self-instruction were available on the pavilions and in the outpatient department (26). The School of Nursing sponsored conferences on administration, study methods, and teaching, which attracted students from teachers colleges and other institutions. Reciprocal agreements were initiated that enabled two supervisors from the Henry

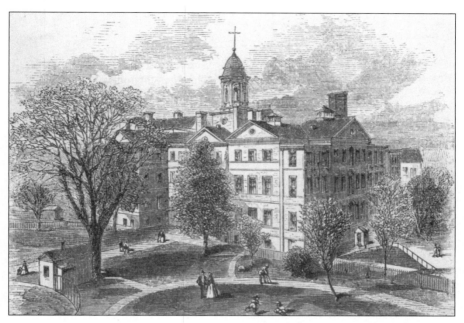

New York Hospital, 1775–1869

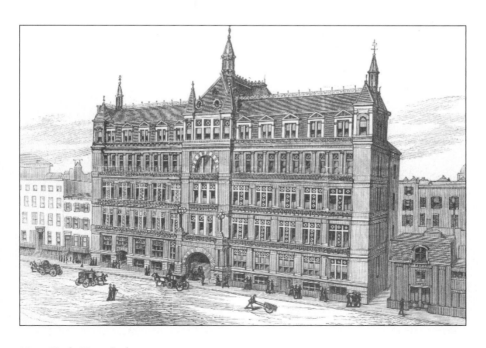

New York Hospital, 1877–1932

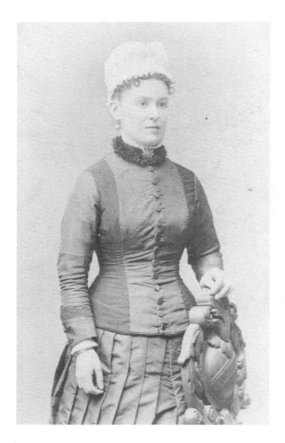

Jennie Baker, Class of 1878
Photo by James Bostwick

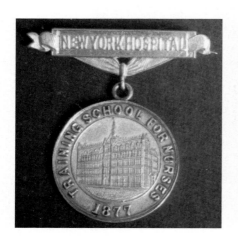

School pin, 1883–1934

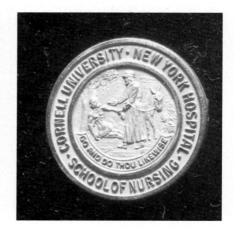

School pin, 1943–1979

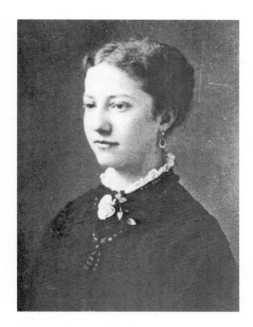

Clara Weeks Shaw, Class of 1880

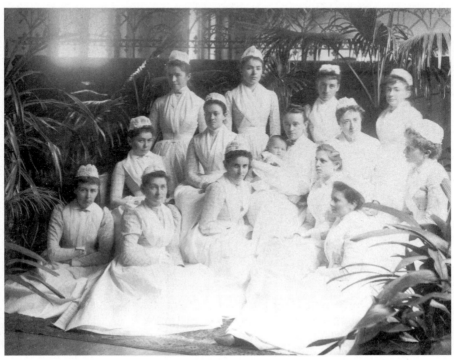

Class of 1890 with Irene Sutliffe (center) holding baby Laura York

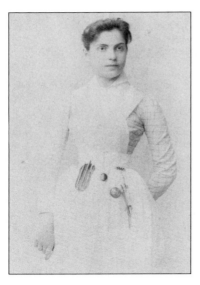

Lillian Wald, Class of 1891
Photo by Hargrave & Gubelman

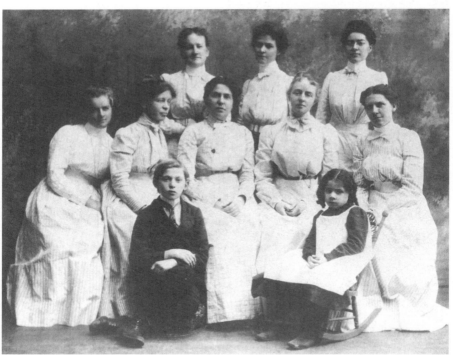

Lillian Wald (seated center) and the Henry Street "family" in 1906; Jane Hitchcock (standing left) is also a graduate of The New York Hospital Training School for Nurses; the little girl, Florrie Long, is the cook's daughter; the relationship of the boy, Sammie Brofsky, is not known
Courtesy the Visiting Nurse Service of New York

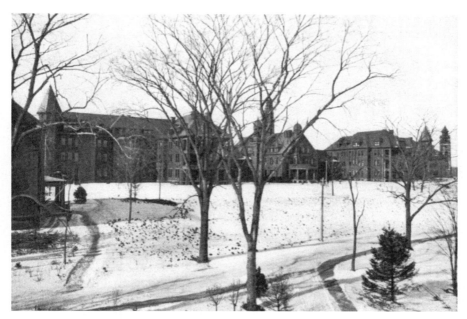

Bloomingdale Asylum, White Plains, 1894

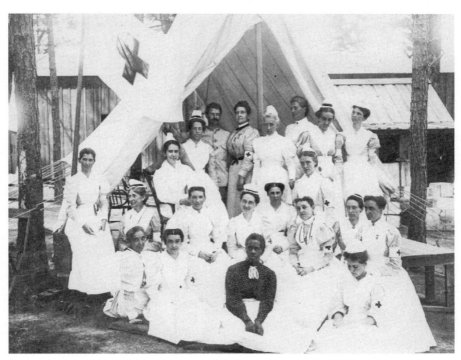

Nurses at Camp Thomas, Georgia, during the Spanish-American War, 1898

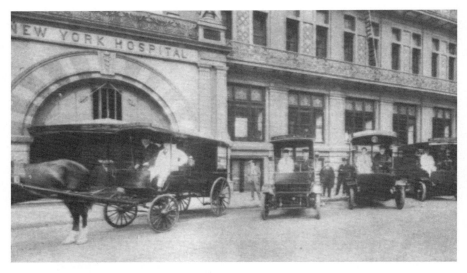

New York Hospital horse-drawn and mechanical ambulances, ca. 1910

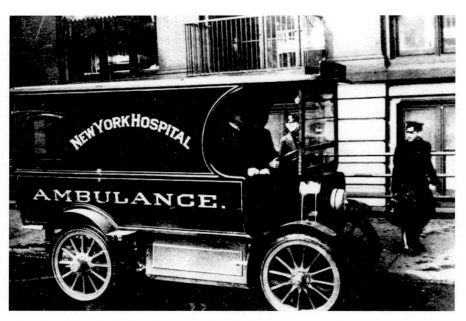

New York Hospital electric-powered ambulances, ca. 1925

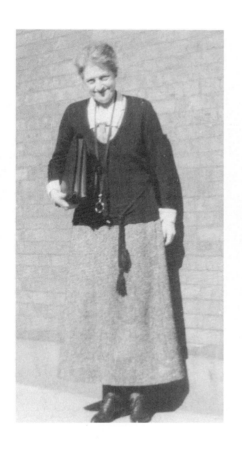

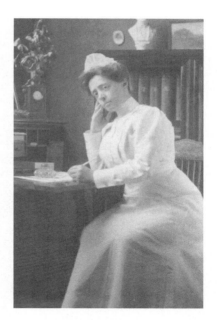

Above: Adeline Henderson, Class of 1892, superintendent of The New York Hospital Training School for Nurses, 1907–1914

Left: Annie Goodrich, Class of 1892, superintendent of the School, 1902–1907
Photo by Amy Bardens

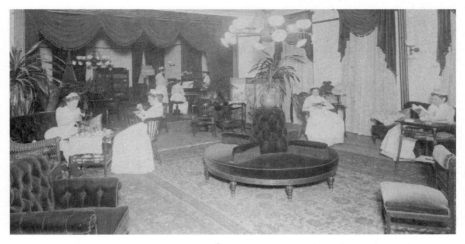

Nurses residence lounge, 6 West 16th Street, 1890s *Photo by Pach Brothers*

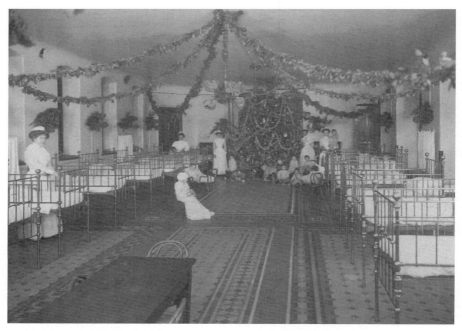

Christmas tree in children's ward, New York Hospital, ca. 1912

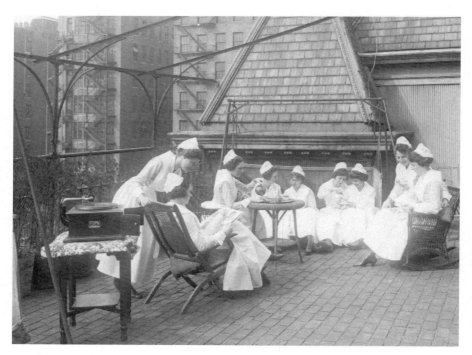

Roof of nurses residence, 6 West 16th Street, 1920s

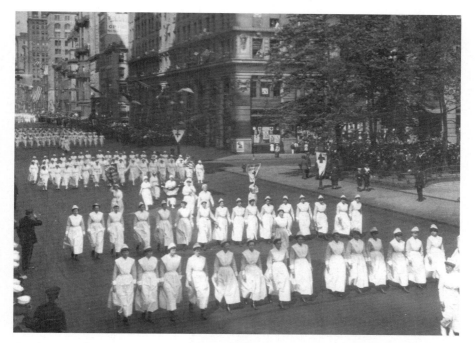

Graduates of The New York Hospital Training School for Nurses join the American Red Cross parade, World War I

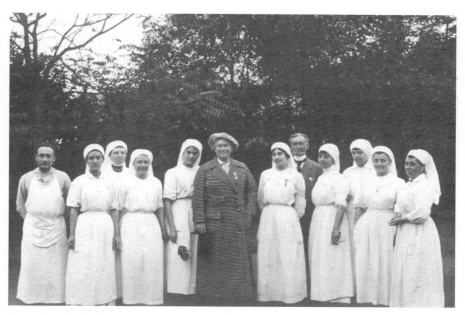

Base Hospital No. 9 Red Cross nurses and volunteers, 1917–1919

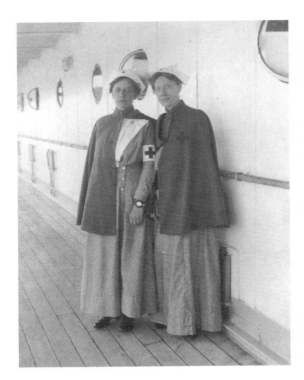

Anna Reutinger, Class of 1904 (left) and Robert Lee Cromwell, Class of 1909 (right)
Photo by Underwood and Underwood

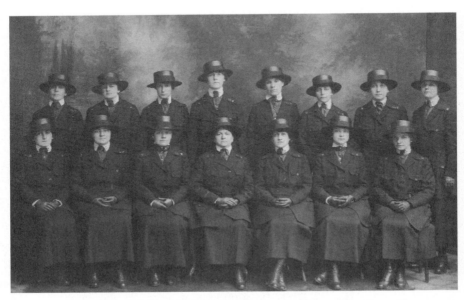

Nurses assigned to the World War I hospital unit directed by Percy Turnure, M.D., associate attending surgeon at New York Hospital, 1908–1931

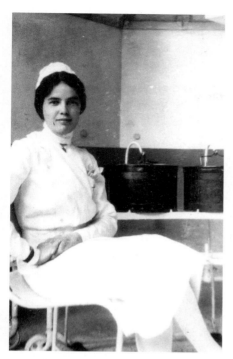

Marie Troup, Class of 1926, later became chief nurse of the Ninth General Hospital Unit in World War II

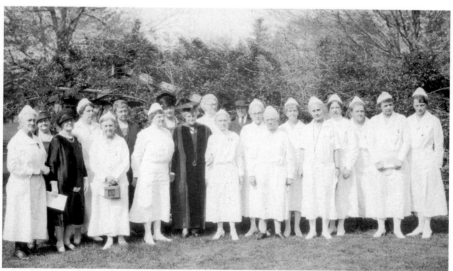

Distinguished Alumni at the 50th anniversary of the School, May 1927, left to right: Isabella Walton, Ida Nudel, Anna Duncan, Alice Ellison, Annie Rykert, Mary Beard, Minnie Jordan, Katherine Sanborn, Annie Goodrich, Katherine Hearn, Irene Sutliffe, Florence Johnson, Mary Samuel, Marianna Wheeler, Mary Vroom, Mary Smith, Anna Reutinger, Emma Golding, Ohle Gill, Bertha Lehmkuhl

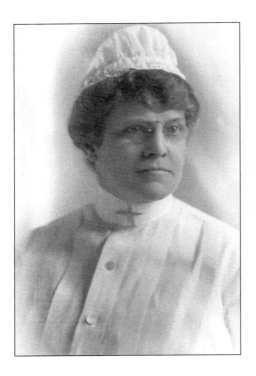

Minnie Jordan, Class of 1902, directress of the School and head of nursing services at The New York Hospital, 1916–1932
Photo by Holmo

Livingston Farrand, president of Cornell University, 1921–1937

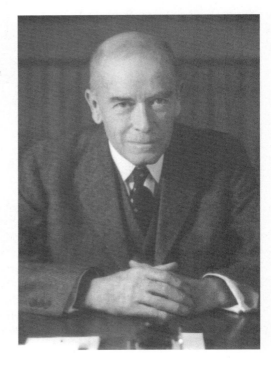

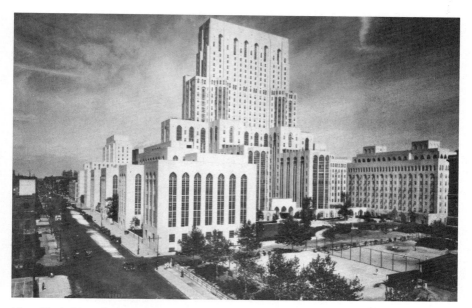

New York Hospital-Cornell Medical Center, 525 East 68th Street, 1932
Photo by William Frange

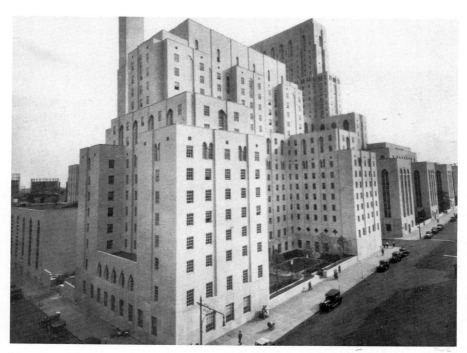

Nurses residence, 1320 York Avenue, 1932 *Photo by William Frange*

Lydia E. Anderson, Class of
1897, taught at The New
York Hospital Training
School for Nurses and the
School library was named
in her honor in 1933
Photo by Mayinie

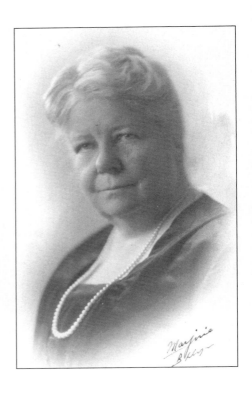

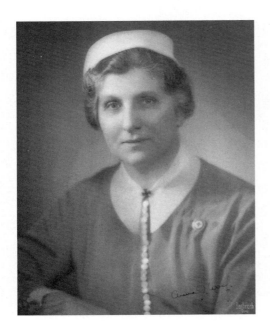

Anna D. Wolf, first director
of the New York Hospital
School of Nursing, 1931
Photo by Bachrach

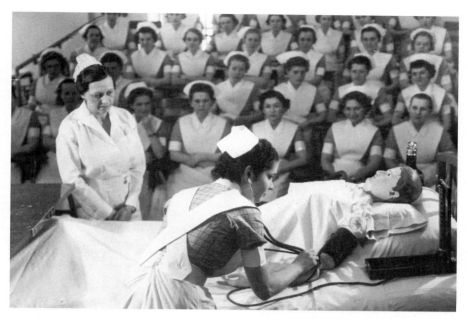

Practicing blood pressure measurement in Nursing Arts class, 1930s
Photo by Paul Parker

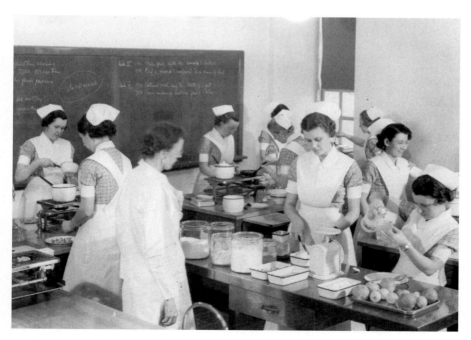

Hendrika Rynbergen supervising nutrition laboratory, 1940
Photo by Paul Parker

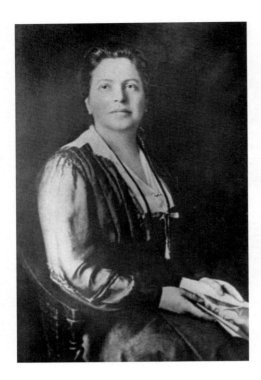

Lillian Wald, Class of 1891, founded the Henry Street Settlement House and Henry Street Visiting Nurse Service

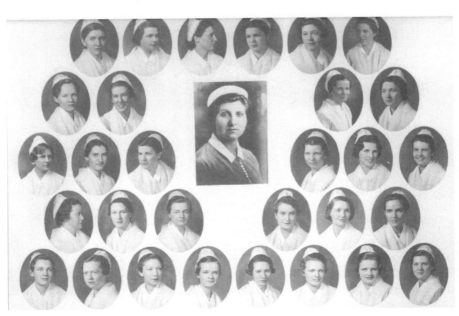

Class of 1935 and School director Anna D. Wolf

Street Nursing Service and East Harlem Nursing and Health Services to pursue various clinical specialties in the nursing program (27).

To help graduate nurses make up deficiencies and become eligible for state registration, Wolf scheduled courses provided by the School (28). As part of the staff education program, she instituted clinical and management courses that were attended by 73 nurses in the fall of 1937 (29). She was determined to foster greater cooperation between nursing committees and their medical counterparts in the various departments. Designed to streamline existing practices, the Committee on the Principles and Practice of Nursing and the advisory medical committee conducted periodic reviews of nursing procedures (30).

Staff nurses welcomed the policy of establishing an eight-hour, six-day workweek for all nursing personnel and eliminating the 12-hour duty for night nurses (31). As of December 31, 1937, full-time employees included 131 head nurses and assistant head nurses, 257 general-duty staff nurses, 107 attendants, 45 clerical workers, and several supportive ancillary workers (32). With the addition of postgraduate and affiliating students, nursing care was administered on a ratio of one registered nurse to two patients. Pleased with the results, the medical director at the Westchester Division commented that "having all nursing care provided by our own personnel rather than nurses employed by friends or relatives has continued" (33).

More good news reached the Board of Governors when they were informed of the declining deficit in the past three years. Murray Sargent, administrator-in-chief, alluded to the increasing problem of overcrowding and stressed that hospital admissions were intended for acutely ill patients and not the chronically ill. "But we are always prepared to care for emergency cases," he added (34).

A highlight of 1937 was the 60th Anniversary of the School's founding, held on June 9–10 in conjunction with graduation exercises. Over 300 alumnae registered for the celebration, which included the oldest alumna from the class of 1882 (35). Greatly missed was Lillian Wald, who had retired in 1933 to the "House on the Pond," her home in Westport, Connecticut. Presiding at the convocation, Annie Goodrich read a June 4 letter to the alumnae from Wald, who wrote with some nostalgia about an earlier period: "Though there are omissions . . .revered at the time, there was an abundance of sympathy and

sweetness and kindness and thoughts of each other and most important of all for the welfare of the patients entrusted to us" (36). Wald
closed her letter with a more poignant thought:

> Mingled with the gladness with which we meet today are sad
> memories, and we know that mourning for those who have
> gone, the best that they had and the best that they gave are
> imperishable. They are with us today, rejoicing in the fulfillment
> of many things that might have seemed impossible in the long
> ago (37).

The alumnae festivities opened with greetings by Hazel Emmet,
the Association's president, followed by Annie Goodrich's historical
narrative of the School of Nursing (38). In his address, Livingston
Farrand emphasized the contribution of nursing to public health (39).
The occasion was particularly moving because of his imminent retirement as president of Cornell University, and a long, supportive relationship with the School. At the closing ceremony, the alumnae established a fund in memory of Irene Sutliffe, who died on December 30,
1936. The fund was initiated with a donation of $1,500 from the
Association, to be earmarked for the advanced preparation of the
School's graduates (40). By honoring Sutliffe in this way, the alumnae
showed their recognition of a great nursing leader whose vision and
influence at The New York Hospital were exceeded only by an unfalter-
ing devotion to her profession.

When Anna Wolf accepted the appointment in 1932, she stated
that her primary aim was to establish a professional school and "not
one in which by the exploitation of students we try to care for a large
number of patients" (41). Throughout her tenure, she devoted her
efforts to changing the educational direction of the School and
strengthening patient care services with the best standards of nursing
care. After Livingston Farrand retired from Cornell in 1937 with the
title of president emeritus, Wolf wrote to his successor, Edmund Ezra
Day, inviting him to serve on the Council of the School of Nursing
(42).

As a new member, Day expressed enthusiasm about a potential relationship between the School and the University. He suggested that Mary Beard and Mary Roberts, who served on the Council, work with Wolf in drawing up a plan detailing all aspects of an affiliation with Cornell. Speaking candidly, he pointed out that many of the problems affecting the nursing program were due to the lack of a close university association with administrative privileges (43).

In January 1939, Wolf presented the plan accompanied by an organizational chart, and identified several of the more compelling issues to be considered. She cited the advantages and disadvantages of the two types of programs suggested: (1) two years of general education with possible prerequisites leading to a baccalaureate degree, and (2) four years of general education with possible prerequisites leading to a master's degree. Areas to be explored included the goals of the program, expectations of the graduates, the budget and financial arrangements, and the relationship of the Alumnae Association to Cornell University (44).

The following April, Day appeared optimistic when proposing a four to five-year combined program of college and nursing courses to qualify for a recognized degree. As for the intricate matter of funding, he noted that the Hospital's Governors would have to support the change to university affiliation and work out the financial adjustments with Cornell (45). He reminded the Council that its purpose was to function in an advisory capacity and not as an administrative body, and that the lines of authority rested with the Joint Administrative Board (JAB) (46).

Deliberations about the School's future intensified in meetings of the Executive Committee of the Board of Governors, which disputed the Council's recommendation that the School's administration be transferred to the University. Committee members asserted that retaining the program's operation within The New York Hospital would be more beneficial in attracting better qualified students and graduates, and ensuring the appointment and tenure of able faculty (47). On June 6, 1939, the Governors approved in principle the Council's recommendation that Cornell University be asked to assume responsibility for the School of Nursing, and that the Hospital would be willing to guarantee financial support, provided on the same basis as at present for a period of five to seven years if some other funding could not be obtained (48).

Later that year, Wolf informed the Governors of a survey of the School's graduates from 1932 to 1938, which revealed that 178 preferred to receive an academic degree and 53 acquired advanced preparation since graduation (49). The findings reinforced her conviction that applications to the School would increase and the student body would be enlarged by a closer university affiliation—"the trend in the best schools of nursing today" (50).

While negotiations were underway, news of the death of Livingston Farrand on November 8, 1939 reached The New York Hospital community. After retiring from Cornell, he continued his involvement with the Hospital as a member of the Board of Governors and the School's Council. Among the numerous tributes to him, *The New York Times* described Farrand as "a man of power and a man of the world." One of his chief characteristics was his ability to harmonize diverse human elements (51).

Wolf and her faculty had great affection for him and sent a resolution to his widow expressing their condolences. In her note, Margaret Farrand responded as follows:

> The resolution touched me deeply. The warmth and affection of the wording coming from the women of a profession so greatly honored . . . I am constantly supported by the nearness of Dr. Farrand's own valiant spirit and ever heartened to keep my faith and courage by his words spoken shortly before he died, which I pass on to you – "It is never the time to be afraid" (52).

During 1939, the New York's World's Fair increased the visibility of the Medical Center, which drew 1,248 visitors from 43 states and 38 foreign countries (53). That same year, the Governors announced the opening of Memorial Hospital at its new site, and lauded the affiliation with Cornell Medical College that "brings in a welcome addition to the several, separate institutions which make an effective Medical Center" (54). Among other institutions, they cited the Rockefeller Institute and Hospital, and the Kips Bay-Yorkville Health and Teaching Center (55). The facilities and clinics under the management and control of the Society of The New York Hospital included the Women's Clinic Lying-in Hospital, Payne Whitney Psychiatric Clinic, Departments of Medicine, Surgery, and Pediatrics, and The New York Hospital-Westchester Division. The Hospital was also associated with the Manhattan Maternity Center and the New York Nursery and Child's Hospital (56).

The issue of university affiliation for the School of Nursing attracted wide interest throughout The New York Hospital-Cornell Medical Center. At the fall 1937 meeting of the Council, Dr. George J. Heuer, surgeon-in-chief, reported on a study of the School's curriculum and nursing service. As chairman of the study committee, he noted the cooperation of the nursing faculty in following through on all courses, hours of student service and their grades, and alumnae data (57). When the Executive Faculty of the Medical College met in December, the members expressed almost unanimous opposition to the idea of the School of Nursing affiliating with Cornell. During a heated discussion, they claimed that the improvement of nursing practice did not depend on higher education and the proposed affiliation would "not be on an adequate educational basis equivalent to the collegiate standards of a university" (59).

At a meeting of the JAB later that month, President Day commented on the "wide divergence of opinion among the heads of departments in the Medical College regarding the purpose to be served by nursing education" (60). In light of these differences, he decided nothing would be gained at that time by presenting the matter formally to the University Trustees, and suggested appointing a subcommittee to study the entire subject (61).

In March 1940, when Wolf announced her intention to resign, it came as a surprise to the Hospital community, but not to some of the nursing faculty. Marjery Trieber Overholzer, a faculty member, later expressed what she believed was Wolf's reason for leaving: "Although Miss Wolf found the president of Cornell [Day] supported the university affiliation, my understanding was that the physicians at the Center at the last minute blocked it. The staff trusted her integrity and were upset when she left. Some of the faculty sensed her bitterness but she didn't want them to say anything to damage the future development of the school" (62).

In a letter to the Alumnae Association, Wolf indicated her gratitude to the Board of Governors for their guidance. She noted that her decision to resign was extremely difficult as "my work has meant so

much to me" (63). Throughout her eight and a half years at the
Medical Center, she had welcomed the Alumnae Association's involvement, and enjoyed a strong, harmonious relationship with both
Presidents Farrand and Day. Since Day's arrival at Cornell, they conferred often, and she characterized him as a "great administrator and
someone who understood nursing. We worked together like a team to
prepare the school of nursing to become part of the team" (64).

In the spring of 1940, the Executive Faculty of the Medical
College discussed a memorandum from Dr. Eugene Dubois describing
the advantages of establishing a nursing school on a collegiate basis.
He explained that after the Council had appointed him chairman of a
committee to explore the matter, he concluded from subsequent fact-
finding that the Executive Faculty had not been given sufficient information in advance of their previous meeting (65). Dubois also
revealed a disturbing impression outside the Medical Center, intimat-
ing that "the doctors of Cornell University Medical College and New
York Hospital are opposed to advances in nursing education. As a
result, it may be difficult to recruit the best person for the school" (66).

Dubois also concluded that nursing students in the School compared favorably in appearance, attitudes, and intelligence with students
in the women's colleges, and with graduates seeking master's degrees in
nutrition at Teachers College and Pratt Institute (67). He urged the
Executive Faculty to reconsider their earlier position, emphasizing that
"we have an opportunity for establishing a leading school of nursing
with a retention of all the best features of the ordinary three-year
course" (68).

At the commencement exercises of the class of 1940, Barklie
Henry, president of the Board of Governors, cited Wolf's pending
departure in July as a "heavy loss. I have valued her as a friend and as
a person of unusual intellect, ability, and grace. I have admired her professionally" (69). During her tenure at the School of Nursing, Wolf
could claim a record of accomplishment in curriculum development,
faculty productivity, democratization of administrative methods, and
recruitment of superior students. She also instituted a more efficient
organization of nursing services that resulted in personal and individualized patient care (70).

Wolf had faced many challenges over the years that she met with
determination and an enduring faith practiced throughout her life.

Although her hopes for university affiliation were not fully realized, she laid the foundation despite differing voices echoing from the Hospital's Medical Board and the Executive Faculty of the Medical College, which included some of the same people. After leaving The New York Hospital, her commitment to collegiate education continued when she became the fifth dean of the Johns Hopkins School of Nursing and director of the hospital's nursing service (71).

By the late 1930s, the nation had come through a decade of marked change influenced by the economic and social climate. The Great Depression was ending, but World War II had begun in Europe. On September 1, 1939, Nazi Germany invaded Poland, and by all accounts the aggression was beginning to intensify. In the nursing profession, one of the major issues concerning its leaders was the need to consolidate the national organizations, an issue raised frequently in the past (72). In January 1939, the ANA's Board of Directors appointed a special committee to examine the matter and consider the possibility of one organization (73). That action eventually led to a major study in the 1940s, whose results would revolutionize the structure of organized nursing.

At The New York Hospital School of Nursing, Anna Wolf was succeeded by Bessie A. R. Parker who accepted the appointment on an interim basis in the summer of 1940 (74). A loyal colleague and admirer of Wolf, Parker first came to the Medical Center shortly after it opened in 1932. A graduate of the Rhode Island Hospital School of Nursing, she studied at Teachers College before becoming evening administrative assistant. As assistant director of nursing and head of the medical-surgical department, she worked closely with Wolf beginning in 1936. The Alumnae Association heartily endorsed her appointment (75).

Well liked by the nursing community, Bessie Parker had excellent interpersonal skills, but lacked the in-depth knowledge and conceptual ability of her predecessor. Yet, she competently administered the nursing program and earned the respect of the hospital hierarchy. It was to her credit when hospital administration and the department heads invited her to their weekly meetings and, in time, she became a regular member (76). However, some of the nursing faculty had reservations about Parker's tendency to comply with questionable decisions of the Governors that affected the School. One faculty member recalled it this way: "Bessie had a good vision . . . different from Miss Wolf. But she built on what had been established" (77). Another colleague stated it more succinctly when characterizing her as "old school" (78).

From the outset, Parker had to deal with the serious problem of turnover in nursing services. In early 1940, Major James C. McGee, surgeon general of the U.S. Army, wrote to the president of the Hospital and the dean of the Medical College, suggesting that the Ninth General Hospital Unit be organized in the event of a national emergency (79). The Hospital rapidly set up the unit, which required a minimum of 45 doctors under age 55 to report for duty, and before long the number tripled (80). A call for military service from the American Red Cross (ARC) prompted 39 nurses to consider enlisting if and when the Ninth General Hospital Unit began to mobilize (81). In the fall of 1940, the ARC expressed its appreciation to the Hospital for recruiting donors to give blood plasma, which was sent to Great Britain (82). Throughout the country, preparations for the war effort involved organizing salvage drives, planning for blackouts and disaster units, and developing methods to protect the patients in case of bombings.

Parker's immediate concern was maintaining adequate staffing since many nurses volunteered with the Army and Navy while others spent their off-duty hours assisting the ARC (83). Under the government's National Defense Program, arrangements were made to offer funding for refresher courses of 8 to 12 weeks to inactive graduate nurses (84). The New York State League of Nursing Education would participate in the refresher program by assisting in hospital and home nursing if the army called for over 4,000 nurses to its service by July 1941 (85). In her annual report, Parker announced that the School was introducing a 12-week refresher course to prepare registered nurses for staffing the Hospital if needed (86).

On September 1, 1940, the nursing profession mourned the loss of one of its great leaders when Lillian Wald died after a long illness. President Barklie Henry announced to the Governors that a memorial service would be held in November at Carnegie Hall, and urged them to attend. On the day of the event, hundreds of dignitaries and admirers of Wald filled the auditorium, including a large contingent of Henry Street nurses looking impressive in their dark blue uniforms. Mary

Beard and Alfred E. Smith were among the speakers who had known or worked with Wald and shared some special remembrances of her contribution to the world (87).

By the end of the year, Parker had been head of the School for five months, and although her focus had been primarily on meeting nursing service needs, she was not unmindful of the educational program's future direction. At a meeting of the Medical College's Executive Faculty on June 4, 1941, the members continued to voice their reluctance to approve the proposed affiliation with Cornell unless the School of Nursing could be placed on an educational basis equivalent to the University's standards (88). They also questioned the availability of funding required for such an undertaking. A few months later they softened their position when the JAB recommended to the Governors that the Society of The New York Hospital assume the total cost of the School (89).

In early 1942, the JAB submitted a plan to the Council and Board of Governors describing the administrative and fiscal arrangements proposed for the affiliation. Murray Sargent, administrator-in-chief, pointed out that the expenses incurred in the new arrangement should be borne by the Hospital since it benefited from the admission of a greater number and better type of nursing student. "The University cannot justify absorbing part of the costs," he stated (90). Within a few days, he changed his mind about proceeding with the affiliation, claiming that there would not be sufficient time to organize the School and publicize it to potential candidates. He also anticipated a smaller rather than larger group of applicants (91).

Annie Goodrich, who had replaced Mary Beard on the Council, challenged Sargent's observations by contending that it was a strategic time to proceed "since high school students are being taken in larger numbers into various kinds of work for larger salaries. College women, especially those in junior colleges, would be drawn to nursing and become prepared for military emergency situations" (92). William Harding Jackson, who succeeded Barklie Henry as president, concurred with Goodrich, indicating the risk would not be too great and that it would be more difficult to effect an affiliation after the war (93).

On January 15, 1942, Jackson wrote to President Day in Ithaca, expressing the interest of the Society in a formal association with Cornell and the School of Nursing. He enclosed the plan and rationale for the affiliation and highlighted the trends in nursing education toward university control, the potential for recruiting a superior group of students, and the present difficulty in attracting applicants who measured up to high scholastic standards for the School (94).

Later in the month, President Day appeared before the Trustees of Cornell University and presented the recommendation of the Board of Governors for an affiliation with the School of Nursing of The New York Hospital (95). He shared with them the 12 statements approved by the JAB and the Executive Committee that detailed the provisions of the proposed agreement between the two institutions (see Appendix C). Day spoke convincingly of the School as "an important part of the Medical Center project that the University must support," and added that the financial responsibility would be assumed by the Hospital and not the University (96).

During the next few months, a spirit of excitement permeated the Medical Center as planning moved forward on the affiliation arrangement. On February 17, 1942, the Governors recommended to Cornell's Trustees that the new program be named the Cornell University-New York Hospital School of Nursing (97). Also recommended was that Bessie Parker be appointed director of the School and nursing service for one year pending further review (98). In May, Day announced that the University's Trustees granted formal approval of the request for affiliation (99). With the School's establishment imminent, the JAB terminated the Council and delayed forming a new one until after appointing a nursing dean (100).

The long-awaited affiliation became official on July 1, 1942 (101). According to the agreement, the School required applicants to have two years of college work at institutions that would be acceptable to Cornell. On completion of the program, they would be awarded a bachelor of science degree in nursing from the University as well as a diploma from The New York Hospital. The entire cost of the program, amounting to about $200,000 a year, would be underwritten by the Hospital (102). Reporting to the Board of Trustees, Day lauded the alliance and declared that "this move further cemented the excellent relationship which the University has had with the Hospital for many years in the operation of the Medical College" (103).

The transition in progress from a deeply ingrained traditional system to a modern one offering a fresh direction marked the beginning of a new era in nursing education at The New York Hospital-Cornell Medical Center. Bessie Parker and her corps of faculty, staff, and students would have many challenges to face in the coming years with a nation already at war.

CHAPTER 7

Time of Transition: War and Peace

The ferment created by the social and political climate of the 1940s presented the nursing profession with one its greatest challenges. Aware that they had to find a means of securing quick, decisive action to meet military and civilian needs, the national organizations established the Nursing Council for National Defense (NCND) to unify all nursing activities and to act as a clearinghouse for nursing affairs (1). Through the efforts of the NCND, chaired by Julia Stimson, legislation was enacted in July 1941 that authorized funds to registered nurses for advanced educational and refresher courses (2).

The following December, when the Japanese bombed the U.S. Navy Base at Pearl Harbor, President Franklin D. Roosevelt described the horrific event as "a date which will live in infamy" (3). In Ithaca, President Edmund Ezra Day addressed the Board of Trustees and summed up his reaction in this way: "As in the life of the nation as a whole, at Cornell the year 1941–42 broke sharply in two parts—before Pearl Harbor and after Pearl Harbor" (4). The signing of the Declaration of War on Japan on December 8 and Germany and Italy on December 11 portended a difficult period for the nation, requiring sacrifice and an unfailing patriotic spirit.

After the United States declared war, the NCND expanded its focus as well the membership, and changed its name to the National Nursing Council for War Service (NNCWS). Among the group's responsibilities were recruiting nurses for the armed forces, allocating resources for the civilian population, increasing schools of nursing, and accelerating nursing education programs (5). Anna Wolf served as chairman, beginning in 1942, and continued as a member until the NNCWS was dissolved six years later (6).

On July 14, 1942, the Governors of The New York Hospital and Cornell University's Board of Trustees sponsored a farewell dinner party at the Hotel Roosevelt for members of the Ninth General Base Hospital Unit, who were scheduled to leave for active duty. President Langdon Marvin noted that the occasion "embodies the spirit of all other New York Hospital groups which have served well in every American War since 1776" (7). Other speakers included Bessie Parker and Marie Troup, a 1926 graduate of the School of Nursing and the new chief nurse of the base hospital unit (8).

On their arrival at Fort Devens, Massachusetts, the staff consisted of 51 doctors, 105 nurses, and a large contingent of nonprofessional personnel (9). In her letter of August 10, 1942 to Troup, Parker expressed the following thoughts: "I have been thinking about all of you many times and wondered if you are comfortable and happy . . . I hope they [the nurses] are surviving their vaccines . . . They will soon be outfitted with those swanky uniforms!" (10).

While stationed at the camp, the nurses shared some amusing anecdotes with readers of *The Alumnae News*. A communication from one young recruit mentioned the recent wedding of a colleague. "Cupid has been darting about from person to person," she wrote enthusiastically. "We will have to keep an eye on Miss Troup because she caught the bouquet!" (11). As it turned out, however, the words were not prophetic—Marie Troup never married.

In the summer of 1943, the unit was shipped to Australia for a brief time before being transferred to more permanent headquarters at a hospital "somewhere in the South Pacific" (12). Some months later, when Parker received a letter from Troup, she surmised from the contents that it might have come from New Guinea:

> Someday you will know the details of the struggle with the treacherous Kumae grass, a sea of mud, endless days of teeming rain, tropical diseases, insects of all kinds, and very limited construction. This Pacific Isle edition of The New York Hospital is a far cry from the parent institution, but rough and unstreamlined as our plight may be, our patients are receiving excellent care and leave the hospital with real respect for the nurses, doctors, and corpsmen (12).

Toward the end of the letter, Troup added that "Muriel Carbery and Colonel Ralph F. Bower constructed and organized the O.R. set up in the Southwest Pacific and they have trained a first class staff of corpsmen" (13).

With the war intensifying in the European and Pacific Theaters, hospitals in the United States had to develop emergency measures in preparation for any pending disaster. The New York Hospital attempted to do its share as the District Hospital Control Center, which covered the entire mid-Manhattan area from 42nd to 86th Streets, and from the Hudson River to the East River (14). Equipped with telephones connected to police sites and local hospital districts, the main Control Center was staffed by volunteers, including nursing and medical students, ready to direct emergency squads and ambulances in the event of air raids (15). Cognizant of the need to provide a safe and protective environment for the patients, Hospital officials had a system in place that involved the use of emergency field units and evacuation plans. The Executive Committee assured the staff that the operating rooms, emergency department, and engine rooms would be sufficiently lit (16).

At a meeting of the Governors on November 9, 1943, President Marvin introduced Alta E. Dines, chairman of the NNCWS in New York State. In light of the existing shortage of staff nurses, Dines informed them that the War Manpower Commission discouraged the employment of private-duty nurses except in cases of dangerously ill patients (17). Dines pointed out that because hospitals were staffed largely by nurses ineligible for the army, nurse's aides, and other volunteers, some nursing procedures and routines would have to be eliminated (18). During this period, Henricus Stander, the medical director, noted that in spite of the large number of nurses who had signed up for military service, a high level of efficiency, morale, and loyalty existed among the remaining staff (19).

Parker's hopes for filling the numerous vacancies were realized to some extent with the hiring of practical nurses and nurses from the registry, which had transferred its offices to the nurses residence at 1320 York Avenue (20). The addition of 697 volunteers and part-time workers helped to stabilize the staffing following a 120% turnover of non-professional personnel and 90% of staff nurses (21). Parker believed that improvements in the situation would occur with a 48-hour workweek operating for all nurses and a more liberal policy toward requests for living-out privileges (22). Another inducement to maintain as well as attract nurses was the increase in monthly salary from $75 to $85 and the possibility of an additional $5 in six months (23).

Even with the critical depletion of nursing and medical staff, The New York Hospital managed to continue operating most of its services, and at the same time carry on significant medical research. In May 1941, Lederle Laboratories awarded the Hospital a $7,000 grant to conduct a study on the use of sulfonamide therapy, an event hailed by the Executive Committee as "an extremely promising new field of research with great clinical value" (24). Another remarkable development occurred in 1944 with the establishment of the first eye bank in the country, which made it possible to collect and store human corneal tissue for use in transplant surgery (25). That same year, the institution was honored by Sister Kenny's visit to a young patient with a severe case of infantile paralysis (26).

The decade evolved into an increasingly fertile time for The New York Hospital with the introduction of new procedures that included the use of penicillin, administering electric shock therapy for mental disorders, performing grafts for nerve injuries and burns, and reconstructing torn arteries with vitilium tubes (27). In 1945, the discovery of the Papanicolaou smear for the detection of cervical cancer in women created worldwide attention (28). With the advent of technology in the post-war era, a number of "firsts" took place in the medical community. During the convention of the American College of Surgeons in 1947, operations performed at The New York Hospital were televised to various sites in the city where members of the organization held their meetings (29). The success of this dramatic demonstration illustrated the potential of television as an effective teaching mechanism in medical education and marked the beginning of the electronic age in health care.

In her dual administrative position, Parker faced the parallel responsibilities of maintaining nursing services and guiding the development of the new Cornell University-New York Hospital School of Nursing. As awesome as the task appeared, she welcomed the changing status of the School and viewed it as "a wonderful venture which preserves the traditions of The New York Hospital School of Nursing and combines them with the opportunities offered to us through the medium of a great university" (30). Her comment showed a resoluteness that offered a needed assurance in times of war.

On August 5, 1942, the Executive Faculty Committee of the School was formed as a policy-making body to further the program's aims, foster interdepartmental relationships, and stimulate general interest in the welfare of the Hospital, students, and graduate staff (31). Members consisted of the dean and associate director of the School, department heads, the president of Cornell University and his administrative assistant, two Cornell University Medical College faculty, and one representative of the nursing faculty (32). At the second meeting in September, Parker appointed a committee to revise the Faculty Bylaws (33). Except for instructors in the sciences and nonclinical areas, all full-time faculty held dual positions at the School and in nursing service.

When 77 students registered for the nursing program in the fall of 1942, Parker described them as "the largest class ever admitted, and contrary to our policy of recent years, we plan to admit a second group in February" (34). The increase in enrollment was facilitated by federal aid from the U.S. Public Health Service that supplemented instructional costs and provided a limited number of scholarships for tuition (35). The Joint Administrative Board (JAB) supported the recommendation to accept applicants for a February class, but with the understanding of admitting no more than 25 students and no fewer than 20 (36).

After the university program opened, the School continued a policy established earlier in the spring that would be in effect for the duration of the war, and that permitted the acceptance of applications from married women with husbands in military service (37). Senior students in the third term were also granted permission to marry before graduation. Parker dourly noted, however, that in some cases there were students who married secretly and did not disclose the information until their last day in the School (37).

Eager to recruit qualified students, the nursing program circulated promotional material titled *Announcements* that defined the School's purpose as preparing selected students in the fundamental principles of nursing and its various clinical aspects as applied to the hospital, home, and other areas in the community (39). Another aim was to develop the individual student as a responsible member of civic and social life (40). The information cited the School's accreditation status accorded by the National League of Nursing Education (NLNE) in 1941 and specified the subjects required prior to admission as well as a personal interview with the nursing director (41). An important criterion for admission was the student's performance on the test administered by the Psychological Corporation of America (42).

The *Announcements* included: the course of study leading to a baccalaureate degree, scholarship and loan aid, free maintenance, recreational activities, the faculty of the School and Medical College, department heads, and costs of the program (43). Students were expected to pay a $100 tuition fee at registration, followed by $50 for each of the second and third years (44). The total amount for the entire period, which covered additional fees such as the health service, laboratory, and library, was estimated to be at least $300 but not to exceed $500 (45). Also mentioned were the agencies for student affiliations such as the Henry Street Visiting Nursing Service, where the student experience had recently been reduced from two months to two weeks of observation due to the demands being made on the Settlement's staff (46).

The early years of transition from a hospital school to a university program did not come easily, particularly since the difficulties were compounded by the onset of World War II. The students, some with only a high school diploma and others with college preparation, tended to create stress on the faculty, who were trying to teach at a university level. A pressing concern was the need to appoint a permanent dean for the School who would direct the nursing service. In February 1943, President Day and Henricus Stander, chairman of the search committee, announced to the JAB that they were "very favorably impressed" by two of the candidates interviewed (47). The next month, the JAB recommended Lucile Petry, a well-known educator and prominent member of the nursing profession, for the appointment (48). After approval by the Board of Governors of The New York Hospital and Cornell University's Board of Trustees, Petry accepted the position and indicated her intention to relocate in September (49).

Petry's association with The New York Hospital-Cornell Medical Center was short lived when Dr. Thomas Parron, surgeon general of the U.S. Public Health Service, selected her to administer the newly formed Division of Nurse Education (50). In the middle of 1943, the 78th

Congress passed the Nurse Training Act (Public Law 740) to "assure a supply of nurses for the armed forces, governmental and civilian hospitals, health agencies, and war industries" (51). The legislation created the U.S. Cadet Nurse Corps and was also known as the Bolton Act after the Ohio congresswoman who introduced the bill in the House of Representatives (52). Administered through the Division of Nurse Education, the Cadet Nurse Corps was directed by Petry, who worked closely with an advisory committee consisting of nursing and hospital leaders (53).

The Cadet Nurse Corps provided tuition and fees, uniforms, and monthly stipends for students enrolled in approved schools of nursing, and offered financial assistance to nurses for postgraduate study. Under the provisions of the Bolton Act, participating schools were required to accelerate their programs from three years to 24 to 30 months. Examinations developed by the new testing service of the NLNE became a useful tool for identifying qualified applicants (54).

During the fall of 1943, Parker described the early impact of the Cadet Nurse Corps on the School of Nursing: "The new plan functions through federal appropriation and in our school the cost is approximately $1500 per student, which covers fees and other expenses," she explained to the Board of Governors. "The student receives a small monthly stipend for 30 months and the Hospital is obligated to pay a monthly stipend of $30 for the remaining six months of the course" (55).

Parker noted the high morale of the faculty, whose responsibilities had doubled with the dramatic increase in the number of students. The School's enrollment figures reached 207 in September 1943, including 157 members of the Cadet Nurse Corps (56). By the following year, 88% of all students in the School belonged to the Cadet Nurse Corps and among them, 80% had at least two years of college (57).

With such a large group, a solution was needed to alleviate an already existing shortage of staff nurses. To make up for the loss, the Hospital developed a unique plan to recruit New York businessmen to serve as volunteer orderlies in their spare time. The nursing alumnae newsletter lauded this effort as inspirational, commenting on the "the spirit of these men—executives, bankers, museum curators, decorators, research experts, and others who gave up their leisure to the lowly and sometimes not too pleasant duties of an orderly for the relief of the sick in this time of critical personnel shortage" (58).

In 1944, the revised bylaws of the Society of The New York Hospital placed the professional conduct of the nursing program under the control of the Medical Board, and the administrative conduct under the Executive Committee and the School. A new amendment stipulated that the director of nursing service would be responsible to the Medical Board and would report on all nursing policies affecting the care of patients (59). Further, the title of the administrator-in-chief of the Hospital was changed to executive director (60).

During a meeting of the Governors in March of that year, President Day reactivated the search committee to find a successor to Petry (61). With the increase of students in the Cadet Corps and expanded teaching facilities, Parker's workload had intensified. Although marked growth occurred in operating expenses, they were offset by the government's contribution of $28,000 (62). However, ever since the School became part of the University system, Parker had to deal with the time-consuming task of submitting two separate annual budgets. The fiscal year for the School operated on an academic schedule from July 1 to June 30, whereas the budget for nursing services was on a calendar year from January 1 through December 31 (63).

In a communication to Parker on June 26, 1944, Cornell's Board of Trustees announced the establishment of a Council for the School of Nursing (64). The recommendation, which originally stemmed from the JAB, was consistent with the University's bylaws authorizing the formation of an advisory council for the individual school or college (65). Composition of the group would include two members each of the Board of Governors and Board of Trustees, the deans of the School of Nursing and the Medical College, the Hospital's executive director, the president of the Medical Board, and two representatives of the Alumnae Association (66). Under President Day's chairmanship, the new Council aimed to reaffirm the goals of the School of Nursing.

World War II spawned what will probably go down in history as the nursing profession's greatest recruitment effort with the creation of the U.S. Cadet Nurse Corps. With climbing enrollments in the School of Nursing, Parker observed that despite the added workload, faculty accepted their responsibilities with an "excellent spirit and without noticeable impairment of service" (67). She also praised the medical faculty "whose support made it possible for us to admit a second large class during the year and assure them a good teaching program" (68). On June 22, 1944, President Roosevelt signed an important piece of legislation titled the Servicemen's Readjustment Act, popularly known as the G.I. Bill of Rights. Among its provisions, the law provided funding to returning veterans, including nurses, who wished to pursue educational opportunities in colleges and universities (69).

The following January, when Roosevelt issued a proclamation to draft nurses for military service, its effect spurred voluntary recruitment to the point of filling the quota without requiring Congressional action (70). During the year, a $600,000 reconstruction program of The New York Hospital took shape with the expectation of increasing patient capacity and improving the operations of the clinical departments (71). At the time, President Langdon Marvin raised the question about the type of medical care to be provided in the future, asserting that whatever might occur, the Hospital would meet the needs of patients requiring diagnosis or treatment (72). Concerned about the possibility of new state or federal initiatives, Henricus Stander stated that the greatest problem confronting the medical profession and particularly the teaching hospital was the "threat of socialized medicine" (73).

On August 14, 1945, victory over Japan brought closure to a devastating war (74). The following month, the first post-war graduation of the Cornell University-New York Hospital School of Nursing took place in the auditorium of the Nurses Residence. As keynote speaker, Dr. William F. Russell, dean of Teachers College, Columbia University, addressed 51 new graduates, many of whom he had known while working as a volunteer orderly at the Hospital along with other professional men. He urged the young women to remember and retain in their nursing care the personal service that was often neglected during the war due to stress and staff shortages (75). When the ceremony concluded, each graduate received the traditional badge displaying a new look that showed the seal of the Society and the name of the School (76).

In October, Parker received a letter from Troup aboard a hospital ship that she described as "rocking quite a bit from bucking strong winds. So please excuse the scrawl. Two years spent on isolated jungle islands have been a long, lonely stretch. But every one of our girls has been a great soldier" (77). Troup noted that some of the nurses with the Ninth General Hospital remained in Okinawa to treat American soldiers held as prisoners of war in Japanese camps (78).

By the end of 1945, about 70,000 of the 250,000 active nurses in the United States had served in the armed forces (79). A study of the short-term effect of the war did not reveal a positive outcome in regard to meeting civilian demands. Most of the young women wanted to continue in the field, but with a marriage boom sweeping the country, many took the "big step" and left the profession (80). Some of the nurses who returned to their former jobs became disenchanted with low pay and status, menial work, lack of Social Security and retirement benefits, the autocratic administration, and limited opportunities to advance (81). A large number, however, took advantage of the G.I. Bill and pursued advanced education where clinical and technical specialization had begun to flourish (82).

In the immediate post-war period, great changes were already visible in the pattern of life and work on college campuses throughout the nation. At Cornell University, President Day described the war years as "one of the paradoxes of our history that a great university founded by a Hicksite Quaker and dedicated to ways of peace, should find itself converted into an intensely active center of war research" (83). He pointed out that since 1940, nearly 4,500 undergraduates left Cornell to enter military service before completing their studies (84). By the end of 1946, Day presented a graphic picture of what was happening when the American soldier returned as the American student:

> ...the year when housing in the University community proved woefully inadequate; the year when classrooms and laboratories began to have night shifts to accommodate the increasing load; the year when applications for admission increased threefold; the year when operating costs soared and the student body approached peak enrollment; the year when the University was confronted with the necessity of expanding its facilities during a period of scarcity of labor and materials—in short, it was a year when the University shared with other corporations, both great and small, the headaches of reconversion (85).

In the fall of 1945, a total of 979 doctors, nurses, lay personnel, and five members of the Board of Governors returned to The New York

Hospital. Returning physicians outnumbered nurses because many nurses elected to seek new career directions in nursing, pursue university studies, or marry (87). These factors intensified the shortage of nurses, which prompted the president of the Medical Board to comment that "far from being reduced after service, problems became even more serious than at any other time during the war" (88).

During the spring of 1945, the Committee on Deanships unanimously recommended Virginia Matthews Dunbar for the position of dean of the School of Nursing and director of nursing service (89). However, it would be another year before Dunbar could officially begin her duties because of her commitments as administrator of the American Red Cross Nursing Services in Washington, D.C. With the war in progress, she had a responsibility to fulfill that involved enrolling nurses in the Red Cross Nursing Reserve, directing them in disasters, and overseeing courses on home hygiene and care of the sick (90).

Years earlier, before entering the nursing program at Johns Hopkins, Dunbar had earned a bachelor's degree from Mount Holyoke College in South Hadley, Massachusetts, and like Anna Wolf who followed a similar pattern, she expressed strong views on the values of a liberal arts education and their application to the practice of nursing (91). On March 1, 1946, when she assumed her new position, the School of Nursing was in the process of implementing President Day's recent directive to require two years or more of college work prior to admission (92).

When first approached by the search committee, Dunbar had reservations about the combined post of education and service. She sought the advice of Annie Goodrich who convinced her of the advantages of the dean having a close connection with the Hospital (93). "It was the thing I talked most about with Miss Goodrich," she later recalled, "but to my surprise she wasn't alarmed at the prospect" (94). At the time of this remark, Dunbar had retired to "Far Hills," her home in Westchester County Center in Colchester, Connecticut (95).

On February 26, 1946, more than 400 nursing leaders and dignitaries, representing numerous organizations and groups including the Rockefeller Foundation and Yale University, attended a dinner at the Waldorf-Astoria Hotel to honor Annie Goodrich and to commemorate the eight decades of her illustrious life. She was presented with eight long-stemmed red roses and a gold-embossed blue leather-covered book containing hundreds of tributes from admirers throughout the world (96).

After arriving in New York, Dunbar began the formidable task facing her with an orientation to the Medical Center and meeting with key people in the organization. Receptive to the recommendation of the JAB, she retained Bessie Parker as assistant dean and assistant director of nursing service (97). From previous contacts and her wide experience in nursing, Dunbar was familiar with the reputation of The New York Hospital and knew Anna Wolf whom she described as a "brilliant woman" (98). While at the American Red Cross (ARC), Dunbar had served on an advisory committee of the nursing program at Johns Hopkins when Wolf first went there as dean (99).

From the beginning, Dunbar perceived the identity of the School to be a serious problem affecting both faculty and students (100). Four years had passed since the transition to university affiliation, but she found little difference in the conduct of the program. What distressed her was that most of the faculty did not seem to know who or what they were, which gave the impression that they were still functioning under the old pattern of the hospital apprenticeship system (101). To remedy the situation, the faculty and students needed to be educated about university procedures and to understand the role of the baccalaureate-prepared nurse in a major medical center (102).

Dunbar had been an instructor and assistant director of the University of California School of Nursing at San Francisco from 1930 to 1938. On a leave of absence in 1935, she became the first nurse in the United States to receive a scholarship from the ARC for advanced study at Bedford College in London and the Florence Nightingale Foundation (103).

Dunbar believed in the importance of building a strong faculty, which she viewed as the greatest single factor contributing to the reputation of the School (104). Eager to institute faculty reforms, she was disturbed to find minimal involvement of the instructional staff in decisions affecting the School (105). Discovering that the Executive Faculty had determined most of the policies, she enlisted President Day's support to to include the participation of the entire faculty (106). It was heartening when Day attended every meeting, which increased faculty interest and motivation (107). According to Veronica Lyons, who later became associate dean, "Miss Dunbar was a very democratic person involving the faculty in policy making and even the youngest person there would have her say" (108).

In the spring of 1946, another policy change indicated that only applications for admission from single or legally separated women would be considered for the future (109). There was a disclaimer, however, for students in the 1946 and 1947 classes, who, with permission from the dean, could marry in the third year. Those already married were expected to continue living in the Nurses Residence (110).

Reporting on the status of admissions to the September 1946 class, Dunbar indicated the acceptance of 39 students, all with two years of college preparation (111). "This number is approximately 60% of what we had hoped to admit, having planned for a class of 60 to 70 students," she said, pointing out that 69% of the total admissions since 1942 included students with two or more years of college as compared with 45% prior to the School's association with Cornell (112). The entering students came from 39 states and 6 countries, with 90% previously prepared in senior colleges or universities (113).

At a meeting of the Governors in October 1946, Dunbar informed them of the problem of recruiting staff nurses, which made it impossible to open additional patient units at the Hospital. When the Governors asked her to consider opening a school of practical nursing, she immediately rejected the idea and asserted that hospitals should not assume that responsibility (114). Instead, she insisted, every effort must be made to encourage graduates of the School to remain at the hospital. "This will mean shorter hours and further attention to salaries" (115).

Later that month, Dunbar met with the Council and stressed the importance of reaffirming the purpose of the School as well as how to adapt to conditions in the coming years. One of the most pressing challenges related to balancing the instructional needs of the students and the service needs of the Hospital (116). Speaking passionately about the matter, Dunbar declared that there was a "crying need for schools of nursing to disentangle the preparation of students from the needs of the particular hospital to which it is connected" (117). She believed that assignments in the clinical area should build on the student's preparation and not the repetitive duties involving excessive hours of experience. Above all, she emphasized that the student must have "time to think if she is expected to assume her full duties as a graduate nurse" (118).

As the end of Dunbar's first year approached, all but 14 of the 228 basic students in the School were enrolled in the Cadet Corps. After October 1945, admissions to the Corps had been discontinued, but as long as students remained until September 1948, the accelerated program would be operating for these classes (119). The dean's leadership had been taking shape with a motivated faculty and new appointments, qualified students with college background, and a curriculum beginning to undergo revision.

Keenly aware of the need to give visibility to the nursing program, Dunbar conferred with the School's public relations department, which introduced several successful activities. She was determined to establish communication with various groups at Cornell University and began by speaking to women students in Ithaca to elicit their interest in the nursing program (120). By invitation, the president of the Federation of Cornell Women's Clubs and the vice president of the Cornell Alumni Association visited the School of Nursing. Through them, Dunbar obtained the cooperation of the affiliating clubs located throughout the country as a resource for disseminating information abut the nursing program (121).

Among other activities, Dunbar maintained an active correspondence that included a letter of August 7, 1946, appearing in *The New York Times*, about opportunities provided by the nursing profession for young women (122). *The Cornell Alumni News* carried an article describing the faculty and students in the School (123). In addition, Dunbar held a press conference for women editors of local newspapers and national wire services, and was instrumental in having stories about students in the graduating class sent to hometown newspapers (124).

The mid-1940s marked the beginning of postwar America, creating both good and bad times for the nursing profession. Most alarming was the pervasive shortage of nurses in the service setting, which had progressed to a chronic state. Other concerns related to the dearth of federal funding for nursing education with the imminent termination of the Cadet Nurse Corps (125). Another problem was the reluctance of directors of hospital diploma programs and their graduates to move into the system of higher education (126).

Some positive outcomes emerged, however, when nursing organizations such as the NLNE developed a position statement in 1947, defining principles on the administration and control of nursing programs by educational institutions (127). Significant studies also were published, with similar observations and suggestions for change. By the end of the decade, a major report on the structure of organized nursing was nearing completion that offered hope for a unified profession (128).

Dunbar continued to be involved with professional organizations while serving as the first dean of the Cornell University-New York Hospital School of Nursing. With an inspired faculty, she would bring a fresh vision to the nursing program, enhancing its reputation worldwide during an impressive reign over the next 12 years.

CHAPTER 8

A New Dean:
Challenges and Change

When appropriations ceased by 1948, 124,000 students in the Cadet Nurse Corps had graduated from basic schools of nursing, and over 10,000 graduate nurses had benefited from federal aid for advanced study (1). At Cornell University-New York Hospital School of Nursing commencement exercises held in September 1946, the 59 new graduates represented the largest number in the School's history (2). As part of a six-month learning experience, 16 student cadets were sent to Veterans Hospitals, one to the Office of Indian Affairs of the U.S. Public Health Service, and three to the Visiting Nurse Service of New York (VNSNY) (3).

In 1947, the School of Nursing re-instituted the two-month affiliation with the VNSNY that had lapsed for a period of six years. The arrangement was considered essential to meet the requirement for joint accreditation from the National Organization for Public Health Nursing (NOPHN) and the National League of Nursing Education (NLNE) (4). Virginia Dunbar and the faculty initiated discussions of the process and looked ahead to two years hence when the self-study report would be submitted (5). During that period, for the first time, the School admitted African American students who enrolled as cadets in the program in 1947 (6). Dunbar noted that the three young women were "very good students," from Meharry College, an excellent black school in Nashville, Tennessee (6). Later, she appointed one of the graduates to the faculty (7).

Prior to 1949, few hospitals in New York City employed qualified African American nurses in nursing service. That barrier was broken when The New York Hospital hired Constance Derrell, a master's-
prepared nurse-midwife, who joined the nursing staff in the obstetric
service of the Lying-in-Hospital. Within 10 months, she became a head
nurse and two years later was offered a dual appointment as clinical
instructor in the Cornell University-New York Hospital School of
Nursing (8).

In preparation for the 75th Anniversary of the School of Nursing
and its fifth year as part of Cornell University, the School conducted a
survey of graduates between the years 1878–1946 (9). Of the 1,434
alumnae surveyed, 733 responded; 483 were reported as deceased.
Married nurses comprised 41% of the sample,which included 37%
who described themselves as housewives. Fifty-three percent remained
single, representing the largest number of active members in the alumnae association. In the employment arena, the graduates held positions
in institutional nursing (42%), private duty (22%), and public health
(21%). The greatest shift occurred as a decrease of 50% of private nursing over a 20-year period. A smaller number of nurses worked in teaching positions in schools of nursing, physicians' offices, and other areas
(10).

In 1947, the School was accepted as a member of the Association
of Collegiate Schools of Nursing (ACSN) (11). Thirty university schools
belonged to the organization, but only 17 offered a basic nursing
course. Mary Beard, a strong ally of Virginia Dunbar ever since they
worked together at the American Red Cross (ARC), had been one of the
ACSN's earliest advocates. In 1944, she resigned from the ARC due to
ill health, but before her death she contributed her papers and books
to the Lydia E. Anderson Library at the Cornell University-New York
Hospital School of Nursing (12).

A firm believer in providing proper counseling in the School,
Dunbar assigned the task of guiding students and the less experienced
faculty members to Veronica Lyons, her new assistant dean (13). When
the faculty suggested that it might be beneficial to employ a full-time
non-nurse counselor to advise the students, faculty, and staff in nursing service, Dunbar consulted with Lucile Allen, who provided student
advisement on the Ithaca campus. After spending a few days at the
School of Nursing and the Hospital, Allen offered the following suggestions to strengthen the counseling area:

- Implement personal selection of all employees
- Lengthen the orientation for several weeks
- Increase contact with the parents of students
- Provide more adequate placement to guide students
- Increase recognition to head nurses and guidance in relating to personnel
- Foster democracy in the social life between students and their professors
- Schedule shorter work hours to prevent fatigue and discouragement
- Initiate personal counseling (14)

In September 1948, the School employed Victoria Frederick, a former assistant counselor at the University, as a full-time faculty member (15). Over time, her services proved invaluable to the students and less seasoned faculty. Since it was crucial to give visibility to the School and attract qualified students, Frederick formed relationships with counselors in colleges and high schools (16).

When President Edmund Ezra Day resigned on June 10, 1948, for health reasons, Dunbar viewed it as a great loss to the School of Nursing and to her personally. She had enormous admiration for him because of his knowledge and genuine interest in advancing the nursing program. In an interview some time after her retirement, she indicated that his support of her candidacy for the deanship in 1945 was probably an important factor in her being offered the position. "I had been Mary Beard's assistant at the American Red Cross for several years and Mary knew Dr. Day," she explained. "They both had worked together at the Rockefeller Foundation some years earlier" (17). Following Day's resignation as president, the Board of Trustees of Cornell appointed him chancellor and administrative representative. In 1951, Deane Waldo Malott became the sixth president of the University (18).

During the late 1940s, changes were underway at The New York Hospital with Dr. Henry N. Pratt replacing Murray Sargent as the director (former title of administrator-in-chief). In the School of Nursing, Mary Klein became assistant professor of medical and surgical nursing, Edna Fritz became instructor in charge of the program for graduate nurses and in-service education for staff nurses, and Muriel Carbery became assistant professor and head of the operating room in a newly created post. After a two-year leave in Europe with the ARC, Verda

Hickcox returned to her position as associate professor of obstetrical nursing and head of nursing service in the Women's Clinic (19). In a system endorsed by Dunbar, most faculties held joint appointments because she believed that they should have control over the quality of nursing care on units where students had their learning experiences (20).

Deeply involved in all aspects of the nursing program, Dunbar participated in committee meetings of the faculty, whose annual reports included recommendations affecting the school's policies. Several groups functioned in special areas, such as curriculum, student affairs, admissions, nursing service, and the program for graduate nurses (21). The committee structure proved to be a valuable mechanism for keeping the faculty informed of trends in education, nursing, and national issues, and generated thoughtful discussions.

In Dunbar's opinion, committee meetings as well as those of the entire faculty stimulated interaction among the participants. Communication had always been one of her strengths, which she characterized as "thinking together". She contended that "picking people's brains is a highly respectable occupation. The kind of experience I am referring to gives a sense of being close to people you are working with, of seeing people think" (22).

The importance that Dunbar placed on communication extended to her encouragement of faculty to develop writing and public speaking skills (23). In this respect, she herself set an example, having responded to numerous invitations to talk before professional and civic groups. Her initial contact with the Cornell Women's Club paid off with several offers to speak at meetings of six clubs in New York and neighboring states. Commenting on these experiences, she noted that "the sustained interest of such informed groups of women who understood the role of universities preparing for the professions could have a national influence in bringing about better nursing for the country" (24). On April 12, 1947, the Cornell Women's Club of New York sponsored a tea in her honor in the Recital Room of the Hotel Barbizon where she addressed the need to encourage the Cornell alumnae to promote nursing as an outstanding career for women (25).

Cognizant of the School's responsibility to strive toward excellence and enhancement of the curriculum, Dunbar stressed that the faculty must be constantly alert to trends in medical care and what should be included in the student's experience. Among the striking changes occurring in medical practice, she cited the early ambulation of patients after surgery, which required nursing students to be prepared in the techniques of careful observation and patient instruction (26).

In the patient care setting, the termination of World War II and the resulting shortages of staff nurses made it difficult to return hospital service to its previous quality. The decrease in working hours tended to take away nursing time, whereas new medical practices intensified the need. By 1947, the staff operated on a 44-hour week, but it was insufficient to meet the tremendous demand, even with a net gain of 142 graduate nurses as compared with 56 the previous year (27).

On one floor of the Women's Clinic, a new approach was introduced called the case assignment model, in which the same nurse was responsible for the complete care of a certain number of patients (28). Henricus Stander, the medical director, pointed out that the traditional practice of assigning care by functions had its disadvantages for both the patient and the nurse. "One nurse giving all the medications and another the treatments has only confused the patients as to his or her primary nurse and leads one to ask, 'Are you my nurse?'" (29).

In light of the persisting nursing shortage, President William Harding Jackson of The New York Hospital suggested releasing staff nurses from spending time on performing non-nursing tasks (30). Some relief occurred in the fall of 1948 when the Hospital recruited a group of workers classified as aides, specifically charged to assist the nurse in bed baths and evening care of acutely ill patients. Identified by a distinctive gray uniform with the title "Nurses Aide" affixed to it, the new employee received on-the-job training (31).

The following year, the Department of Pediatrics initiated the first series of institutes for graduate nurses and physicians on the care of premature infants. In an arrangement with the VNSNY, the School of Nursing provided a staff education program for 33 nurses to observe medical and nursing practices at the Hospital. Another undertaking, held in conjunction with the New York City Hospital Transport Service for Premature Infants, offered one month of supervised experience to 10 nurses (32).

The demand for nurses with advanced preparation in a clinical specialty represented a growing trend in the nursing community. To meet this need, and in view of the unusual features of the Medical Center, Dunbar asserted that the School 's efforts in graduate education should be directed toward nurses enrolled for academic work in other universities in the metropolitan New York City area (33). At a meeting of the Curriculum Committee, faculty members proposed a new policy that all graduate students be required to take the NLNE Achievement Test in a given clinical area (34). During 1948, 32 graduate students at Teachers College, Columbia University completed clinical course work (35).

In 1949, the Society of The New York Hospital reported some easing of the nursing shortage, which made it possible for the Hospital to open 111 more beds, mostly to care for children (36). Staffing consisted of 617 graduate nurses, 372 supplementary workers, and 101 students in clinical assignments (37). It was a particularly trying time because of concerns generated about a potential outbreak of poliomyelitis. On July 27, the Commissioner of Hospitals in New York City expressed alarm about the increasing incidence of the disease and requested The New York Hospital to be prepared for receiving patients (38).

To cope with the poliomyelitis outbreak and meet the need to accommodate 15 affected children, Hospital officials and nursing administration moved rapidly to develop a plan, and in less than a week everything was in readiness to receive patients. For the treatment of adults, a new 24-bed unit of opened on one of the pavilions that had been previously closed. Dr. David P. Barr, who became the medical director following the recent death of Henricus Stander, characterized the preparations at the Hospital as "a remarkable accomplishment achieved by the efforts of administrative, nursing, and medical staff with the cooperation of the National Foundation for Infantile Paralysis" (39). Barr gave special recognition to Dr. Philip Stimson as a consultant who "gave unstintingly of his time and brought his rich experience to bear in the difficult problems of organization and management" (40).

After World War II ended, the class entering in September 1948 was the last group to wear the blue and white checked uniform that replaced the blue plaid fabric from Scotland, which was not available during the war (41). The postwar era also marked the "demise" of the traditional black shoes and stockings that had been worn for decades by nursing students. Flora Jo Bergstrom, who entered the nursing program in 1924, recalled wearing high-laced black shoes from November to May and black oxfords from May to November (42).

Another graduate, Louise Lincoln Cady, class of 1934, shed further light on the matter when pointing out that the "hated black shoes and stockings" had been made to last until the students were seniors, at which point they were rewarded with a brand new pair of white oxfords and hose (43). When that occasion arrived, the students followed an established ritual in which they marched en masse to the East River and gleefully tossed the worn black shoes into the river. Some years later, Alma Woolley, a 1954 alumna, noted that by then, white shoes and stockings were part of the student uniform. "They were made by a company called Garrods, so that's what we called them," she declared, adding that some of the students disliked the shoes because of the style and "were happy to throw them into the East River after graduation!" (44).

In the fall of 1949, the School of Nursing reported an enrollment of 126 students, of whom 79 were in the entering class (45). A new policy required all applicants to take the pre-nursing test offered by the NLNE (46). Dunbar explained that "the advantage of this test over the one offered previously is mainly that it gives the faculty an opportunity to compare the aptitude of each applicant with those of other students in the first and second year of liberal arts colleges. This is important since we are now recruiting from other colleges" (47). Dunbar also noted that "counselors in those colleges are in need of advice from our faculty relative to the degree of scholastic aptitude necessary for success in this school" (48).

The year marked other notable developments, such as the last group of students in the Cadet Nurse Corps to graduate, and the granting of joint NLNE-NOPHN Accreditation to the nursing program (49). This latter action signified that nurses prepared at the School were qualified to practice both general and public health nursing (50). The formation of the National Nursing Accrediting Service by the six national nursing organizations led to the distribution of a listing of accredited schools of nursing for the first time (51).

For over a year, the hours of student service in the clinical area had been reduced from 48 to 44 weekly, but admissions to the School continued to operate in February and September (52). After applicants were accepted, it was Dunbar's practice to write to the parents and invite them to a brief, informal program and tea at the time of registration. In the letter, she stated that "there will be opportunity to hear something of what nursing has become in these days and also what the day-to-day life of a student is like" (53).

Dunbar's concern for the welfare and health of the students never abated from the moment that she became the dean. In addition to her strong advocacy of the reorganized student association and its fully functioning student government, she supported *The Blue Plaidette*, the newsletter started and staffed by the students (54).

One of her prime interests related to student aid, a problem that intensified when funds provided through the U.S. Cadet Nurse Corps were discontinued. A reconstituted Committee on Scholarships accelerated efforts to acquire funds by initiating a program of annual gifts for student assistance (55).

During this period, considerable activity permeated the hospital. Mary Millar, a graduate of the School in the early 1950s, vividly recalled the satisfaction derived in taking care of patients and being part of a large famous medical center. "We had exposure to the latest diagnostic and medical techniques and the pervasive atmosphere of learning. Most of our clinical experience was spent on the pavilions where all except private patients were cared for" (56). Millar noted that although the nursing students did not have classes with the medical students, they shared the medical library after it was combined with the Lydia E. Anderson Library. Other than working together on the units and attending Grand Rounds, most of the contacts took place informally in dating, parties, and various social activities (57).

In January 1948, amendments to the historic 1927 agreement of the Society and Cornell's Board of Trustees were adopted for the first time (58). The original document had officially established The New York Hospital-Cornell Medical Center Association, but it did not specifically identify the formation of what would become the Cornell University-New York Hospital School of Nursing in 1942. An amendment to Article I enhanced the status of the School by acknowledging it as part of the University system. Another amendment related to the role of the president of the JAB as providing the overall direction of the Center. The JAB had the responsibility of submitting nominations for all positions of the professional staff of the Hospital and faculties of the Medical College and School of Nursing (59).

The amended agreement came at a propitious time in light of the recent appointment of Dr. Stanhope Bayne-Jones as president of the JAB. In his announcement to the Governors, President Jackson declared that "we have obtained the most outstanding man for one of the most important positions in the medical world" (60). Ever since Canby Robinson resigned in 1934, no effort had been made to replace him over the next 13 years. During the interim, the dean of the Medical College and the executive director of the Hospital reported independently to the JAB (61).

Bayne-Jones assumed his new post with a distinguished record as administrative leader, cancer researcher, and author of scholarly works (62). Early in his career, he was a member of the bacteriology and pathology faculties of Johns Hopkins where he received his medical training. In 1932, he joined the bacteriology faculty of Yale Medical School and held that position for the next 15 years, which included five years as dean. A Brigadier General during World War II in the Army Medical Reserve Corps, he also served as deputy chief of the Preventive Medicine Service in the Office of Surgeon General (63).

Reporting to the president of Cornell University in the fall of 1948, Dunbar expressed appreciation for Bayne-Jones' attendance at meetings of the nursing faculty and Executive Faculty soon after his arrival in New York (64). She detailed a number of activities underway in the School, including faculty discussions of a recently released report of an important study conducted by Esther Lucile Brown, a well-known social anthropologist (65). The impetus for the project came from the National Nursing Council, which had approached the Carnegie Corporation for funding. The research aimed to examine the question of who should organize, administer, and finance professional schools of nursing (66).

Throughout the study period, Dunbar, Anna Wolf, and several other prominent nurses had served on the Professional Advisory Committee. William Harding Jackson, president of The New York Hospital, headed the Lay Advisory Group, which consisted of influential community leaders such as Mrs. August Belmont, a board member of the ARC and active supporter of the Cornell University-New York Hospital School of Nursing (67). Some years later, Brown recalled her

impressions of Dunbar, whom she first met at a meeting of the
Professional Advisory Committee held at her apartment:

> Virginia Dunbar talked less readily and was tentative in her judg-
> ments. But her intellectual interest, her great sincerity, her
> searching for a theme and evaluation of past and present devel-
> opments impressed themselves upon me. Afterward and when I
> spent many weeks at The New York Hospital as a patient, I dis-
> covered her essential warmth and understanding (68).

The Brown Report fit into the historical sequence of analyses of
nursing education beginning with the Goldmark Report in 1923 and
the Grading Report by May Burgess in the early 1930s. A review of its
more telling findings reached the conclusion that "the preparation of
professional nurses belongs squarely in institutions of higher learning"
(69). The Report stirred up a rash of controversy within and outside the
profession, posing, in particular, a threat to hospital schools. Fears and
considerable confusion pervaded the nursing community.

Before dissolution of the National Nursing Council in 1948, one
of its last actions was to establish a committee to implement the Brown
Report under the aegis of the NLNE. Represented by all six national
nursing organizations and funded largely by the W. K. Kellogg
Foundation, the committee focused on the improvement of nursing
service and the rebuilding of a system of nursing education (70). The
members approached their task by exploring three phases: study and
analysis of the report in order to identify areas for implementation,
comprehensive planning, and an action plan (71).

Following publication of the Brown Report, Dunbar correspond-
ed frequently with Brown, who directed the Department of Studies in
the Professions at the Russell Sage Foundation. They shared information about projects and other activities underway and exchanged annual reports of their respective organizations (72). In the spring of 1949,
Brown was admitted for surgery to The New York Hospital where she
remained for several weeks in the Baker Pavilion. During her convales-
cence, she received a note from Dunbar who wrote: "I know we are all
very happy that your recovery has been so good, which, when all is said
and done, is a surgical accomplishment quite of its own" (73).

In March 1950, Brown sent a letter to the Board of Governors
expressing perceptions formed during her 10-week hospitalization:

That long enforced visit gave me even more of an opportunity than my two weeks there last spring, to observe something of nursing care and administration. . . . At present we have at The New York Hospital a group of nurses who can render excellent service in making a patient comfortable in a physical and to some degree a psychological way. I sincerely hope that ways and means can be found for attracting increasingly able students to the school on behalf of subsequent benefits to your hospital and to nursing at large (74).

At a National Nursing Planning Conference in January 1949, action taken by the Committee on Implementing the Brown Report led to the formation of a subcommittee to carry out a school data analysis (75). Facilitated through funding from the Rockefeller Foundation, the project produced an interim classification of basic schools of nursing, both degree and diploma programs (76). It was anticipated that the data would be useful for regional planning for nursing service and nursing education, for identifying schools where recruitment efforts would be directed, and for other purposes such as federal aid for nursing education (77). After evaluation, the schools were classified in only three groups, which tended to defeat the study's purpose since the poorest nursing programs were not identified. This limitation and others generated further study that eventually resulted in a system of temporary accreditation (78).

At the November 16, 1949, meeting of the Council for the School of Nursing, attended by Bayne-Jones as a new member, Dunbar presented information about the school data analysis and the high standing of the School of Nursing (79). She also reported on the increase in the number of students admitted with two years of college preparation (80). Cited among other positive developments were the strides made in the counseling program in advising students, providing guidance to their organization, and assisting those who did not adapt or wished to remain in the nursing program (81).

Toward the end of the 1940s, changing neighborhoods in New York City and the spread of hospital insurance produced the first serious decline in the number of pavilion patients at The New York Hospital (82). This development paved the way for the medical staff to use some of the semi-private beds for teaching purposes. It would take another 15 years until the introduction of Medicare and Medicaid to extend the teaching program to the remaining semi-private and private rooms (83).

According to Henry Pratt, director of the Hospital, relationships during the late 1940s were greatly strengthened with Memorial Hospital, the Hospital for Special Surgery, and the Second Division of Bellevue Hospital. In 1947, the Lying-in-Hospital of the City of New York, the New York Nursery and Child's Hospital, and the Manhattan Maternity and Dispensary merged with The New York Hospital (84). When the Sloan-Kettering Institute became a division of the Cornell Medical College for educational purposes, it reinforced the association between two major institutions (85). Continuing its service to the community, the Hospital established more clinics in the outpatient department, the Vincent Astor Diagnostic Service, and a recovery unit in the Department of Surgery. It also acquired extensive subsidies from agencies and individuals to conduct medical investigations (86).

A spirit of optimism pervaded the Hospital with the improved financial situation and the annual income on the rise with large payments by and on behalf of patients. There also were notable returns from investments and Capital Funds, increased contributions from the United Hospital Fund, and membership gifts (87). Hospital services were increased to meet the needs of a growing patient population, more surgical operations, laboratory and X-ray examinations, and in-depth training of interns, residents, and fellows (88).

Although the Hospital's financial picture seemed to predict a rosy future, the School of Nursing did not share such a favorable view about its continuing sources of support. In addition to scholarships, a necessary safeguard for the development and welfare of the School could only be assured through an endowment. Prior to accepting the position of dean in 1945, Dunbar had candidly told President Day that the financial arrangement of the School greatly troubled her (89).

From a historical perspective, Dunbar was not the first nursing leader associated with the School to raise the issue of securing an endowment. Two decades earlier, Annie Goodrich, then the dean of the Yale School of Nursing, wrote to Lillian Wald that with the imminent development of a new hospital center "we have to begin early and until it is an established fact to acquire a two million dollar endowment"

(90). At that time, the joint agreement between Cornell and The New York Hospital had alluded to the eventual establishment of a new school of nursing within the proposed complex.

In a follow-up letter, Goodrich suggested that a request be made to Edward Sheldon, president of the Society, to pledge for a certain amount "on the basis of education always requiring a subsidy and the wrong of imposing the regular education program on the hospital" (91). Wald responded on February 24, 1928, indicating that when she and Mary Beard met with Sheldon, he did not seem to think that the Governors had given much thought to the question of funding. "But we have no idea of allowing it to rest there," declared Wald (92).

During her tenure, Anna Wolf had recognized the need for an endowment, but she had other issues to deal with that related primarily to gaining support for the establishment of a university school. It was not until Dunbar became dean and wrote and spoke about the matter that serious discussions were initiated. When a major fund-raising effort by Cornell was underway in 1948, she approached President Day about including the School of Nursing in the campaign (93). He concurred with her that it should be listed with the other University divisions requesting larger financial support. "Despite the agreement we have with the New York Hospital with respect to the financing of the school's current needs, it would be my idea that the University should make every effort to raise some endowment for the School" (94).

Dunbar acquired strong support from Stanhope Bayne-Jones, who pointed out to the Council in the fall of 1949 that he was well acquainted with the purposes, needs, progress, and accomplishments of the School, and that it deserved a separate endowment to relieve the Hospital of all its expenditures (95). Emphasizing the importance of having unrestricted funds, he suggested collaborating with Dunbar and others in preparing material documenting the importance of an Endowment Fund (96).

In February 1950, Dunbar informed Bayne-Jones that the public relations staff had recently discussed a fund-raising campaign for the School (97). The following May, she attended an organizing meeting of the Greater Cornell Committee in Ithaca, in which the deans of the various University divisions explored urgent needs that included the endowment of professorships, scholarships, and fellowships (98). That

summer, the Board of Governors wrote to Dunbar about action recently taken by the Executive Committee and Membership Committee:

> No fund raising program in the School of Nursing should be
> undertaken separately and apart from a functioning program for
> the Society as a whole, unless as a joint committee for the School
> in connection with Cornell University. The committee felt that
> the problem of raising funds for the Nursing School should be
> considered as part of possible campaign for capital funds of the
> Society or as part of a joint campaign with Cornell University
> (99).

At their meeting in December, the Governors approved the
appointment of Dunbar and Bayne-Jones to the newly formed
Planning and Development Committee, to consider objectives and
ways to raise funds for the School of Nursing (100). In a memorandum
to the dean, Bayne-Jones expressed this thought: "The idea of an
endowment seems to me to be so sound and essential, I think we
should keep on trying to get it" (101).

In the spring of 1951, Willard I. Emerson, vice president of
Cornell, attended a meeting of the Planning and Development
Committee and suggested forming a group to study plans for a fund-
raising effort in connection with the School's 75th Anniversary in June
1952 (102). The event would be an opportune time to promote interest in the Endowment Fund. Movement toward this aim seemed to be
progressing when the Governors recommended that an account be set
up for the School (103). They decided that the Society would be willing to transfer to the account the $1,000 contributed by Anna
Reutinger to the Hospital some years earlier to honor Irene Sutliffe
(104). Dunbar followed through and wrote to Reutinger for permission
to announce at the upcoming anniversary celebration that her gift
would be the first financial contribution to the Fund (105).

In his letter of August 21, 1951, to Deane Malott, Cornell's new
president, Bayne-Jones summarized the main considerations regarding
funding for the School of Nursing. Acknowledging the leadership of
Dunbar, who worked with him in preparing the nine-page report, he
cited the JAB's recommendation that fund raising should be a joint
effort of the University and the Society (106). A total of $46,000 was

accumulated from special funds, but no endowment had as yet materialized (107). Bayne-Jones pointed out that the interests of the School were so distinctive that they could well be presented to possible donors separate from other fund-raising programs at the Medical Center (108). Accompanying the letter, he enclosed a copy of the Brown Report, which he described as follows: "This book may be to nursing education and schools of nursing in the future what Abraham Flexner's book was to medical education and medical schools in 1910" (109).

Later that year, an item appeared in *The New York Times* that gave public visibility to the Endowment Fund with President John Hay Whitney's announcement of a $70,000 gift from the Hiram Edward Manville Foundation. "The importance of endowments for schools of nursing make the designation of this gift probably significant," stated Whitney (110). At the 75th Anniversary Dinner held on June 12, 1952, in New York's Plaza Hotel, Bayne-Jones reported that the sum had reached $75,000 including contributions solicited during the celebration (111).

The news of an Endowment Fund thrilled the more than 400 alumnae who came to the "Big Seventy-Fifth" to rejoice, reminisce, and express their pride in the great traditions of the School of Nursing. During the event, one of the more touching moments occurred when the dean and Annie Goodrich unveiled a portrait of Lillian Wald (112). With her remarkable sense of history, Dunbar revered the past, while recognizing the importance of looking toward the future of the School by ensuring its financial stability and keeping pace with developments on the national scene. Determined to sustain the beginning momentum and expand the Endowment Fund, she would work tirelessly in the coming years to achieve that aim.

The Dunbar Touch:
Striving for Excellence

Since the beginning of the 20th century, phenomenal growth occurred in the nursing profession. In the 10-year period alone, from 1943 to 1953, the number of registered nurses increased by 100,0000, practical nurses more than tripled, and nurse's aides in civilian hospitals rose to almost 200,000 (1). Despite the remarkable increase in nursing personnel, the demands for nursing service following World War II outstripped the supply. Extraordinary advances in medical science, the increase in the number of hospital beds and their use, and expansion of public health and industrial services had all intensified the need. The inadequate supply of nurses deeply troubled nursing leaders, but they viewed the quality of nursing care to be just as crucial. Lucile Petry Leone, chief nurse officer of the U.S. Public Health Service, observed:

> The use of complicated therapies and instruments requires nurses to possess more scientific knowledge and understanding. The extension of health care to include rehabilitation brings new functions to nursing. . . . When medicine advances, nursing takes on new functions (2).

At mid-century, the urbanization of America and a steadily expanding population that began with the "baby boom" of the late 1940s greatly affected the delivery of health care. Specialization opened the door to new clinical knowledge and technical skills, and medical care became more efficient, complex, and expensive. A pattern of health care programs as part of community health was beginning to emerge with the goal of attaining the highest level of quality through a systematic organization of all services by health professionals (3).

The changing lifestyles of Americans brought on by a shift from a rural to urban economy altered patient-care services so that civilian general hospitals, such as The New York Hospital, had to expand and rebuild to meet the needs of a growing population. The fact that people lived longer meant a rise in chronic diseases and other conditions of the elderly, making institutional care more common (4). Scientific and technological advances created the need for new surgical facilities and recovery rooms, and the introduction of intensive care units required equipment and monitoring devices as well as personnel competent to administer and supervise them (5). In the early 1950s, a revolutionary event occurred in medical research with the discovery of the poliovirus vaccine by Dr. Jonas Salk under a grant from the National Foundation for Infantile Paralysis.

At the beginning of the decade and with a nation at war with Korea, President Harry S Truman authorized the sending of a regimental combat team there on June 29, 1950. At The New York Hospital, a small group of nurses and 17 house staff, with 30 more anticipated, awaited orders to be called to service by July 1, 1952 (6). During the three-year conflict, approximately 1,400,000 American soldiers served as part of the United Nations Command (7).

June 1952 sparked a new era for the nursing profession with an historic event culminating in the merger of four national nursing organizations. During a memorable week in Atlantic City, New Jersey, the memberships of the Association of Collegiate Schools of Nursing (ACSN), American Nurses Association (ANA), National League of Nursing Education (NLNE), and the National Organization for Public Health Nursing (NOPHN) voted to support a new structure based on two organizations, the ANA and the National League for Nursing (NLN) (8). Many nursing leaders were disappointed when members of the American Association of Industrial Nurses decided to remain independent after soberly weighing the need for autonomy against the advantages of a merger (9).

Other groups previously associated with the national organizations, including four important committees and the National Nursing Accrediting Service, became part of the new structure (10). A significant development occurred when the National Association of Colored Graduate Nurses (NACGN) voted to dissolve in 1951 with the understanding that its functions would be assimilated into the ANA. This action was consistent with ANA's position in 1946, calling for the "removal as rapidly as possible of barriers that prevent the full employment and professional development of nurses belonging to a minority racial group" (11).

In the early 1950s, the new NLN granted accreditation to 51 of the 126 collegiate nursing programs (12). As baccalaureate education developed, however, the schools tended to lack uniformity with a number of them producing uneven and unsound programs (13). In the consecutive pattern, professional education followed two years of general education conducted on separate academic and medical campuses. The correlated pattern had a different focus, in which general and professional studies were integrated throughout the curriculum, with classrooms and laboratories located together. Another approach, the more common and long-standing affiliate-type pattern, was implemented in the academic setting with college courses either preceding or following preparation in the three-year hospital diploma program. This latter pattern tended to resemble and perpetuate the apprentice-type model of the hospital school (14).

At an October 1951 meeting of the Council of the School of Nursing, Virginia Dunbar shared her concern about the confusing system of nursing education (15). Her observations were echoed by Margaret Bridgman, a consultant to the NLN and a prominent educator who served on President Harry S Truman's Commission to Study the Health Needs of the Nation. When the report of that group was released in 1953, the commissioners concluded that nursing belonged within the general system of education, which would bring it into a position "parallel to medicine, with an academic responsibility resting upon the educational institution and the clinical experience given mainly to the hospital" (16). In Bridgman's view, the purpose of higher education for nurses must be consistent with the general standards of colleges, provide students with the benefit of a genuine college education, and award nursing degrees representative of an upper-division major in the degree-granting institution (17).

While baccalaureate education attempted to gain a stronger foothold in the profession and increase its sphere of influence, associate degree programs emerged in 1952 to become part of the American system of nursing education. Although associate degree nursing education was not conceptualized prior to 1950, about 80 arrangements had been reported between hospital schools of nursing and junior colleges that provided general education courses (18). At the turn of the century, only eight junior colleges existed with 100 students, but by 1958 a total of 653 junior colleges had enrolled almost 700,000 students (19).

The genesis of the associate degree movement in nursing education could be traced to its architect, Mildred L. Montag, who in her doctoral dissertation proposed a new type of technical nursing preparation. The purpose, she stated, was to "plan a program for the preparation of the nurse with predominately technical functions, and to propose a program for the preparation of nurse personnel for faculty positions in these programs" (20). Montag ascribed the functions of the technically prepared nurse to that of an assisting role in the planning of patient care, and providing bedside nursing under supervision. She envisioned a self-contained program, two academic years in length, and leading to registered nurse licensure (21).

Associate degree programs in nursing began as an experiment and continued to grow at a substantial rate. In the academic year 1955–1956, 20 programs existed, and two years later the number more than doubled, with the majority located in junior and community colleges (22). While this type of nursing education increased steadily, baccalaureate education evolved at a much slower rate. A more serious problem concerned the dearth of well-prepared faculty nationwide, revealing that less than 40% in college programs held master's degrees, 51% had baccalaureate degrees, and 13% no degree (23). In her comprehensive study of the origin and development of accreditation in baccalaureate nursing education, Gwendoline MacDonald pointed out that the inadequate supply of qualified faculty had created a chronic situation "that will persist until there are enough graduates from high quality baccalaureate basic programs in nursing with the potential for graduate study and leadership positions to fill the gap" (24).

Well aware of the need for qualified faculty as essential to maintaining high standards in the School of Nursing, Virginia Dunbar encouraged her instructional staff to pursue graduate study, which in some cases meant taking a leave of absence to complete the degree-granting program (25). For some years, graduate nurse students majoring in teaching, administration, and supervision at Teachers College, Columbia University, affiliated at the Cornell University-New York

Hospital School of Nursing for clinical study and practice. Dunbar strengthened the relationship by communicating frequently with R. Louise McManus, director of the Division of Nursing Education, consulting with the faculty, and speaking before various groups at the College.

On one occasion, accompanied by Veronica Lyons, chairman of the curriculum committee, she met with McManus to "explore possible field work opportunities for students preparing to direct curriculum development programs in basic nursing education" (26). Another time, Dunbar and Elinor Fuerst, assistant professor of fundamentals of nursing, joined representatives of nursing schools and hospitals in the Metropolitan New York area at a Teachers College all-day conference to consider the interests and needs for specialized assistance in studying problems in nursing service and nursing education (27). They attended the event at the request of Helen Bunge, executive officer of the Institute of Research and Service in Nursing Education.

In October 1951, Kate Hyden, associate professor at Teachers College, wrote to Dunbar requesting a 12-week experience for graduate students enrolled in an advanced maternity nursing program (28). Hyden had met earlier with Verda Hickcox to discuss student placement in the Hospital's outpatient department and labor and delivery floors. Reciprocal arrangements between Dunbar and McManus were further worked out with several members of Teachers College's distinguished faculty agreeing to offer courses to staff nurses at the Hospital as part of their in-service education program (29). The topics focused on interpersonal relations in nursing, fundamentals of nursing service, administration for head nurses, training in leadership skills at all levels of nursing personnel, and implementation of team nursing (30).

Although the School of Nursing's association with Teachers College proved mutually advantageous, in light of faculty interaction and student participation, the workload of the instructional staff intensified markedly with an increased enrollment and new demands in nursing education and service. Furthermore, faculty members continued their affiliation arrangements for the fieldwork of students from other schools, such as St. John's University in New York and Boston University (31).

Dunbar's emphasis on research in nursing motivated faculty to initiate their own studies and participate in others underway at the Medical Center. Because of her interest in stimulating research activity among the students, an elective was introduced for seniors who indicated a desire to develop projects under faculty supervision (32). Their efforts generated some creative outcomes, ranging from descriptions of surgical experiences to developing an experimental home care nursing and observation guide (33).

In 1951, Audrey McCluskey, assistant department head in medical nursing, chaired a study of the nursing care of patients with tuberculosis, cosponsored with the New York Tuberculosis and Health Association (34). The investigation involved an interdisciplinary committee that aimed to explore appropriate content in the curriculum for teaching patients with the disease. Medical research on the chemotherapy of infectious diseases conducted at the Medical Center led to the admission of extremely complicated and terminally ill patients to the Hospital's tuberculosis service (35). In 1953, Dr. David Barr, president of the Medical Board, reported on the progress of a joint enterprise with the Navajo Medical Board in Arizona. He pointed out that the project combined the resources of a large university medical center, private industry, U.S. Department of the Interior, a team from the Rockefeller Institute, and the Navajos who were afflicted with a high incidence of tuberculosis (36).

Imbued with a long-standing belief that nurses must understand how to meet the special health needs of any group in society, Dunbar was instrumental in promoting faculty participation in the Navajo-Cornell Pilot Project. She believed that the overall purpose of the undertaking was to define the concerns of a health program for people of a different culture, and to seek ways of providing health service in a manner acceptable to them (37). Faculty members who spent time at Many Farms, the site of the project, included six public health consultants and Henderika Rynbergen as nutrition advisor (38).

In May 1955, President Hamilton Hadley expressed the pride of the Society in welcoming the Hospital for Special Surgery "as an associate in our center, a most modern and model hospital with its 170 beds for orthopedic and arthritic patients and its large outpatient clinic" (39). It had taken four years to construct the building in which the architect's design enabled all patient rooms to face the East River (40). Though gaining a close physical and organizational relationship with The New York Hospital, the new facility retained its independent status

(41). In addition to its clinical focus, it was involved in teaching and research.

The year the Hospital for Special Surgery opened between 70th and 71st Streets adjacent to the East River Drive, the Society was involved in other ambitious building projects. Through funding contributed by John D. Rockefeller, Jr., construction of a psychiatric outpatient department began at the White Plains Westchester Division (42). At the same complex, work was completed on the Thomas Eddy Educational Building to be used as a teaching center for students, including those affiliating in psychiatric nursing (43). Henry Pratt, director of The New York Hospital, characterized 1956 as the "busiest year and financially the most successful in twenty five years at our present site" (44). He further noted the incorporation of The New York Hospital-Cornell Medical Association Foundation, which would "enable donors to give funds to support the joint educational, scientific, and charitable purposes of the center" (45).

In 1952, Bessie Parker retired from her position as assistant dean and assistant director of nursing service. In recognition of her contribution, the Governors awarded her a President's Chair, an honor bestowed previously only on physicians and the retiring presidents of the Society (46). *The New York World Telegram and Sun* featured an interview with Parker, in which she reflected with tongue-in-cheek on the years gone by: "A wide broom with the white uniform. . . .I spent more time at the broom than at the bedside. Nurses aren't sweepers today!" (47).

A significant action took place on March 4, 1952, when the Governors approved the recommendation of the Joint Administrative Board (JAB) to separate the positions of the dean of the School and the director of nursing service (48). Stanhope Bayne-Jones initiated the new policy after suggesting it to Dunbar, and she heartily welcomed it (49). The times and demands were different from 1945 when she assumed the dual role at the time of her appointment. Bayne-Jones viewed the change as a constructive move in "strengthening the leadership of the collegiate school of nursing and the hospital's nursing service" (50). As a result, Dunbar became the first full-time dean, assisted by Veronica Lyons as associate dean and Muriel Carbery as director of nursing service (51).

In June 1953, President Hamilton Hadley announced that Bayne-Jones would be leaving the Medical Center for a new opportunity as civilian technical director of research of the U.S. Army Medical and Research Development Program (52). The news disappointed Dunbar because of their five-year productive relationship. She had always found him to be "a very understanding man and on the look-out for us in an inconspicuous way" (53). As Bayne-Jones' successor, Cornell's Board of Trustees appointed Dr. Joseph Hinsey to head The New York Hospital-Cornell Medical Center with the new title of direc-tor (54). On accepting the post, Hinsey agreed to relinquish his pres-ent position of dean of the Medical College and professor of anatomy.

It was important to Dunbar that the School of Nursing's curricu-lum reflect the latest trends in health care. In 1951, the faculty began a revision of course work that resulted in a dramatic shifting of empha-sis in the content. A related effort was a joint project with the NLN to study the teaching of orthopedic, tuberculosis, mental hygiene, and psychiatric nursing (55). Another grant, awarded to the Medical College from the National Foundation for Infantile Paralysis, was designed to offer an instructional program in rehabilitation for nurses (56). As work progressed on the curriculum, the faculty recognized the need to offer a unit on nursing care in long-term illness because of the increase in the aging population and chronic disease (57). They also proceeded with content alterations in obstetrical nursing in light of early ambulation and hospital discharge, and a "rooming-in" program with the mother and infant in the same room (58).

At the beginning of the decade, Dr. Leo Simmons, a sociologist on leave from Yale University, was appointed visiting professor at the Medical College and the School of Nursing (59). With a grant from the Russell Sage Foundation, Simmons hoped to determine what social science could learn from medical and nursing education and, converse-ly, what they could contribute to the field of social science (60). In 1954, the School received funding from the Foundation, which made it possible to employ Frances C. Macgregor, a social scientist, as a full-time faculty member in the School.

Macgregor's task involved exploring content from the disciplines of social anthropology, psychology, and sociology that would be appli-cable to the basic nursing program (61). She participated in curriculum planning and studies of nursing care, and assisted faculty members in strengthening clinical specialties instruction, teaching, and research (62). In 1956, the grant was extended to include human behavior, and concepts and methods that applied to nursing and patient care (63).

With direction from Dunbar, the efforts of the nursing faculty to improve the curriculum represented a notable achievement. The decision to integrate the nursing specialties across the program produced cohesiveness and demonstrated consistency in applying nursing principles (64). The content also showed the relationship of the psychological aspects of growth and development to health and illness throughout the life span. When completed, the revised curriculum presented a new, modern look that reflected the creativity and vision of an industrious, committed faculty.

Without question, students in the School of Nursing underwent a rigorous regimen of classes and clinical experience, but it was not all work and no play. Dunbar encouraged them to become involved in extra curricular activities, such as dramatics, the Glee Club, and student publications. She later claimed that student participation was "carried out successfully in conjunction with graduate nurses and, in a number of instances, with students in the Medical College" (65). In March 1950, 25 senior students signed up for the second annual "get acquainted" weekend on the Ithaca campus (66). A number of them were familiar with the site having spent their first two years in Cornell's undergraduate program. During the weekend, the students toured the surroundings, enjoyed afternoon tea hosted by the women's student association, and attended a dance in the evening sponsored by Psi Upsilon Fraternity (67).

For the first time in its history, the School arranged to send a nursing student as a representative to the 1953 International Council of Nurses Congress in Rio de Janeiro. Four years later, two other students attended the event in Rome, Italy (68). In the mid-1950s, a new Committee on Faculty-Student Rounds helped to stimulate greater interaction between students and faculty (69). Scheduled twice a month on a rotating basis in the various clinical departments, joint presentations featured nursing problems and studies in which the nurses participated. Attendance at the sessions was optional for the student body and graduate nurses, but compulsory for senior students (70).

The year 1954 marked the end of an era in nursing when Annie Warburton Goodrich, one of the most esteemed graduates of The New York Hospital School of Nursing died on December 31. A few years earlier, Esther Werminghaus visited Goodrich at her home in Colchester, Connecticut, and related some touching impressions of that meeting:

A cozy fire crackles merrily on the hearth in the living room where windows open out on three sides toward the far hills. The windows are framed by gold-tinged drapes which accentuate the light streaming in all three directions . . . . Her soft white hair crowns a figure which bends forward ever so slightly. Her delicately shaped yet capable hands are extended and grey eyes speak a very merry welcome. For all its thin etching of tiny wrinkles, her face has recaptured an expression recorded only in portraits of her as a young woman before heavy responsibility and fatigue began to mold her features (71).

In the summer of 1956, the nursing profession's dream of federal funding for nursing education became a reality when President Dwight Eisenhower signed into law the Health Amendments Act (72). Title I authorized the U.S. Public Health Service to establish a program of traineeships for specialized public health training for professional health personnel, including nurses. Graduate nurses preparing for administration, teaching, and supervision were eligible for traineeships under Title II of the Act (73). In 1958, the NLN went on record stating that financial aid to schools offering educational programs in nursing, or financial aid to students, should only be given to NLN-accredited programs (74). Also reaffirmed was a policy stating that a college or university had to be currently approved by regional bodies as a condition of eligibility for NLN accreditation (75).

Among Dunbar's efforts to promote funding for nursing education was her involvement in the founding and incorporation of the Nurses Educational Fund, a scholarship program administered by the NLN (76). During the 1950s, the NLN's Department of Baccalaureate and Higher Degree Programs not only concentrated on baccalaureate education but also accelerated its efforts to improve graduate education in nursing. By the end of the decade, master's programs in 29 colleges and universities had acquired NLN accreditation (77).

Dunbar's determination to seek financial aid for the School of Nursing never waned. She diligently monitored the progress underway in seeking an $8,000,000 endowment. In the spring of 1956, Joseph Hinsey informed the Governors that nursing education should be endowed and approaches made to foundations. He noted that "although our first application to the Ford Foundation has been turned down, we shall continue in our efforts to convince the Foundation of the need of endowed support" (78). At a meeting of the Council in October, the members recommended that a statement be developed for the public to describe the purpose of the School and the importance of establishing an endowment (79). Dunbar explained that the new curriculum changes would help them to interpret how the faculty were exploring needs in the field of nursing and trying to prepare young women to meet them (80).

While an endowment seemed essential to ensure the School's future, the dean also pursued her goal of building a sound scholarship program (81). Grants amounting to $2,550 awarded from the Scholarship Fund in 1950 had grown to $8,684.40 in 1958 to meet the growing number of student requests (82). The increasing demand for scholarships paralleled the rising enrollment in the School.

Following the School's previous accreditation visit in 1949, the faculty had undertaken a rigorous curriculum revision incorporating the recommendations of the National Nursing Accrediting Service. On April 22, 1954, Eleanor Helm, director of the NLN Department of Baccalaureate and Higher Degree programs, informed Dunbar of new accreditation policies (83). While work proceeded on the next self-study report, Cornell University asked the School of Nursing to participate in the re-evaluation process of the Middle States Association of Colleges and Secondary Schools, anticipated in late 1957 (84). In November of that year, a site visit was scheduled to accommodate both the NLN and Middle States site visitors around the same time, which seemed highly desirable.

When the self-study report was completed, Dunbar sent copies to Eleanor Helm at the NLN and a lengthy summary describing the School of Nursing to Lloyd Elliott, chairman of the Middle States Committee of the President's Office, Cornell University (85). Prior to the NLN site visit, Marie Farrell, dean of the school of nursing, Boston University, and one of the evaluators, wrote to Dunbar to discuss upcoming arrangements. She also shared a personal recollection when attending Teachers College some years earlier:

> You may never fully realize the total effect you had on many of us who were privileged to have your course on Ward Management. It has influenced all the teaching I have done since

and I will consider myself highly successful if I have one modicum of success that you achieved for the students in that one
class alone (86).

On the first day of the site visit, which extended from October 30
to November 2, 1957, Farrell and her colleague Edith Oakes, assistant
professor of nursing at the State University of New York in Syracuse,
interviewed Dunbar and selective members of the staff, faculty, and
students. They also met with administrative and medical officials and
the director of the JAB. From November 3 to 6, the visitors conferred
with key people in Ithaca, including administrators and other representatives of the University (87).

At a meeting on December 11, the NLN Collegiate Board of
Review of the Department of Baccalaureate and Higher Degree
Programs granted continuing accreditation to the basic baccalaureate
program with public health nursing offered by the School (88). In the
report of the site visitors, the following problem areas had been identified as requiring clarification as well as improvement:

- Source of financial support for the school
- Long workweek for students having clinical experience
- Number of semester hours of credit
- Basis of maintenance for students
- Lack of clarity between the organization and administra-
  tion of the University to the Joint Administrative Board
- Provision for faculty sabbaticals
- Limitation of library space (89)

The suggestions emanating from the accreditation review provided a stimulus for correcting deficits in the School and maintaining its
reputation. Reporting to the Governors in 1957, Francis Kernan, the
Society's new president, praised the new graduates for their high marks
on the state board licensing examination. "Our students as a group
scored first in medicine, surgery, obstetrics, and pediatrics, and second
on psychiatry" (90).

In the late 1950s, the Governors continued to focus on the need
for hospital expansion to assure the community of adequate services.
Ground was broken to construct the Connie Guion Building, named to

honor the first female clinical professor in the nation and a graduate of Cornell University Medical College (91). The Hospital sought contributions to reach a goal of over $2,000,000 for this new addition to the outpatient department (92). President Kernan lamented the many and varied problems in maintaining a first-class institution like The New York Hospital, which housed more than 1,500 beds with teaching facilities for medical students, residents, interns, nurses, and other groups. He explained that to "support some 250 research programs, all in the field of physical and mental health, to purchase the new equipment which the demands of modern medicine require, add immeasurably to our costs" (93).

As a new undertaking, the Hospital was awarded funding from the New York State Department of Health, in cooperation with the U.S. Children's Bureau, as a first step in establishing a Demonstration Center (94). The project's intent was to prepare staff nurses as leaders of parent groups and offer additional training for supervising other individuals to be group leaders (95). Designed for parents, beginning in pregnancy and extending through the first year of life, the Demonstration Center was perceived as an integral part of a total nursing service within a hospital setting. Professional people could observe, study, and evaluate the organization, implementation, and impact of such a service and adapt the model to their own facility (96).

Progress was also made in the educational program of the School with the addition of a mental health consultant to the faculty on a grant from the National Institutes of Health (97). Nursing students continued their affiliation at the Visiting Nurse Service of New York while arrangements were completed with the Visiting Nurse Association of Brooklyn to accommodate the increased enrollment (98). In 1957, other developments occurred, including a reduction in the length of the program from three calendar years to two academic years and eight months. For the first time, the School held a combined commencement with the Medical College, with graduation scheduled in June instead of September (99).

In the fall of 1956, the School accepted a total of 93 new students, the largest class ever to be admitted in peacetime (100). The group came from 48 different colleges in 15 states and the Canal Zone, with more than half of the students from schools and homes outside of New York State (101). The significance of the large number of students was exceeded only by the news that it would be the second to last entering class for Dean Dunbar prior to her retirement in 1958. During her 12 and a half years of superb leadership, she succeeded in her mission to convert the School of Nursing into one of true university stature that generated respect among the medical, hospital, and nursing community. It came as no surprise that throughout her tenure, she attended the regular monthly meetings of the Medical Board, claiming it was "a privilege which gives opportunity for mutual understanding and full cooperation" (102).

Virginia Dunbar gave an identity to the School while guiding a loyal and inspired faculty to grow professionally by continuing to learn and producing scholarly works. She also encouraged them to establish closer relationships with the students whom she viewed as the best and the brightest. A few months before she officially retired, the senior class presented a portrait of her to the School of Nursing. At a reception in her honor, held in the Nurses Residence, she received many accolades and gifts, including a Revere silver bowl and a new Plymouth automobile from the Society. When presenting the bowl, President Kernan commented on her years of "meritorious service when the standards were of the highest order" (103).

Throughout her administration, Dunbar expressed deep concern about the financial arrangement of the School, whose entire support except for student fees came from the Hospital. Early on she had recognized the importance of obtaining an endowment to expand and improve the nursing program and to keep pace with trends and events in national health care. The launching of the Endowment Fund in 1951 promised a hopeful beginning toward a lofty goal estimated at $20,000,000 to make the School self-supporting. Through Dunbar's unrelenting efforts, contributions came in from alumnae, graduating classes, organizations, and individuals, and by 1958, the Fund reached $138,000 (104).

A letter from Jean French, chairman of the Endowment Committee, requested the Alumnae Association to honor Dunbar by making a gift in her name. She noted that the sponsors of the Fund included officials at the Hospital, physicians in the Medical College, nursing faculty, and prominent persons such as Esther Lucile Brown (105). In its 1958 winter issue, *The Alumnae News* reproduced an excerpt of a letter from Anna Wolf, in which she alluded to the Fund:

Miss Dunbar's contribution to the advancement of nurses' education has been unique. . . . The Dunbar endowment is an appropriate tribute to one who has given such devoted selfless service for the better education of nurses, not only in the school she administered but to other schools she administered loyal service and support (106).

On October 16, 1958, President Kernan announced the appointment of Muriel Carbery as dean of the School and the continuing director of nursing service (107). She would begin her position in a return to the dual role as the 1960s approached, portending a decade of social activism and revolt, and reforms in the nursing profession. The events of the times and their impact on the Cornell University-New York Hospital School of Nursing would test the abilities and vision of its new leader.

CHAPTER 10

A Tempestuous Decade: Patterns and Programs

The 1960s ushered in a new era of fresh concerns as population growth continued, technology expanded, and a surge of social consciousness swept through the country (1). Despair followed the assassination of President John F. Kennedy, and while the nation healed, other events began to capture their attention. Most notable were the rise of the Civil Rights Movement, the reaction against the Vietnam War, and the protests of young people on college campuses toward administrative policies. Reform became the dominant theme of the decade, generating changing attitudes toward traditional values, unconventional lifestyles, and a resurgence of the Women's Movement.

During this period, some of the nation's most progressive health legislation was enacted as the American public became increasingly health conscious and recognized the social and economic penalties resulting from illness. The concept of the right to health care assumed new significance with the Comprehensive Planning Act of 1966, which stated in its preamble that "the fulfillment of our national purpose depends on promoting and assuring the highest level of health attained for every person" (2). Health manpower became a prominent issue on the national agenda with the development of new sources to pay for health services. For over 30 years, the federal government had increased its involvement in health care projects and programs, with its policies and actions viewed as the "most powerful single instrumentality in shaping the manpower resources of the United States" (3).

Mounting health problems and expectations for health care created enormous pressure on health professionals to deliver high-quality services. Dr. William Stewart, U.S. Surgeon General, pointed out that nursing was being severely challenged by a scientific revolution that "has forced an acceleration of specialization requiring professional nurses to take on new and complex responsibilities" (4). The nursing profession welcomed the introduction of clinical specialization in many of the medical and surgical interventions performed in hospitals (5).

Events in the larger society profoundly affected the educational system, particularly at the college and university level. The number of community and junior colleges grew substantially, and state legislation made many state colleges into branch campuses or other integral parts of the university (6). In nursing education, funding from private foundations stimulated the development of experimental graduate-level programs to prepare teachers and administrators for positions in community and junior colleges (7). Nursing educators began to look critically at master's programs, to streamline accrediting procedures, and to identify deficiencies in the non-accredited baccalaureate programs attracting registered nurses (8).

In response to earlier demands from graduates of hospital schools, specialized baccalaureate programs emerged that offered blanket credit to applicants for their previous preparation (9). This practice greatly disturbed the National League of Nursing (NLN) Council of Baccalaureate and Higher Degree Programs, which conducted a survey to determine the procedures used to evaluate these students (10). By 1962, the Council noted movement away from giving blanket credit and toward adopting the policies of the parent institution in awarding advanced standing for other than college education (11).

Leaders in the profession strove valiantly to raise standards in schools of nursing, while organized nursing services had to contend with the continuing shortage of nurses. In most general hospitals, administrators reported that the number of nurse's aides equaled that of staff nurses and the number of licensed practical nurses appeared to be on the rise. By the mid-1960s, 367,250 registered nurses and 277,000 licensed practical nurses were employed by hospitals and nursing homes (12). At The New York Hospital, the per diem nurse became the mainstay of part-time assistance (13).

At The New York Hospital, the census revealed a pronounced increase in the number of seriously and terminally ill patients (14). President Francis Kernan informed the Governors that operating expenses for the year 1959 reached $20,113,437.21, against which the Society's total income from all sources came to $18,704,155.90 (15). The deficit, he soberly reported, was over $1,000,000 and more than doubled the amount from the previous year. Kernan attributed the problem to "the necessity of meeting salary and 'fringe benefits' competition from industry, increased prices in all of our supply items, and the mounting costs of living throughout the country and especially in New York City" (16).

In 1962, the Hospital instituted a charge to pavilion patients for the services of the medical staff (17). The new policy seemed logical since 38% of the patients carried some form of insurance, 45% received payment from other third parties, and 16% paid their own bills in full or in part (18). Henry Pratt, director of the Hospital, pointed out that many of the insured patients could readily afford to pay a professional fee. Furthermore, any additional income from insurance would go "to improve the modest stipends of the hardworking and loyal house staff" (19).

Promising information about nursing services came from the director, Muriel Carbery, who reported that the turnover rate of staff nurses dropped to 36.2% in 1960 from 41.1% in 1959 (20). Surmising that the decline reflected an increase in job satisfaction, she cited such contributing factors as better supervisory techniques, in-service learning opportunities, and staff involvement in patient-care decisions. Boosts in salary resulting from improved personnel policies added to employee morale and security, along with Blue Shield coverage, life and disability insurance, and cumulative sick leave (21).

Reducing nursing staff turnover was essential for providing continuity of care especially with the introduction of more complicated procedures and treatments. Hemodialysis and organ transplant teams were formed in addition to establishing a coronary care unit for the intensive and continual monitoring of patients by nurses (22). In 1963, surgeons at the Hospital performed the first kidney transplant in the metropolitan region, and three years later the number reached 20 operations in which kidneys were transplanted from human donors (23). This surgical innovation prompted the Joint Administrative

Board (JAB) in 1968 to recommend that The New York Hospital be designated the regional center for kidney transplantation in New York State (24).

On the patient-care units, clinical nurse specialists were becoming more visible with some assigned to cardiac and renal teams. Muriel Carbery informed the Governors that nurses had to be prepared for the "next order of the day," in light of the special skills required to handle modern, time-consuming therapeutic equipment. She stated that open-heart surgery, organ transplants, and the use of monitoring equipment for critically ill patients "demanded nursing practitioners with sound scientific background through knowledge of nursing arts and technical skills" (25).

The appointment of Carbery as the head of the nursing service seemed to be a natural choice because she had held the post since 1952 and was delighted to retain it after Virginia Dunbar retired. Her decision to accept the deanship, which meant a return to the dual role, surprised several faculty members including Mary Klein and Edna Lifgren, who believed that it would be extremely difficult to administer both the School and the service area (26). Other faculty speculated that Dr. Hinsey, the director of the Medical Center, did not want to be bothered with a second person (27). When Dunbar learned of the change in policy, she expressed disappointment, especially after the advances made in the nursing program under her direction as a full-time dean (28).

According to Laura Simms, an associate professor and head of the Department of Surgical Nursing, Carbery's joint appointment was probably a question of expediency. "President Malott had no one else and Muriel was available" (29). Although some attempt had been made earlier to recruit Eleanor Lambertsen for the deanship, she decided to accept a position with the American Hospital Association. Simms pointed out that when President Malott tried to explain the reorganization to the faculty, they found his interpretation confusing. He assured them, however, that if the new arrangement proved unsatisfactory, the matter would be reconsidered (30).

The Governors and medical community admired Carbery's competence in nursing service and her long years of devotion to the Hospital. A 1937 graduate of the School's diploma program, she had previously earned a bachelor of arts degree from Hunter College in

New York City with a major in the classics. Except for a four-year overseas tour of military duty during World War II, most of her nursing career was spent at The New York Hospital-Cornell Medical Center. Beginning as an operating room nurse, she went up the ranks in various positions, primarily in nursing service, becoming its director as well as associate professor in 1951, the year she received a master of science degree in nursing from The Catholic University of America (31).

Throughout her professional life, Carbery participated in the work of nursing organizations, such as the American Nurses Association (ANA), the NLN, and the New York State Board of Nurse Examiners. She served on the advisory council of the Veterans Administration, which reflected her continuing interest in the welfare of the military nurse. In 1958, the American Hospital Association invited her to become a faculty member of the Inter-American Seminars on Hospital Administration presented in Bogotá, Colombia, and Montevideo, Uruguay (32).

On January 23, 1960, Cornell University's Board of Trustees amended the bylaws, which directly affected the School of Nursing. President Malott recommended that Muriel Carbery and Henderika Rynbergen be elected to nontenured positions with the title of professor of nursing, to become effective on July 1 (33). Another amendment stated that all academic appointments, regardless of grade, should not exceed one year, except in the case of individuals elected to the rank of associate professor or professor with indefinite tenure (34). In the spring of 1962, the University authorized sabbatical leave for faculty in the School of Nursing and Medical College (35). That year, the Army Nurse Corps Reserve honored Carbery by promoting her to colonel, the highest rank in the ANC (36).

Throughout her administration, Carbery delegated a major part of the School's administrative responsibilities to Veronica Lyons, the associate dean, who knew the program intimately after a long and productive association with Virginia Dunbar (37). A veteran of 30 years nursing experience, Lyons earned the respect of the faculty and students for her knowledge and excellent management skills. She enjoyed a harmonious relationship with the dean, who depended upon her increasingly to deal with the more pressing concerns affecting the nursing program. Another member of the administrative team was Louise

Hazeltine, a graduate of the class of 1949, who had worked intermittently in both nursing education and service until her appointment as assistant to the dean (38).

In 1959, Carbery described the visit of three officials of the Division of Nursing Resources, Department of Health, Education, and Welfare as the "highlight of the year" (39). The representatives, Polly Adams, Helen Belcher, and Ellwynne Vreeland, met with the nursing staff and faculty to learn about their efforts to improve patient care. They expressed interest in interdisciplinary planning, structured research, and the materials prepared for patient teaching. The visitors also shared information about the resources of the Division, including $1,000,000 available in grant money to stimulate studies on nursing care. They indicated that the clinical and academic climate of the Medical Center appeared unusually promising for carrying out investigations, and encouraged the faculty to apply for grants in their areas of expertise (40).

Several faculty members were already involved in research initiated during Dunbar's administration. As principal investigator of one study, Doris Schwartz, assistant professor and public health nursing coordinator in the Comprehensive Care and Teaching Program, was completing the final phase of her project on the nursing needs of chronically ill ambulatory patients (41). The National Institutes of Health awarded the original grant to the Medical College where Schwartz held an academic appointment (42).

In 1959, the Public Health Association of New York City presented its annual award of merit to Schwartz in recognition of her innovative program for nursing students that emphasized the principles of nursing care for the ambulatory patient (43). During her long tenure at the Medical Center, she became an effective advocate of the School, addressing various groups about the progress underway in nursing. She also traveled to Ithaca with Vera Keane, another faculty member, to speak at a program for students enrolled in Cornell's College of Arts and Sciences (44).

Another study in the realm of public health nursing, funded by the Rockefeller Foundation, focused on nursing students and how experiences in the field enhanced their emotional and intellectual development. That investigation was conducted by Frances McVey, who worked with Dr. William Glaser and a research associate at Columbia University on the three-year project (45). In other research, Frances Macgregor completed her report titled "Social Science in Nursing," which described the integration of social science concepts and methods in the curriculum and clinical areas (46). In April 1962, she pursued a two- to four-year pilot project on research training seminars for students proposed by the American Nurses Foundation. The next month, Macgregor reported that the Foundation agreed to fund $6,000 for the research, which would involve approximately five nursing students in the School of Nursing (47).

In late 1964, Frederick Trask, the new president of the Society, informed the Board of Governors that construction would begin soon on a 35-story building to house a large numbers of medical, nursing, and administrative staff and their families (48). Trask also updated the Governors on developments at the Hospital's Westchester Division, staffed by 70 physicians and housing 350 beds. Almost 90% of the patients discharged during the year had benefited from treatment (49).

The following year, Trask announced that the Westchester Division, which previously did not have university affiliation, was functioning as an integral part of the Department of Psychiatry of the Medical Center. It "now functions as a teaching hospital for Cornell residents, comparable to the Payne Whitney Psychiatric Clinic of The New York Hospital" (50). The Clinic was one of the first private facilities of a general hospital that evolved into a comprehensive center. Trask also noted that Dr. E. Hugh Luckey would succeed Joseph Hinsey as president of the Medical Center. Relinquishing his post as physician-in-chief, Luckey would be both vice president of the Hospital and vice president for medical affairs of Cornell University (51).

At the beginning of the 1960s, the School's Curriculum Committee determined that it was timely to initiate a detailed evaluation of the present program (52). As chairman, Veronica Lyons appointed subcommittees on mental health, community nursing, growth and development, and clinical practice to explore and experiment with new methods and content in the months ahead (53). While the groups proceeded with their task, Carbery indicated her expectation of introducing the new material to the entering class of students in September 1962 (54). At the outset of the revision, she reiterated the need for major changes, pointing out that when the School converted to university status, it retained two prominent characteristics of the former traditional diploma program: (1) emphasis on prolonged practice and (2) student nurses earned their maintenance by giving nursing service beyond the level of education required. "Ours is one of the very few remaining baccalaureate programs in the country which has not changed in these two respects," she asserted (55).

In her annual report, she described the course content, placement, and teaching methods proposed in the three-year program. The Curriculum Committee had focused on streamlining the program, eliminating unnecessary repetition, collaborating more closely with representatives of various clinical departments, and improving the basic courses in the natural and social sciences as well as fundamentals of nursing offered in the first year (56).

When the new proposals were submitted to the Executive Faculty in January 1962, the members compared the course offerings with those suggested in the *Guide for Evaluating Professional Nursing Programs*, issued by the New York State Department of Education (57). Aware that the proposed revision contained course content which exceeded the minimum amount stipulated in the *Guide*, they believed that the selected curriculum pattern required a larger foundation for the preclinical period and the quality of the product should not be sacrificed (58). The dean commented on the recommendation that students should pay for their room and board, while observing that most young people in college programs were eager to earn more to meet educational expenses, especially with well-established jobs available to them. "Such an arrangement is feasible on this campus," she stated, adding that within the laws governing professional practice in New York State, the School could permit nursing students "to earn by giving care to patients in an auxiliary capacity" (59).

On May 8, 1962, Carbery wrote to Arthur P. Jones, assistant commissioner for professional education in Albany, requesting approval to make changes in the nursing program as currently registered (60). "We wish to offer three academic years plus one four-week intercession during the first year. Students will have 15 weeks of vacation each year that includes two weeks at Christmas, one week in the spring, and 12 weeks each summer" (61). In addition to requiring a total of 60 credits for admission to the entering class, graduation exercises would be scheduled early in June of the third year (62).

The following September, Carbery met with the Executive Faculty to review the new curriculum and the recommendations for change. The program provided for the summer quarter to be free for students except in cases requiring makeup practice relating to clinical courses. Without classes in the summer, the nursing faculty would also have more opportunity to evaluate their teaching program, complete their records, and prepare for the coming year (63). During the meeting, President Malott voiced his disapproval of the long summer vacation, declaring that the pattern was "contrary to current thinking which emphasized the need in American society to make optimum use of time in the calendar year of education" (64). He also was highly critical of the reduced time suggested for the nursing practice of students (65).

Malott's response may have been well intentioned, but it was not the first time that the faculty questioned his attitude toward the nursing program. In a retrospective interview, Veronica Lyons Roehner spoke of Dr. Day as "thoughtful and quiet and so easy to get along with, but Malott was completely different and you could never feel quite sure about him" (66). Another faculty member, Laura Simms, recalled Malott as not being very supportive. "When I first came to Cornell, Bayne-Jones always attended faculty meetings. Dr. Hinsey who succeeded him was a bit paternalistic but I felt he saw the need for a school of nursing as part of the medical center" (67).

In January 1963, more opposition to the new nursing curriculum came from the Medical Board a few months after the proposed changes were introduced (68). Subsequently, Carbery informed Cornell's Board of Trustees that in an evaluation session involving the entire faculty, there was concurrence on the program's objectives as having been successfully met during the first year (69).

Despite the adverse reaction from some in the medical and hospital community, nursing faculty and students welcomed the revised curriculum. A policy affecting married students that had been adopted soon after Carbery became dean, continued to be popular and may even have stimulated recruitment into the program, with 93 new registrants in the fall of 1962 (70). Young women in this category were now permitted to make their own living arrangements instead of adhering to the previous requirement of living within walking distance from the Hospital (71). The increase in married students in each entering class prompted Carbery to explore the possibility of housing couples in small apartments similar to those available to medical students and those being planned for house staff (72).

A major feature of the revised educational program was the elimination of many nursing service-centered activities that reduced student hours in the patient-care setting (73). Another policy change related to discontinuing the School's coverage of maintenance for students, requiring them to pay for their own room and board like other college students (74). Cognizant of the need for financial assistance, the dean and her staff developed a plan with nursing service to initiate a student work program. The idea of preparing nursing students to qualify as auxiliary staff members in the Hospital seemed to have merit once they learned technical skills early in the program (75).

At the beginning of the second term in January 1963, 60 students began their employment in the Department of Nursing on a schedule of eight hours a week during the academic year. In the group, 50 expressed a desire for full-time work during the summer months, and a year later the number grew to 87 for four to ten weeks (76). Stringent policies were implemented that included working on inpatient units and the outpatient department under the supervision of a clinical nurse or senior staff nurses. Identified as nursing assistants, the students wore a specially designed uniform to distinguish them from other nursing students on the units. They were not allowed to take orders from physicians or to administer or assist in the preparation of medications (77). Another option for earning extra income opened up when the State Education Department issued a policy permitting nursing students completing their second year to take the licensure examination for practical nursing. By 1965, Carbery reported that "forty students thus licensed have been employed for the summer months in The New York Hospital" (78).

In the mid-1960s, shortly after affiliations ended for students from Skidmore College and Burbank College, the Cornell University-New York Hospital School of Nursing assigned a small group of first-year students to clinical laboratory practice at the Hospital for Special Surgery. Another new arrangement was established with the Department of Hospitals of the City of New York, which provided a four-week experience in nursing chronically ill and handicapped patients at Goldwater Memorial Hospital (79). Carbery noted that beginning in September 1965, the semester plan for the School, encompassing course work and affiliations, would conform to the same dates scheduled for all programs of the University (80).

An issue that had surfaced periodically since the end of World War II was the acceptance of male applicants, who in the past had been referred to other schools of nursing (81). Discussing a reversal of this policy, the Executive Faculty considered the selection process of suitable candidates, employment opportunities for male nurses, and earning potential, especially for those with family responsibilities (82). When the number of inquiries began to increase, the School of Nursing's Faculty Admissions Committee decided to investigate the matter and make recommendations on an individual basis. Depending on the findings, they would determine whether to admit to the baccalaureate program qualified young men interested in a nursing career (83). In the fall of 1967, the first male student was enrolled in the School of Nursing, and a year later five more young men were admitted in the entering class (84).

Throughout the decade, student life at the School flourished with annual visits to the Ithaca campus, and some nursing students participated with peers in Cornell University programs, such as a summer experience in Honduras and Guatemala, sponsored by Cornell United Religious Work (85). For the first time, one of the nursing students joined several groups from colleges and universities on the project titled "Crossroads Africa" (86).

The Student Organization, represented and conducted by elected officers, continued to function effectively through an executive committee, judicial council, and standing committees (87). A full-time counselor-in-residence was available as well as a social director to assist with planning special events and acquiring resources. Each female student had a "big sister," who contacted her prior to arrival and provided helpful information about the nursing program (88).

Informal meetings sponsored by the Student Organization and the Faculty Committee on Student Affairs helped to strengthen relationships between the two groups. In February 1963, the Executive Faculty recommended that student representatives be appointed to certain faculty committees (89). Dean Carbery informed Denise Skelly, president of the Student Organization, about the committee's action and asked her to name the students to serve on the Student and Staff Health Committee and the Library Committee (90). In 1962, the Lydia

E. Anderson Library had merged with the Medical College library, with both transferring their holdings to the new Samuel J. Wood Library Building (91). Offering extensive and up-to-date collections, the library became one of the most valued and widely used resources by students and faculty in the School of Nursing and Medical College as well as staff of The New York Hospital, Sloan-Kettering Memorial Hospital, and the Hospital for Special Surgery (92).

With the next accreditation visit due in 1964, work on the self-study report was already underway. Prior to the site visit scheduled for October 19–23, the Executive Faculty reviewed the 1957 report from the NLN Collegiate Board of Review and Middle States Association of Colleges and Secondary Schools (93). After discussing the recommendations, the members agreed that significant progress had been made. The policies and practices of the School of Nursing conformed in most respects with other schools in the University system (94).

The NLN selected two evaluators from different institutions in Cleveland, Ohio: Dorothy Brinker, associate nursing dean at St. John's College, and Jean Stair, associate professor of public health nursing, Frances Payne Bolton School of Nursing, Case Western Reserve University (95). Following the visit, the School received a favorable report from the NLN Collegiate Board of Review and was awarded continuing accreditation (96). Changes were suggested in the following areas: (1) independent support of the School of Nursing; (2) increased faculty participation on university committees; (3) better curriculum balance between the biological and social sciences, with improved (decreased) teaching load for the science faculty; and (4) increased elective courses in the curriculum (97). The NLN requested that a progress report on follow-through of the recommendations be submitted in the fall of 1968 (98).

The growing responsibilities of faculty during this period required a firm commitment to balance their academic workload with the changing demands in the patient-care setting. Nine members of the faculty took the initiative when they volunteered to participate on the Hospital's Nursing Service Committee, which provided leadership in the planning and administration of nursing at the Medical Center (99). The majority of faculty continued to function in a teaching-supervisory capacity as they guided students in their clinical learning experiences.

An important addition to the complement of nurses working in the Department of Surgical Nursing was the clinical nursing specialist.

Through the vision of Laura Simms, associate professor and head of the department with an earned doctorate, a new role was created to help patients experience a more personalized and improved quality of care. Simms pointed out that unlike the legal and medical professions, which emphasized practice, nursing appeared to place a higher value on teaching and administration. Determined to change that attitude, she introduced the clinical specialist in her department to prove that a demonstration of expertise in nursing practice could merit the same prestige and salary accorded to administrators and teachers (100).

Simms envisioned the role of the clinical specialist along the lines of an independent practitioner, salaried by the Hospital's nursing service, and assuming the responsibility for the quality of care administered to the patient. She began her experiment by employing a clinical nurse specialist in the field of cardiac surgery, who provided individualized care while operating free of the institution's structure. When approached in 1966 by Virginia Dericks, a master's prepared nurse with a long-time interest in the care of ostomy patients, Simms believed that people with this health problem could benefit from a similar arrangement (101). Dericks accepted the position of clinical specialist, in which she would be responsible for the care of all patients at the Medical Center who had or would undergo ostomy surgery.

Dericks came to her new post with several years of experience in staff nursing, supervision, and teaching in the areas of medical-surgical nursing, chronic disease, rehabilitation nursing, and public health nursing. "What troubled me most in the past was my struggle to remain in close touch with the patient," she explained. "Promotions and higher salary seemed to take me farther away from direct involvement in patient care" (102). With the opportunity provided by Simms and supported by Carbery, the director of nursing service, Dericks was eager to step into her challenging new role.

At the outset of the ostomy care program, she requested that her office be located in the Department of Surgical Nursing in the main building, because of its accessibility to patient units, clinics, and physicians' offices. She had the freedom to plan her own time and work and to cross departmental lines to visit ostomy patients housed on other units. "In the beginning I found my 'patient practice' by consulting the operating room schedule and making rounds," she declared. "Referrals eventually came from head nurses, staff nurses, doctors, social workers, visiting nurses, and sometimes the patients themselves" (103).

Early on, Dericks acquired a large telephone clientele calling in to share their progress as well to discuss concerns. As her practice grew, she continued to carry out the main functions of the program, which included physical care of the patients, psychological help, teaching the nursing staff as well as patients and their families, and developing a long-range plan. She was also available for consultation whenever requested, in addition to her involvement in empirical research. When her caseload became unusually heavy, nursing personnel assisted in the care of ostomy patients. Toward the end of the decade, Mary Ann Schmidt joined the program as a full-time clinician. By that time, clinical nurse specialists at The New York Hospital-Cornell Medical Center had become quite visible with their services in pediatrics, mental health, kidney dialysis, heart disease, rehabilitation nursing, ostomy care, and a special project to study the nursing needs of ambulatory patients in the outpatient department (104).

While innovative patterns of nursing care delivery were underway at The New York Hospital as well as new developments in the School of Nursing, a series of dramatic events emerged in the nursing profession that dominated the entire decade. In March 1963, the faculty discussed the implications of the recently released report of the Surgeon General's Consultant Group on Nursing (105). Two years earlier, Luther Terry, U.S. Surgeon General, had appointed prominent leaders in the health and education professions to advise him on nursing needs and "to identify the appropriate role of the Federal Government in assuring adequate nursing services for our nation" (106). When the Consultant Group completed its investigation, it cited the shortage of well-prepared faculty in nursing schools and the disproportionately high percentage of auxiliary nursing personnel as the most serious concerns facing the profession (107).

The 20 recommendations contained in the report covered a wide spectrum with particular emphasis on the urgent need to expand and improve the quality of the educational programs (108). In December 1963, Mary K. Mullane, chairman of NLN's Council of Baccalaureate and Higher Degree Programs, wrote to Dr. Terry and stated that college and university nursing programs held the key to carrying out most of the recommendations, and that financial support would greatly expand the preparation of nurses at the collegiate level (109). The following month, Lucile Petry Leone, chief nurse officer of the U.S. Public Health Service, and a former member of the Consultant Group, announced pending Congressional legislation to implement the recommendations (110).

In March 1964, Carbery informed the faculty that she had requested copies of the bill and would explore the possibility of funding (111). A major breakthrough for the nursing profession occurred when President Lyndon B. Johnson signed into law the Nurse Training Act of 1964 in September. While several nursing dignitaries stood at his side on this historic occasion, he stated that the Act was "the most significant nursing legislation in the history of our country . . . . This is truly a notable achievement toward raising the standard of health care in the nation" (112).

An important feature of the Nurse Training Act was the public recognition it gave to national accreditation standards, and that accreditation by the NLN was a condition of eligibility for funds to be dispensed (113). Congress had authorized $283,000,000 over a five-year period for grants to schools of nursing, loans and traineeships to students, and nursing school construction (114). In addition to the eligibility requirement of NLN accreditation, federal funding for nursing education under the Nurse Training Act was contingent upon schools complying with Title VI of the Civil Rights Act of 1964, which barred any school practicing discrimination from receiving financial assistance (115). When Carbery met with the faculty, she urged them to suggest projects applicable to the provisions of the legislation (116). The development of creative undertakings would enhance the quality of the nursing program, increase its visibility, and make it more attractive to obtain grants from other sources.

The availability of traineeships was designed to encourage graduate nurses to seek higher education to prepare them for positions in clinical practice, teaching, and administration. Funding under the federal program also made it possible for nurses with master's degrees to pursue full-time doctoral study. It seemed reasonable to assume that more faculty of the Cornell University-New York Hospital School of Nursing would take advantage of this opportunity, since only a few were prepared at the doctoral level.

In January 1965, the School began participating in the Nursing Student Loan Program (117). The funds could not have come at a better time in light of the increasing costs of nursing education, which reached $6,000 for the three academic years, including room and board (118). Since about a fourth of the students sought financial aid, the federal loan program and assistance from New York State helped to sustain them for most of the nursing program. Further encouraging news came from the dean, who announced that the Committee on Scholarships had passed a milestone during the year with its 18th annual gift of $10,000, to be added to the cumulative amount of $105,300 (119).

The generous allocation of federal funds for nursing schools suggested the potential for an expansion of programs that had implications for the School of Nursing. By demonstrating that faculty credentials could be strengthened, highly qualified students would be recruited, and exciting outcomes generated by innovative projects; the stature of nursing at the School and the contributions of nurses to clinical practice would be indisputable.

While a spirit of optimism pervaded the nursing community, the Hospital was in the throes of a massive fund-raising campaign, having experienced a serious deficit at the beginning of the 1960s. The School of Nursing expected to benefit from the drive and add to the Endowment Fund initiated more than a dozen years earlier. Although a sense of security endured, and even comfort in some cases, the fact remained that financing of the nursing program remained under the control of the Hospital. This ongoing arrangement had been repeatedly mentioned with some dismay in the reports of accrediting bodies.

To ensure the independence of the School and free it financially from the Hospital, it would be up to an energized leadership, an informed faculty, and supportive alumnae to achieve this aim. The remainder of the decade represented a critical period for them, requiring collaboration and perseverance to reach the goal of a substantial endowment for the Cornell University-New York Hospital School of Nursing.

CHAPTER 11

Muriel R. Carbery: Insider at the Helm

The **1963 report of the Surgeon General's** Consultant Group on Nursing accelerated a period of marked activity, characterized by both advancement and bitter controversy in the nursing profession. Concerned with the chaotic state of the educational system, the group recommended that a broad study be undertaken to explore the problem (1). Three years later, the National Commission for the Study of Nursing and Nursing Education was formed with President Allen Wallis of the University of Rochester as chairman and Jerome P. Lysaught appointed to direct the investigation (2). When the commission's report was published in 1970, titled *An Abstract for Action*, its conclusions appeared consistent with positions on nursing education enunciated earlier by the American Nurses Association and the National League for Nursing (NLN) (3).

In the spring of 1965, the NLN had approved Resolution #5 as its first official position advocating college and university education for the preparation of nurses (4). The statement preceded the ANA position paper distributed in December of that year (5). Although the two statements espoused similar views on nursing education and produced a strong image for the profession, the victory was short-lived. Overwhelming pressure from NLN's Council of Diploma Programs, the American Hospital Association, and the American Medical Association weakened the resolution.

An unrelenting opposition exploded following the release of the ANA statement, which proclaimed that all education for those who work in nursing should take place in institutions of higher learning within the general system of education (6). The most vocal adversaries included hospital administrators, physicians, licensed practical nurses, and thousands of registered nurses who remained loyal to the traditions of hospital schools. In 1966, 85.7% of employed graduates of diploma nursing programs had not progressed beyond their basic level of education (7).

New hope came to proponents of collegiate education when the National Advisory Commission on Health Manpower recommended that formal education for all health professionals should be conducted under the supervision of universities (8). Appointed by President Lyndon B. Johnson in 1966, the commission was charged "to develop appropriate recommendations for action by government or by private institutions, organizations, or individuals for improving the availability and utilization of health manpower" (9). The findings concluded that the country was undergoing a critical time, in which health care costs had increased at twice the rate of overall prices and an enormous dissatisfaction existed with the unavailability of professional services (10). These factors had implications for health manpower, particularly nurses who represented the largest group of health care providers.

The year 1965 might be best described as "transitional" because of the pending impact of the nation's most important health legislation. The recent passage of the Social Security Amendments represented a major legislative milestone in giving the federal government responsibility for the financing of health care (11). On February 24, 1966, The New York Hospital invited a representative of the Social Security Administration to speak on the benefits provided under Medicare's Title 18 and Title 19 of the Medicaid Program designed for low-income persons in need of medical care (12). In his report to the Governors later that year, Henry Pratt, director of the Hospital, presented the provisions of the amendments, which included prepaid hospitalization on a private basis to citizens over age 65, low-cost insurance for care by doctors and other services, and aid to dependent children and their indigent relatives with the implementation of state laws (13). He also announced the formation of a Committee on Medicare at the Hospital to deal with these developments (14).

Pratt pointed out that when Medicare and Medicaid became effective in July 1966, the added flow of federal funds would provide

42% of the income for in-patient services. As a result, the deficit that the Hospital normally sustained because of housing patients in the pavilions would be substantially reduced (15). Although the legislation appeared to alleviate some of the problems of financing the voluntary hospital, he observed that it tended to create other concerns:

> One is the probability of more extensive governmental regulation of health services . . . the ever-present danger of stifling initiative which has been the main source of progress in the field. The specter of over regulation looms larger on the horizon because of the almost inevitable rise in hospital costs (16).

In order to implement the Medicare and Medicaid programs and maintain teaching facilities at the Medical Center, the Board of Governors and Cornell's Board of Trustees formed the Cornell Medical Group as a mechanism to oversee the provisions of medical care (17). They believed that establishing a central administrative service would help free physicians to spend their time on other responsibilities (18). Membership in the group, chaired by Dr. Frank Glenn, included the heads of clinical departments in the Hospital and Medical College who were salaried physicians engaged in patient care, teaching, and research (19).

Changes in the patterns of health delivery, symbolized by the theme of "total patient care," accelerated the activities of nurses and doctors at the Medical Center (20). The Governors approved the construction of a new recovery room and a pediatric clinic research center, and moved ahead with the installation of a comprehensive electronic data processing system with access to Memorial Hospital, the Sloan-Kettering Institute, and the Hospital for Special Surgery (21). In addition to the rise in the number of kidney, heart, and corneal transplants, open-heart operations increased to 203 in 1968 from 75 performed the previous year (22).

Affiliations with other institutions also increased, with agreements signed between the Medical Center and the Manhattan Eye, Ear, and Throat Hospital, North Shore University Hospital in Manhasset, Long Island, and the Burke Rehabilitation Center in White Plains, New York. Although no formal affiliation had been established with Rockefeller University, close contact and cooperation continued with the Center's famous neighbor (23).

Despite the expanding services and personnel, an underlying uneasiness plagued Hospital officials with the annual deficit reaching almost $2,000,000 in 1960. The following year, the deficit was reduced to $463,314 (24). Conscious of mounting financial needs of The New York Hospital and Cornell University Medical College and their combined responsibilities, the University's Trustees and the Society's Governors decided to launch a major campaign in 1961 for capital funds (25). Studies showed that within the next three years a total of $54,700,000 would be needed, and by 1971 the figure was estimated at $80,200,000 (26). Prior to the 1960s, no major effort had been undertaken to obtain outside support for the capital needs of the Medical Center (27).

Toward the end of June 1961, the Fund for Medical Progress was launched with a steering committee chaired by President Frederick Trask and an executive committee to oversee and guide the operations of the campaign (28). When the faculty of the School of Nursing met in the fall, they learned that two fund-raising campaigns had been proposed, with one conducted by The New York Hospital-Cornell Medical Center, and the other in preparation for the Cornell University Centennial (29). The following month, the Governors, Trustees, and alumnae representatives announced unanimous support for the School of Nursing and the Medical College, emphasizing that their needs be reflected in both campaigns (30).

At an elaborate ceremony held in the Grand Ballroom of New York's Waldorf-Astoria Hotel, the Fund for Medical Progress officially opened on December 7, 1961 with John Hay Whitney, the general chairman, presiding (31). Muriel Carbery and Veronica Lyons served as hostesses at the event attended by about 1200 guests including Virginia Dunbar, former dean of the School of Nursing. Highlighting the salutary effect of the new undertaking, Pratt claimed that it lifted the spirits of the nursing, medical, and administrative staff, and "reinforced their faith in the continuing growth of the institution" (32).

A goal of $54,000,000 was established for endowment and construction projects to ensure that programs in teaching, research, and patient care would continue on a superior basis (33). In January 1962, President Malott of Cornell explained to the Executive Faculty that any donation to the School of Nursing would fit into the category of a *restricted gift*. He pointed out that it was not the policy of the University to provide financial support from the general funds to any of its schools having either an endowment or state funding (34). In April, Helen Berg, a faculty member, and Louise Hazeltine, assistant to the dean, were appointed to work with a faculty committee to develop a two-year plan proposing a specific financial goal (35).

At the outset of the drive, an endowment of $10,000,000 was proposed for the School of Nursing (36). In his preliminary report to the steering committee, Tozier Brown, project director, revealed some discouraging news concerning early efforts to seek contributions. Representing Mertz and Lundy, the consulting firm hired by the Society to conduct the campaign, Brown pointed out that as yet no foundation and relatively few individuals appeared interested in contributing to an endowment, but he hastened to add that "the major donor list has by no means been exhausted" (37). The main obstacles included the limited resources of the nursing alumnae and the sizeable number of groups whose interests lay principally with the Hospital and the Medical College. Furthermore, there did not appear to be any leadership demonstrated at the Governors' and Trustees' level in relation to securing endowment funds (38). Several recommendations were offered to stimulate more involvement from the dean, faculty, and alumnae.

Brown's findings evoked considerable discussion when the steering committee met on July 8, 1963. The members agreed that a rigorous approach had to be applied to effect a more vitalized program. It was noted that the "point of emphasis for the School of Nursing must be on its educational program and responsibility and not the deficit it produces in the operation of the hospital" (39). At another meeting later that month, the steering committee tentatively endorsed a proposal that focused on public health and the behavioral sciences in the School's curriculum, and reflected the thinking of Dean Carbery, Veronica Lyons, and Henry Pratt (40). The members suggested that the document be shared with James Perkins, Cornell University's new president, who knew Emory Morris, general director of the W. K. Kellogg Foundation in Battle Creek, Michigan (41). Perkins followed through and on October 22, 1963 wrote to Morris:

> Dear Emory: I am sending you a request for support of the School of Nursing at the Cornell University-New York Hospital. I am quite clear that the School . . . is a first class show and badly

in need of help. I hope you will give this application your most
serious consideration. If there is anything I can do or my colleagues in New York to answer questions on your mind, we are
of course ready and willing (42).

Perkins subsequently visited Morris in Battle Creek where they
had a productive meeting. In a letter that December to Perkins, Morris
indicated that he had spoken with Mildred Tuttle, who administered
the nursing grants program for the Foundation, and expressed interest
in becoming familiar with the School of Nursing in the near future
(43). When Brown shared a copy of Morris' letter with Carbery, she
contacted Tuttle to arrange a meeting "to discover what we are doing
and why we are seeking funds. We offer you the hospitality of our residence and medical center" (44). Tuttle responded by informing
Carbery of an upcoming visit to New York in May and a willingness to
meet at that time (45).

In the meantime, John Hay Whitney suggested to the steering
committee that a direct approach regarding an endowment be made to
U.S. Representative Frances Bolton, whom he recently learned had
donated $1,000,000 to support nursing education in the Cleveland
area (46). He alluded to the Nurse Training Act and the possibility of
funding coming from that source. The committee requested that
Carbery confer with President Trask and schedule a visit with Bolton in
Washington, D.C. (47). The meeting eventually materialized, and
although it was characterized as "unusually pleasant," the
Congresswoman expressed doubts as to whether federal money would
be available for the School's purposes other than for scholarship aid.
She offered, however, to use her contacts in seeking potential donors
(48).

On March 2, 1964, President Perkins presented background
information relating to earlier discussions with the Kellogg people. He
explained that it was critical to explore ways of developing a more firm
appeal to the Foundation, which had recently awarded a health education grant of $1,000,000 to the Hospital Research and Educational
Trust of the American Hospital Association (49). Described as the
largest single grant ever made by Kellogg within the hospital field, it
covered a five-year period and aimed to improve and expand educational opportunities in the field (50).

At Brown's suggestion, Carbery agreed to revise the previous presentation to Kellogg and highlight the uniqueness of the nursing program and the need for well-prepared nurses during a time of a serious shortage. The steering committee stressed that it was important for her to learn firsthand from Tuttle what the Foundation's interests were that "will lead to better pleading our case" (51). Reporting to the executive committee on May 11, Carbery shared the results of her three-hour meeting with Tuttle in New York, also attended by Veronica Lyons. She appeared to be "greatly encouraged" having acquired the necessary information to formulate a new proposal. Brown stated that he and Trask were eager to hear her recommendations and rationale for making another approach to Kellogg (52).

During the fund-raising period, other efforts underway for the School were brought to the attention of the campaign's executive committee. Trask suggested to Carbery that she invite Katherine Hadley to lunch at the Hospital. He indicated that Hamilton Hadley, one of the Governors, had mentioned that his wife, who was president of the Rubicon Foundation, expressed a desire to "give away all of the capital and a project in nursing might interest her" (53). Mrs. Hadley's interest stemmed from a close association with Lillian Wald and the Henry Street Settlement. In the spring of 1964, she met with Carbery and Trask in her home and urged Carbery to request a grant from Rubicon to support a professorship in the School of Nursing (54).

Meanwhile, the charge to Carbery to work on the revised presentation to the Kellogg Foundation appeared to be moving slowly, which concerned the Executive Committee (55). Not until March 1965 was the subject again broached when Pratt announced that the dean was preparing a proposal on postgraduate training. As it turned out, the Foundation was not interested, which prompted Trask to consider contacting Morris about submitting another application. Before proceeding, however, he decided to meet with Carbery to see if she had a special appeal in mind (56).

Earlier in the year, the dean learned at an Executive Faculty meeting that the Fund for Medical Progress was close to achieving its goal, which had been increased to $60,000,000 the previous year. She noted the lack of success in convincing large donors to contribute to the endowment for the School of Nursing. Present at the meeting, Laura Simms urged that the issue be discussed with the entire faculty (57). To attract contributors, the School was involved in several fund-raising activities, such as distributing brochures to give visibility to the nursing program and highlight its achievements. Another effort involved the promotion of a new 20-minute documentary film to be shown at special meetings. A positive feature of the campaign was the separate fund initiated by the Alumnae Association whose gifts from members surpassed the goal of $50,000 by 40% (58). "It remains to be seen," declared Carbery, "whether we are successful in reaching the $10 million endowment to support our nursing program" (59).

On January 1, 1966, the Society welcomed its new president, Kenneth Hannan, succeeding Frederick Trask, who had been an active participant in the campaign (60). The next month, Carbery wrote to Hamilton Hadley concerning a note she had received from Stanhope Bayne-Jones describing an appeal he made to Mrs. Eugene Meyer for the School's endowment (61). As a recent donor of $12,000,000 to the George Washington University Hospital, Mrs. Meyer informed him that if she had any money left when completing her responsibilities, "I shall keep your request for the Endowment Fund of the Cornell-University-New York Hospital School of Nursing in mind" (62).

In her message to members appearing in the February issue of *The Alumnae News*, the dean invited them to join the Annual Giving Campaign to increase the endowment. "In order for the School to maintain its leadership position, we must continue to seek independent resources to ensure future strength in nursing education," she asserted (63). The newsletter also contained the report of Gladys Jones, chairman of the Endowment Committee, who pointed out that when the drive began in 1952, alumnae and friends had pledged a total of $75,000. "As of this date, they have paid $68,000 . . . . I wish to thank all of you for your loyal and generous support to your school" (64).

On June 29, 1966, when the Fund for Medical Progress concluded, along with the dissolution of its committees, a new mechanism was instituted to secure the financial needs of the Medical Center. In 1967, the Joint Administrative Board created the Capital Gifts Committee to assume long-term responsibility for obtaining the necessary funding to support present and future needs of the institution (65). The first fund-raising campaign had surpassed its goal and produced a remarkable financial upsurge that would hasten the growth of programs and projects at the Medical Center. However, the outcomes anticipated for a sizeable nursing endowment fell far short of the mark, which led to the sobering realization that a dramatic change was indicated to ensure the future stability of the School.

During the next two years, the Executive Faculty explored long-range planning for the nursing program that included an informal needs assessment and the financial implications. The members expected a rise in student enrollment, with class size reaching as much as 400, while projections for additional faculty were kept to a minimum based on the assumption of "implementing a program using new technology and an improved teaching plan" (66). They predicted that the baccalaureate would be a prerequisite for admission to the program and that its length would be reduced to two years.

Cognizant of the changing patterns in nursing education, the Executive Faculty could foresee the need for a more flexible program which could be adapted to the needs of individual students (67). They also anticipated introducing more specialized and short-term courses for graduate nurses in light of the trend toward continuing education. Identified as another important need was new housing for the School to replace the deteriorating building at its present site constructed more than three decades earlier (68). In October 1969, the Board of Governors appointed an ad hoc committee to develop a long-range planning program for The New York Hospital-Cornell Medical Center (69).

Following the retirement of Veronica Lyons in early 1965, Ruth Lundt Kelly succeeded her as the associate dean (70). Fresh out of Teachers College as assistant professor of nursing, she had an earned doctorate from the Harvard School of Education. Only one other nurse on the 65-member faculty held a doctoral degree at a time when a growing number of collegiate programs in the nation sought and employed nurses with earned doctorates. Among the remaining 63 Cornell faculty, 56 had master's degrees, 6 had bachelor's degrees, and 1 had no academic degree (71). The faculty included 2 full professors, 11 associate professors, 1 visiting associate professor, 28 assistant professors, 13 instructors, 7 assistants in instruction, and 3 nonprofessional administrative faculty.

The academic qualifications of the nursing faculty ranked lower than those of other faculty members in the University. These figures appeared to remain constant throughout the decade in spite of the federal traineeships available to nurses seeking higher degrees. According to the School's records, there was no evidence of educational leaves requested by faculty during the 1960s, which seemed to indicate that they did not seek financial aid provided by the government to apply for full-time advanced study, especially at the doctoral level.

Through their participation in workshops, seminars, and short-term courses, many of the faculty kept up-to-date with advances in the profession and particularly in their area of expertise. Mary Millar, a graduate of the School with a master's degree who taught fundamentals of nursing, later recalled Carbery's encouragement when she decided to enroll in a summer course on programmed instruction at the University of Rochester in New York. The dean granted her a short-term leave of absence along with paid tuition and a full salary (72). "It was a wonderful learning experience, and by the end of the eight weeks I had produced a unit on salicylates," declared Millar. "In addition to continuing to develop the pharmacological units, I was a consultant to others on the staff and made in-service presentations on this new approach to learning" (73).

Shortly after Kelly's arrival, Carbery assigned her the task of chairing a committee to advise on the future disposition of the Research Training Seminars (74). For several years, Frances Macgregor had conducted the program, that operated under a grant from the American Nurses Foundation, which intended to discontinue funding in 1966 (75). The dean believed that the faculty had to determine the content in the basic curriculum "to prepare nurses to understand, evaluate, and use research appropriately" (76).

The School was heartened by the award of two grants in 1967. The grant from the National Institute of Mental Health provided five-year funding for the appointment of a full-time mental health-psychiatric nursing faculty member and an assistant on a half-time basis (77). The other grant, a $20,000 award from the Rockefeller Foundation, was designed to implement a program operating through the Sealantic Fund as the Nursing Education Opportunities Project (78). As a participant, the School was expected to identify individuals for nursing from disadvantaged groups that demonstrated academic potential. During the first year of the grant, more than half of the candidates were adults employed in auxiliary positions at the Hospital, but by the second year, high school students became the prime audience in the project (79).

In December 1968, the project director, the director of admissions, and a black nursing student met with groups of high school students (80). "We are working with the Julia Richman and Benjamin Franklin High Schools in this endeavor," stated Carbery in a periodic progress report to the Rockefeller Foundation. "One of the objectives is to admit a limited number of high risk students to the Cornell University-New York Hospital School of Nursing" (81).

Kelly was fairly new in her post when echoes of discontent began to rumble throughout the School. Ever since the last curriculum revision, problems gradually surfaced relating to the dual role of the faculty (82). Prior to 1964, joint appointments applied to all faculty members except those teaching in the areas of public health and chronic diseases. As the time for clinical supervision of students increased and workloads intensified, suggestions were offered to develop alternative patterns of appointment (83). A few of the faculty formed teaching teams, while others taught only clinical courses on a full-time basis. When the dual arrangement was eventually terminated, it generated complaints from some members who claimed that it was the uniqueness of the joint appointment that first attracted them to the School (84).

At a meeting of faculty in March 1965, Trude Aufhauser, an associate professor of pediatric nursing and department head, led a heated discussion about the lack of uniformity in academic appointments (85). Carbery responded by stressing that "faculty responsibilities and assignments should be the basis for appointment patterns and without regard for nursing service" (86). More debate ensued, especially on the relationship between the clinical and nonclinical faculty as well as inconsistencies regarding academic and calendar year appointments (87).

The ending of dual appointments created unexpected consequences, diminishing the role of nursing service and the visibility of the department heads. In the aftermath of the curriculum revision, course chairmen had assumed total responsibility for student assignments in the clinical area, which automatically decreased the involvement of the heads of departments and led to confusion about the place of nursing service in the organization of the School (88). Laura Simms, a department head at the time, who also served as a liaison between the Curriculum Committee and nursing service, remembered the dissension well. "The course chairmen began running the School, and the department heads no longer comprised the executive faculty," she explained. "Prior to that time, all the curriculum changes were approved by department heads but when the course chairmen formed a curriculum committee, the nursing department heads took a back seat" (89).

A memorandum of June 20, 1967 to the dean from Dorothy Ellison, head of the operating room department, spelled out the concerns of other department heads, who wanted to participate in course development and "contribute to the teaching in a manner in keeping with their responsibilities" (90). A few months later, she noted that some faculty members no longer shared this view, which caused deterioration in communication "to the point that isolation from the program in the School and its implementation is almost complete" (91). Ellison cited as examples the exclusion of department heads from the student handbook and the list of faculty telephone numbers, and the organizational chart showing them in a dependent box located far from the top administrative level.

When the furor continued, the dean clarified her perception of the role of the clinical department heads. "They are responsible for controlling the quality of patient care in their clinical areas and hence need to be consulted in the assignment of students and faculty to their areas for learning experiences," she asserted. "The department heads also wish to participate in the development of course content" (92). But the issue continued to rankle until a Faculty Council was proposed to serve as a channel of communication between the teaching staff and nursing administration (93).

Established as a forum to deal with the more compelling issues, such as the organization of the School, procedures for contracts, and access to the dean, the group consisted of five faculty with two selected by their colleagues, two by the dean, and the fifth by the other four members (94). With Ruth Helfferich as the chairman, the Faculty Council forged ahead in its work to resolve problems and produce harmony in the program (95). She announced at the outset that meetings would be scheduled regularly with the dean and closer contact maintained with the entire faculty. Helfferich also emphasized that the

Council was not designed to provide counseling on an individual basis (96). After the first year of operation, she stated that it "served a vital role in bettering communication between faculty members and also with the administration" (97).

While the Faculty Council proceeded with its task, Carbery reminded the teaching staff that the NLN Collegiate Board of Review expected a progress report of the School's action on recommendations offered at the time of the last accreditation visit (98). Although the faculty corrected most of the problem areas, some required further study. A troubling issue cited in every report was the dependence on the Hospital for financing the nursing program.

During 1965 when Cornell University was planning for its upcoming Centennial, faculty members of the School of Nursing, assisted by the Alumnae Association, attended a luncheon at Lincoln Center to highlight the occasion (99). A few years later, they participated in another festive event, the 200th Anniversary of The New York Hospital, scheduled for the spring of 1971. The celebration opened with a Sunday service at Trinity Church, followed by a host of activities including scientific sessions and a variety of programs. The nursing faculty were delighted to do their share having been invited to arrange a symposium featuring distinguished alumnae and leaders in the profession (100).

***

During the late 1960s, advances in health care and new directions in nursing education propelled the School of Nursing to undertake an in-depth exploration of the curriculum and evaluate its effectiveness in light of changing needs and demands. One of the important issues requiring study was the optimum length of the educational program to prepare a beginning professional nursing practitioner (101). Another area of high interest related to the feasibility of developing an experimental program for applicants with a baccalaureate in a non-nursing discipline (102). For some time, a number of requests had been brought to the attention of nursing administration from college graduates eager to pursue a career in nursing. Registered nurses, who did not have a baccalaureate degree in nursing, also expressed a desire for the School to initiate a program that would help them to achieve this credential (103).

A broad study was subsequently initiated in September 1967 to identify areas of potential change in the curriculum and to determine if the basic program could be shortened (104). An ad hoc committee proceeded with the task, and a course of study was developed covering four semesters and requiring 63 academic credits. The plan included one summer session on psychiatric nursing and a redistribution of content in the last semester to focus on the area of leadership (105). Applying a thematic approach, the new streamlined curriculum, known as Program I, featured major health problems in place of the traditional focus on medical specialties. It was implemented in the fall of 1969 for basic students, who had to meet the admissions prerequisite of 60 credits of completed college work. In the meantime, any hopes of moving ahead with an RN-baccalaureate completion program were diminished, at least temporarily, when the U.S. Public Health Service rejected the School's proposal for funding (106).

The revamping of the School to produce structural changes also led to the introduction of Program II, designed to recruit college graduates interested in the nursing field. After the State Education Department approved the curriculum, the pilot program of four semesters began operating, and in September 1968, 11 students were admitted to the first class (107). When officials from the nursing division of the State Education Department visited the School the following spring, they commented on the high interest in the project because of the expressed need of the college graduate seeking preparation in nursing (108). Observing the students enrolled in Program II, Dean Carbery noted that the majority "exhibited considerable self direction in learning and the more mature student has provided a challenge for the faculty. Both were 'learners' this past year" (109).

The development of Program II not only strengthened the School by broadening its base, but it was a forward-looking step toward the professionalization of nursing. In one sense, pre-professional education for undergraduate programs prior to nursing preparation could be viewed as a throwback to the beginning of modern nursing. Lest it be forgotten, many of the early graduates of The New York Hospital Training School for Nurses, as exemplified by such prominent leaders as Annie Goodrich and Julia Stimson, had acquired a firm liberal arts foundation before entering nursing.

The implementation of Programs I and II evoked an enthusiastic reaction from the nursing students, whose interest in the new structure prompted a revision of the bylaws of the Student Organization. An ad hoc group composed of faculty and students collaborated on the effort that included guidelines for the Judicial Committee relating to a code of ethics and penalties for violations (110). As the governing body, the Student Senate had a number of unresolved issues to deal with, including the increasing demand for scholarships.

The student enrollment increased beyond the 250 mark, showing little change in the geographic distribution of the students who continued to represent several states in the nation. The majority claimed home residences in New York State and the northeast region, but the innovative nursing programs also attracted international students. A notable development during the 1960s was the diversity of their ethnic and minority backgrounds, with an increasing visibility of black and Asian students as well as young men interested in nursing.

At the beginning of 1968, the dean announced that Sigma Theta Tau, the national honor society of nursing, had approved the School's application for a charter (111). A prestigious event as only collegiate schools of nursing were eligible for membership, the installation of Alpha Upsilon Chapter took place on Sunday, March 3. Eighty-two members, consisting of 50 alumnae, 19 students from the classes of 1968 and 1969, and 13 nursing faculty, were inducted into the new chapter (112).

During the year, the Committee on Scholarships informed the dean that contributions over the past two decades had reached a total of $145,900 (113). By this time, the financial assistance program of the School had adapted the University's model and an analysis of parents' confidential financial statements. "These were the tools used to evaluate the financial necessity of students requesting assistance," explained Carbery (114). Describing another source of aid, she cited the annual fund-giving campaign spearheaded by the Alumnae Association in November 1967. With a goal of $18,000 set for the first year, 29 alumnae agreed to serve as a sponsoring committee and contributed $50 each (115).

According to the dean, the amount of $40,000 would be required for the 1969–1970 academic year to accommodate 30% of students requesting some form of financial help (116). At meetings of the Financial Assistance Committee (formerly the scholarship committee), the members authorized a total of $102, 857 in the form of grants to be administered by the School, New York State, and foundations, as well as student loans (117). Among the factors influencing the need for student funding, Carbery identified the increase in tuition fees, the program's attempts to recruit applicants from a broader socioeconomic base, and the mounting interest of college graduates seeking admission to Program II (118).

The costs of the School of Nursing became a topic of increasing frequency at meetings of the Governors, and in June 1968, they appointed a standing committee "to be concerned with possible extension and evaluation of sites comparable to those of other institutions around the country" (119). The composition of the new Committee on Nursing included three Governors, the director of the Hospital, and the dean of the School. On August 28, R. Palmer Baker, Jr., one of the Governors, informed Carbery that he intended to present to the committee a draft of a report on the functions and future of the School (120). He summed up the financial problem in this way:

> I think that we must consider how long the Hospital is likely to be able to pass along the cost of the School of Nursing to its patients – which means principally to the Government today – and make some judgment as to whether this is sound in principle. In this connection it would be helpful to know what other hospitals do (121).

When the Committee on Nursing met the following February, it concluded that the costs of the School would be carried by the Hospital, which reaffirmed the policy of continuing financial support, although the members were not unaware of the pending reduction in monies from the federal government (122). In the fall, Carbery informed them of the School's inability to meet its financial obligations to students who anticipated assistance unless it borrowed from the Bundy Plan Fund, set up to offset the cost of the dean's annual salary (123). She also introduced the idea of possibly taking approximately $10,000 from the Endowment Fund to be used temporarily for scholarship assistance (124). The other people on the committee supported her suggestion, but the matter was tabled when they learned that $29,000 had been donated from another source (125).

The dean's willingness to dip into the Endowment Fund seemed contradictory to her past assertions on the importance of the School becoming independent. Perhaps she justified the gesture as appropriate in light of the growth expected in student admissions, which implied a greater demand for financial assistance. Unlike an endowment, however, scholarship aid could not meet the critical goal of ensuring the School's future. During a meeting in December 1969, Carbery mentioned that she was working on studies of costs (126).

When it came to budget matters, the dean assumed complete control and shared a minimal amount of information with the faculty. Recalling her tenure as associate dean until the mid-1960s, Veronica Lyons Roehner believed that the faculty did not realize the seriousness of the financial situation. "But Miss Carbery did," she added, "because she sat in on those meetings that had to do with the budget" (127). Helen Berg, an alumna and former faulty member, later declared that most of the faculty did not know that the Hospital financed the School (128). One of the more revealing comments came from Laura Simms when she stated rather bluntly that "Muriel was always of the opinion 'you don't look a gift horse in the mouth.' If you were given the money without any strings attached to it, then use it!" (129).

As the Cornell University-New York Hospital School of Nursing moved toward a new decade, the Endowment Fund had reached the amount of $330,774.29, which was a far cry from the optimistic expectation of a $10,000,000 goal established in 1961. In 1969, however, other important issues arose as Carbery 's tenure as dean was ending and a new perspective emerged on the dual role. She would continue at the Medical Center as the director of nursing service, a role that she obviously preferred and had earned her the admiration of the medical and hospital community and the nursing staff. In that position, she could claim some impressive accomplishments.

In the academic setting, Carbery did not appear to exhibit a similar interest or the expertise required of the dean of a program in a major university. Despite this limitation, partially created by the split in the dean's administrative responsibilities, some notable achievements occurred that could be attributed primarily to the efforts of a creative and industrious faculty. The School, however, lacked the inspirational direction and vision of a leader required to move more aggressively toward securing a stable financial base, and taking advantage of opportunities available in a decade of unprecedented governmental funding. The times could not have been more opportune for the School of Nursing, especially when other higher-degree programs in nursing were beginning to flourish throughout the nation.

CHAPTER 12

Troublesome Times:
The Changing Climate

The protests that marked the 1960s produced a counter culture of American youth that rejected traditional values and affected every college student in some way. Although the majority of students did not share every aspect of the culture, most of them participated to some degree. The height of the revolt occurred around the same time as the buildup of the Vietnam War between 1965 and 1968, and the climax of racial confrontation from Selma, Alabama, to the assassination of Martin Luther King, Jr.

By 1970, three-quarters of college students believed that changes in administrative practices were needed and aggressively pursued reforms by engaging in demonstrations both violent and nonviolent. Hugh Luckey, who succeeded Joseph Hinsey as president of The New York Hospital-Cornell Medical Center, observed that student unrest and anxiety became evident in 1967 when an entirely new attitude emerged among students in the Medical College and the School of Nursing. Student concerns, he pointed out, centered around three areas: (1) the relevance of their curriculum to other important health issues of the day, (2) increased direct involvement of the Center's institutions in community service, and (3) student participation in governance (1).

Responding to an unprecedented request from Provost Dale Corson, the faculty of Cornell passed several resolutions on March 13, 1969. Corson, who would become the University's eighth president in July, had urged the faculty to react to incidents on the Ithaca campus that he characterized as "possessing the potential for the University's destruction" (2). At a meeting in Bailey Hall, 600 faculty members reaffirmed certain principles fundamental to maintaining the University as a center of free inquiry, scholarship, and teaching. They also determined that unique authority would be granted to the institution's Faculty Council to assist the administration in dealing with the problem of student unrest (3).

In a memorandum to the faculty, administrative and nonacademic staff, and the Student Body, Corson informed them of recent action taken by the Executive Committee of the Board of Trustees. Regulations had been adopted on July 15, 1969, to ensure public order on university premises as required by the newly enacted Section 6450 of the New York State Education Law (4). They consisted of a statement of principles, freedom of speech and assembly, applicability, enforcement of penalties, and other actions (5).

Corson shared with the academic community his despair over the broadening of the war in Southeast Asia, particularly the invasion of Cambodia and the renewed bombing in North Korea. He had joined with several other college and university presidents in sending a telegram to President Nixon that expressed the extraordinary apprehension occurring on college campuses (6). At a meeting on June 5, 1970, the Faculty Council of the School of Nursing discussed the war and especially the tragic events that occurred on the campus of Kent State University the previous month. The members declared their support for the rights of students to dissent and to participate in nonviolent activities (7).

The extension of the Vietnam War and continuing protests on college campuses prompted 114 nursing students in the School to sign a petition requesting a week to participate in political campaigning (8). On June 12, 1970, the University and the Medical College agreed to give students two weeks off to campaign (9). When Dean Carbery met with Dr. Luckey after faculty approval, they agreed to close the nursing program on certain days in October and November (10). During the year, the Office of Student Relations sponsored lectures and symposia featuring experts to discuss campus unrest and the precipitating factors (11).

While concerns about the Vietnam War dominated the national scene and students responded *en masse* with their demonstrations, The New York Hospital-Cornell Medical Center concentrated on a number

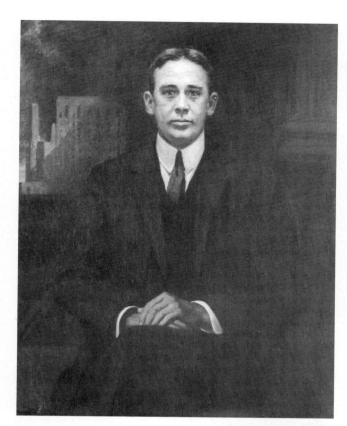

Payne Whitney,
Board of Governors,
1912–1927

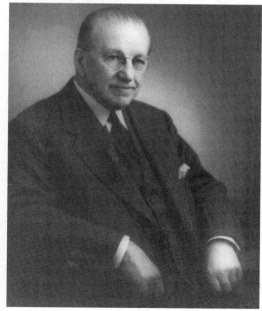

G. Canby Robinson, director
of the medical center and
head and professor of medicine at the medical college,
1928–1934

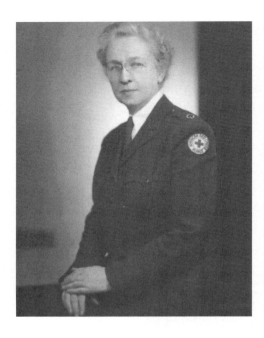

Mary Beard, Class of 1903,
director of American Red Cross
Nursing Service, 1938–1944
Photo by Harris Ewing

Bessie A. R. Parker,
director of New York
Hospital School of
Nursing and Director
of Nursing Service,
1940-1946, and assis-
tant dean of Cornell
University-New York
Hospital School of
Nursing, 1946–1951
*Photo by Atelier Von
Behr*

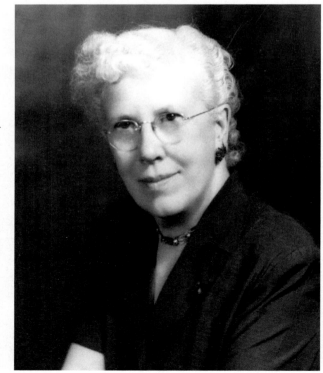

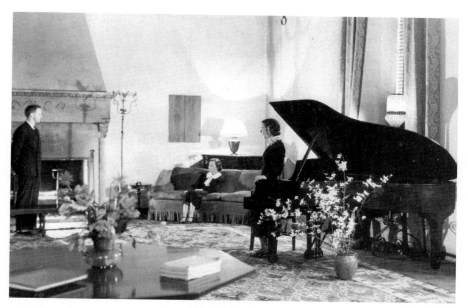

Nurses residence reception room, 1937 *Photo by Paul Parker*

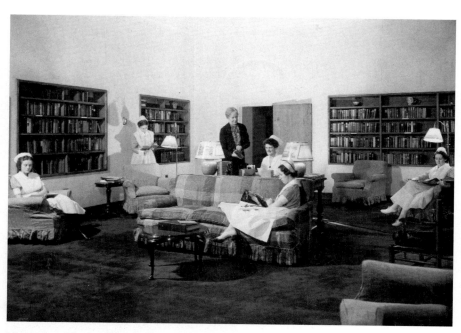

Nurses residence library/lounge *Photo by Paul Parker*

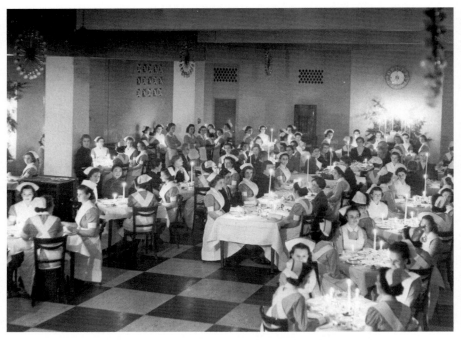

Nurses residence dining room, 1938 *Photo by Paul Parker*

Julia Stimson, Class of 1908

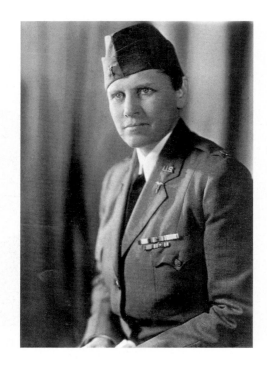

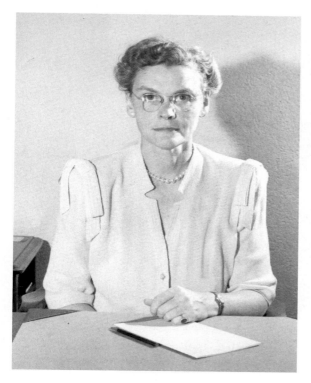

Virginia Dunbar, dean of Cornell University-New York Hospital School of Nursing, 1946–1958 and director of Nursing Services at New York Hospital, 1946–1952

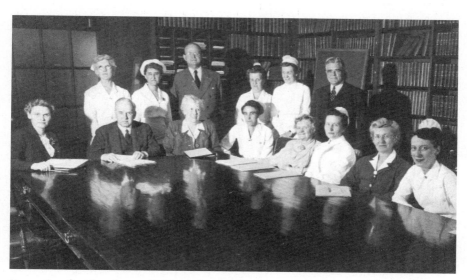

Executive faculty: (seated) Virginia Dunbar, Dr. Edmund Day, Bessie Parker, Agnes Schubert, May Kennedy, Elizabeth Moser, Margery Overholser, Veronica Lyons; (standing) Olive Reed, Mary Klein, Dr. Joseph Hinsey, Carolyn Sprogel, Alice Moffatt, Dr. Henricus Stander, 1946

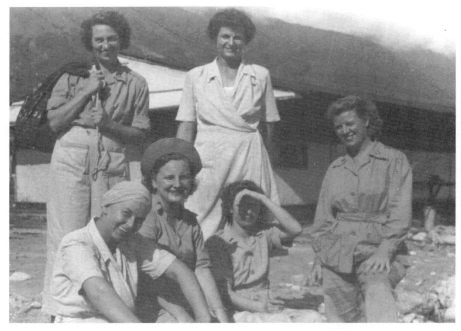

Ninth General Hospital nurses at Goodenough Island, New Guinea, 1943–1944

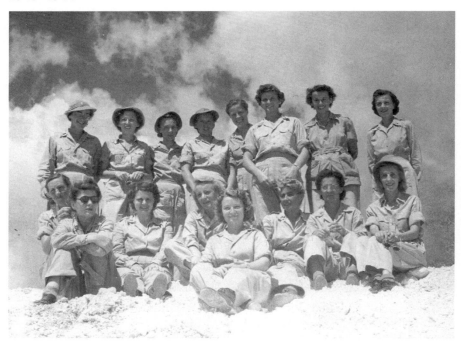

Ninth General Hospital nurses at Biak Island, 1944–1945

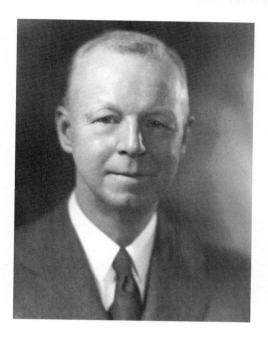

Stanhope Bayne-Jones,
CEO/president of the Joint
Administrative Board and the
medical center, 1947–1953
*Photo by Underwood and
Underwood*

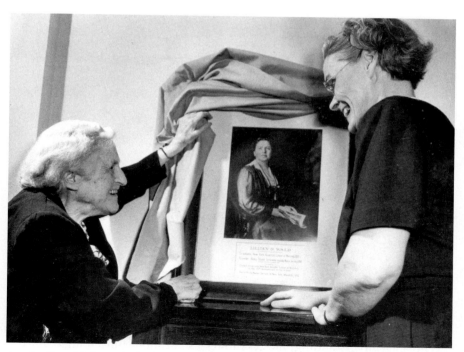

Annie Goodrich and Virginia Dunbar unveil Wald's portrait during the
school's 75th anniversary, 1952 *Photo by the New York Times*

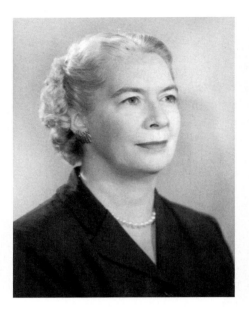

Muriel R. Carbery, Class of 1937, director of Nursing Services, 1952–1974, and dean of the School, 1958–1974
Photo by Paul Parker

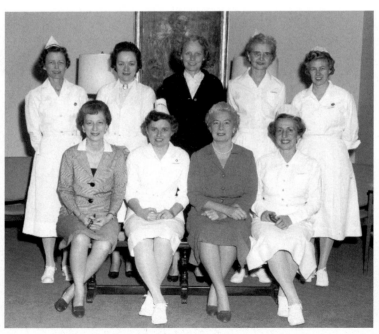

Executive faculty: (standing) Elizabeth Brooks, Eleanor Muhs, Margie Warren, Helma Fedder, Audrey McCluskey; (seated) Veronica Lyons, Dorothy Ellison, Muriel Carbery, Trude Aufhauser, 1961

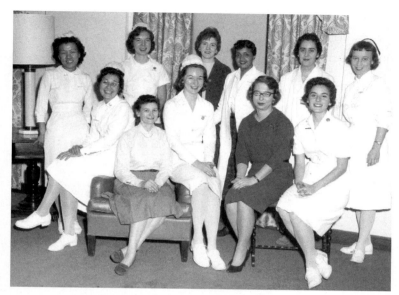

Pre-clinical faculty: (seated) Helen Berg, Ann Hahn, Mary Millar, Darlene Erlander, J. Taylor; (standing) Edna Lau, Evelyn Tychsen, Marjorie Miller, Carol Fray, Anne Donnelly, C. Kay, 1961

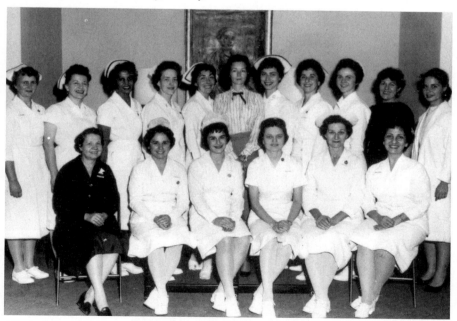

Clinical faculty: (seated) Ethel Tschida, Mary Bielski, Marie Russo Carter, Barbara Jones, Anna Ondovchik, Lena Saffioti; (standing) Virginia Dericks, M. Ahlen, Carol Fripp, Marjorie Nebesky, G. Movizzo, Jeanne Sherman, G. Fox, Nina Argondizzo, P Baldridge, Phyllis Schlags, June Weinstein, 1961

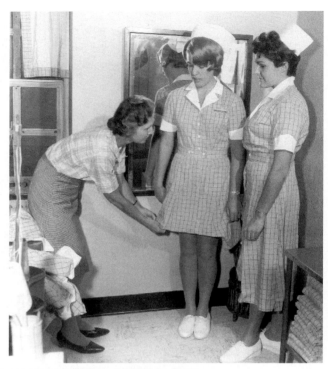

Updating the hemline of the student uniform, 1968

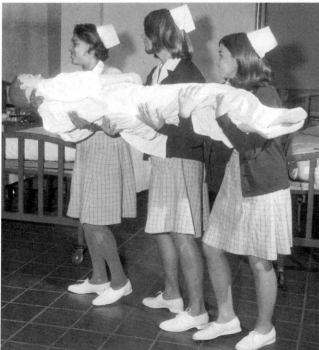

Students practice moving a patient in Fundamentals of Nursing laboratory, 1968

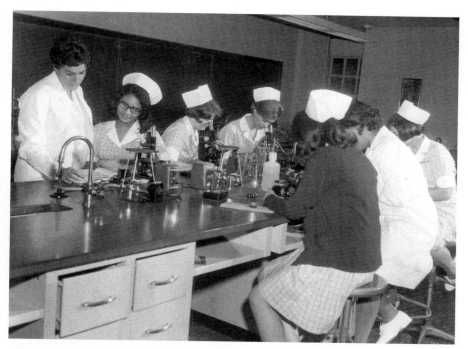

Science laboratory, 1968

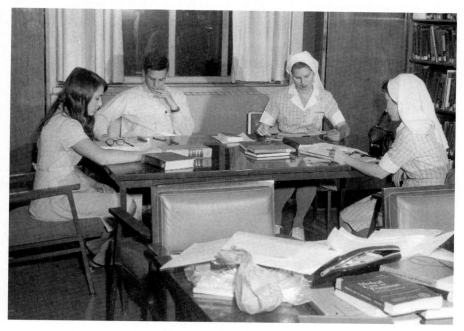

Studying in the Lydia E. Anderson Library, 1969

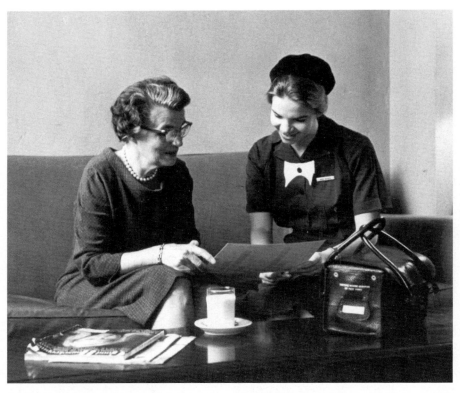
Student making a home visit during public health experience, 1960s
Courtesy WernerWolff/Starphoto.com

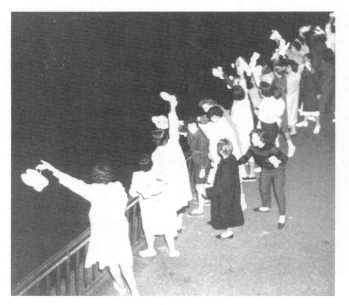

Graduating seniors observe the long-standing tradition of throwing their student uniform shoes into the East River

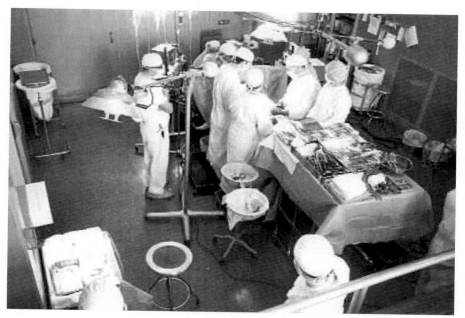

Kidney transplant operation, Department of Surgery, 1968

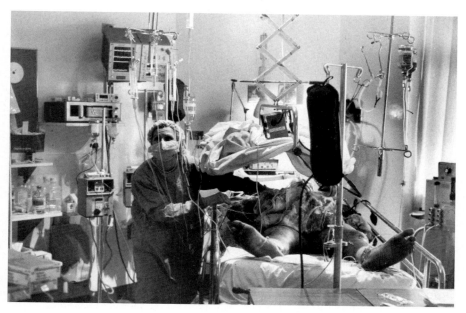

Patient care in the Burn Center

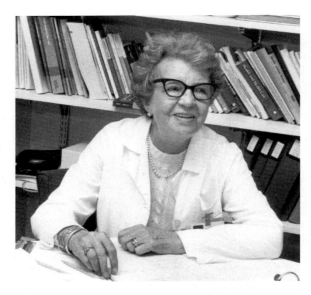

Eleanor Lambertsen,
dean of the School of
Nursing, 1970–1979
Photo by Susan Lukes

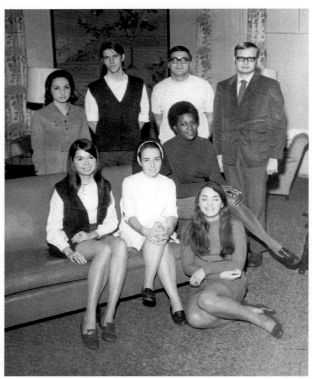

Student Senate (standing) Anne D'Atri, David Humes, Charles Sardegna,
Jeffrey Hill, (seated) Virginia Harrett, Maureen Neus, Denise DiMarco,
Florence Clark, 1970

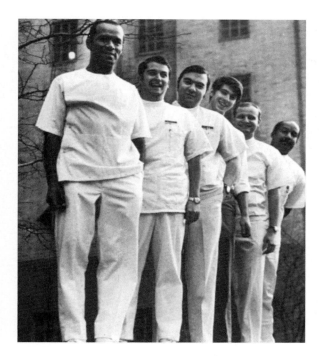

Male students in the Class of 1971 (from left) John Jenkins, Anthony Amodia, John Campo, David Humes, Jeffrey Hill (Class of 1970), Captain Gaillard

Student nurse and patient in the nursery, 1975

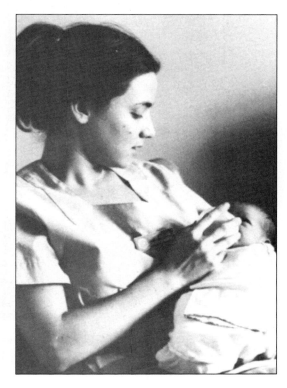

Students consulting patient charts at the nurses station, 1976

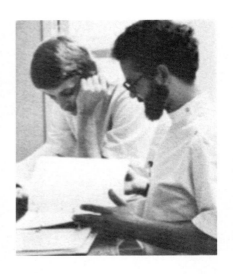

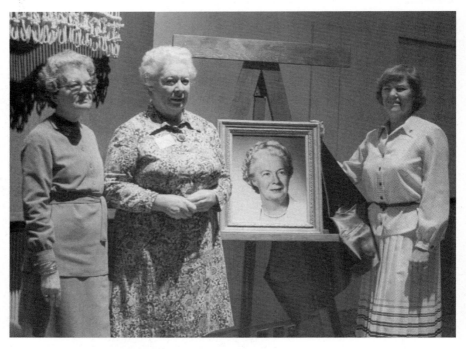

Eleanor Lambertsen, Muriel Carbery, and Jeanne Dorie unveil Carbery's portrait during the School's 100th anniversary, 1977
Photo by William Feig

of other issues. In the School of Nursing, the Executive Faculty began to explore future needs in light of an anticipated enrollment growth with the implementation of new programs. They also raised questions about the existing pattern of dual administration (12). When discussing the matter with Luckey in February 1968, they acknowledged that the personality of the incumbent and the organization's expectations had an impact on the activities and beliefs about the combined role. The importance of communication and human relationships was also recognized (13).

The Executive Faculty's interest in assessing the joint arrangement occurred at a most propitious time. A new trend in the profession was beginning to surface in which the nursing dean served as the chief of nursing practice in the teaching hospital (14). Designed to unify nursing education and service, the dual position appeared to hold great promise for improving patient care. Following a visit with Rozella Schlotfeldt, dean of the Frances Payne Bolton School of Nursing, Case Western Reserve University in Cleveland, Laura Simms shared her observations of how the new administrative pattern was operating in that institution (15). "In this organization there has been an attempt to put all aspects of teaching, research, and the direction of nursing practice under one person," she explained. "The director of nursing would then be responsible for the clinical teaching program and would report directly to the dean." Simms added, however, that because faculty members involved in undergraduate teaching did not realistically have time for research, it was necessary to have a sufficient complement of faculty so that some might be released periodically to pursue special projects (16).

In early 1969, a situation arose involving a faculty member and nursing administration that led to serious repercussions affecting the University. At an evaluation conference in January, attended by Muriel Carbery, Ruth Kelly, and Joseph Musio, an associate professor of science in the School, the dean stated her intentions not to renew Musio's contract for the coming academic year. Challenging her assertions of unsatisfactory performance, Musio referred to previous evaluations, particularly the last favorable one from Kelly in 1968 (17). On February 21, Carbery informed him that his appointment would be terminated and he could resign immediately (18). In a letter three days later, he indicated his refusal to resign and requested a hearing in accordance with provisions of the Faculty Handbook of Cornell University and the 1940 *Statement of Principles of Academic Freedom and Tenure* (19).

When Musio brought his case before the Faculty Council, the group requested more information from the dean (20). Subsequently, he retained an attorney who communicated the problem to James Perkins, Cornell's president at that time. The American Association of University Professors (AAUP) was also contacted, and sent telegrams to Perkins and Carbery urging the "immediate restoration of Professor Musio to his academic duties and adherence to Association standards in any contemplated dismissal proceeding" (21).

Protesting the treatment of Musio, many of the nursing students threatened to stage a boycott. In February 1969, Carbery wrote to the Student Organization and explained that his dismissal had been based on the "unusual number of low grades and this gave us some concern" (22). After hedging several meetings scheduled by the Student Senate, she notified its president of instructions "to reinstate Musio for the balance of the academic year and to give him an assignment pertinent to the needs of the school" (23).

On March 3, six students representing the classes of 1969, 1970, and 1971, reported to the Student Organization their observations of a meeting with Carbery. They pointed out that her reasons for terminating Musio were unrelated to low grades and that the School's officials asked her not to discuss the matter (24). Furthermore, her perceived reluctance to respond to communications from the Student Senate was due to their "misinterpretation and I will not meet with students if I feel the time is inappropriate" (25).

The following June, Musio complained to the AAUP about receiving a letter from Carbery indicating that his appointment would not be renewed. The Association questioned her action because she had been told in February that the final date for notification of renewal to a faculty member in the second year of service should have occurred two months earlier on December 15 (26). According to the organization's policy, that date had been established and was cited in the AAUP's *Standards for Notice of Nonreappointment*. Therefore, Musio could expect to be reappointed (27).

Eager to end the dissension, Cornell responded through its assistant legal counsel, who pointed out that the University had never agreed to Musio's right to renewal of his appointment. Despite the AAUP's persistence to secure a satisfactory resolution, a letter from Dale Corson in October 1969 stated that "it would not be in order for Cornell University to make any other accommodation for Professor Musio and the matter was closed" (28).

Musio resigned his position during the controversy, but questions persisted about his faculty status. He believed that the reason for his dismissal was because nursing administration resented his participation in institutional affairs, as well as the criticism he expressed about the dated practices of the School, particularly in regard to curriculum reform (29). He also claimed that the termination of his services violated considerations of his academic freedom. The AAUP disputed this contention, pointing out that no machinery existed in the School of Nursing to afford due process when academic freedom and tenure were at stake (30).

The strongest advocacy for retaining Musio on the faculty came from the nursing students. According to Louise Hazeltine, assistant to the dean at the time of the furor, Musio was an outgoing, social person who related well to them. "Perhaps he was a bit unorthodox in approaching his content but he was a good teacher and the students loved him. It probably irritated some of the more traditional faculty and particularly Ruth Kelly, who had recruited him in 1967 and then changed her attitude" (31). Recalling that she saw nothing inappropriate about his behavior, Hazeltine stated that she did not know the basis for Carbery's decision, but it may have been more personal than professional (32).

When the student yearbook, *The Blue Plaid*, was published by the Class of 1970, it carried a glowing dedication to Joseph Musio, excerpted below:

> He'd talk with a small group of you and set our minds spinning . . . . His bag was ecology – of Existence, Being, and Purpose. His dynamism took you outside of yourself for a while. No question was too stupid, no opinion too ridiculous. . . . We think of Joe now, quietly in our heads and smile to ourselves for what he meant to us each – individually (33).

The significance of the Musio case was that it demonstrated the weaknesses in the School's policies, or lack thereof, in relation to due process, tenure, and adequate provisions for reappointment. In a letter of May 1, 1969, to the dean, Sister Marcia, president of the Student Senate, requested a meeting to discuss due process as it related to the "termination of an associate professor of science" (34). After some delay and unanswered communications, Carbery met with the students in the fall to explore academic freedom, due process, and Cornell University's adjudicatory system for student conduct (35). These were compelling issues that would continue to be addressed for some time.

Toward the end of the 1960s, the School of Nursing assumed a new direction when the Governors announced that Muriel Carbery intended to retire on January 1, 1970 (36). Finding it difficult to cope with increasing demands in both education and nursing service, she also asked to be relieved of her position as dean. In the fall of 1968, Hugh Luckey sent a letter to the nursing faculty indicating Carbery's pending retirement and the appointment of a Committee on the Deanship to study the organization of academic and service activities in nursing at the Medical Center (37). As chairman, he expected the committee to recommend the names of potential candidates for the position of dean. Also, he asked the nursing faculty for their views on the selection process, the dean's role, the evolution of nursing education and practice during the next decade, the organization of the School of Nursing, and the professional experience and qualities required of a dean (38).

The following January, Luckey reported on the committee's progress, which included a series of meetings and consultation with the Executive Faculty, who were clinical department heads of the Hospital's nursing service, the Student Senate, and other groups (39). Letters were sent to faculty and nursing service people for suggestions about potential candidates. When nursing students were queried on their opinion of the dual pattern of administration, the consensus favored the single role of the dean because of the personal connection and greater accessibility (40).

In their deliberations, the Committee on the Deanship concluded that the dual position of the dean and nursing service director carried too heavy a responsibility for one person to do justice to either role, and that the Office of the President of the Medical Center should serve as a coordinating point (41). On approval from the Joint Administrative Board to separate the roles, the Governors recommended that Carbery be offered the position of director of nursing service beginning January 1, 1970 (42). She accepted the appointment and agreed to continue in her present dual role until a permanent dean arrived.

With a new decade approaching, changes occurred in the organization of the faculty and the extension of more liberal policies to students. Agreements were established with five accredited institutions in Manhattan, which allowed students in good standing and with advisor approval to register for courses without having to adhere to the admission procedures of the particular school. The arrangement provided them an opportunity to take electives in general education at Fordham University's School of Education, the New School for Social Research, Pace College, Hunter College School of General Studies, and Marymount College (43). During the academic year, the school calendar was planned for a 16-week semester for the entire student body to be consistent with the University's schedule.

Most faculty members worked full time during the ten-month academic year. Dean Carbery appointed the chairpersons for a two-year term with an option for renewal if indicated (44). She delegated the administration of the curriculum to the associate dean, Ruth Kelly, who acted as a conduit for relating the concerns of the faculty. The heads of clinical nursing departments held joint appointments in the School and contributed to course content in their respective areas (45). In March 1969, the dean announced to the Executive Faculty her intention to select faculty members to represent nursing on standing committees of the Hospital's Medical Board (46).

During Carbery's administration, efforts to promote closer interaction between nursing and medical students in the academic setting appeared promising after the faculty discussed the desire expressed by both groups to attend classes together (47). Although they recognized that formal agreements often existed between institutions in offering different teaching opportunities, in this situation few areas existed in the curriculum for sharing a common core of information. As separate schools with their own faculty and incorporation, one offered graduate education while the other functioned at the undergraduate level. Some accommodation was made, however, when a faculty member of

Cornell University Medical College informed Carbery that he would open his elective course on "population" to a limited number of nursing students (48).

Through Eleanor Taggart, president of the School's Alumnae Association, other attempts were made to strengthen communication with the medical community. In the fall of 1969, she responded enthusiastically to an invitation from Albert Rubin, president of the Medical College Alumni Association, to participate in the upcoming combined Alumni Day (49). At a medical school reunion to be held at a later time, Rubin encouraged nursing alumnae to attend the event (50).

The School of Nursing was greatly honored in 1969 when the Committee on Alumni Trustees Nomination of Cornell University endorsed Helen Berg as one of the four candidates to be elected to the Board of Trustees (51). A graduate of the class of 1951 and an associate professor, Berg had been president of the Alumnae Association from 1960–1964. Formed in 1940, the 17-member nominating committee that submitted her name had added a nursing representative to its roster in 1950 (52). The process for selecting a candidate began each spring with a ballot sent to every nursing graduate to vote for two alumnae to serve on the Board of Trustees. Berg's appointment was touted by the Medical Center as a "first" for the School's alumnae (53).

In March 1970, President Corson met with the Faculty Council and other senior faculty to inform them that the search committee recommended Eleanor C. Lambertsen to be the next dean of the School and professor of nursing (54). The group unanimously endorsed the recommendation, which received further approval the following month from the Society's Board of Governors and Cornell's Board of Trustees (55). Dr. Lambertsen's salary would be entirely paid by the Bundy Fund administered through the State Education Department (56). Under provisions of the Fund, which was an outcome of a study directed by MacGeorge Bundy, president of the Ford Foundation, New York State had agreed to reimburse a given school according to the number of academic degrees awarded annually.

In the new administrative arrangement, Lambertsen was scheduled to begin her appointment on July 1, 1970, with Muriel Carbery continuing as director of nursing service and Louise Hazeltine as assistant dean (57). No evidence was available to show whether Ruth Kelly had expressed interest in applying for the position of dean or was considered for it. During her four-year tenure at the School, she had shown leadership in the development of new programs and projects, but her rather abrasive manner tended to antagonize a number of the faculty (58). She worked part time in 1970 until resigning to accept a position in another institution.

Lambertsen's appointment to head the School of Nursing was hailed as "quite a coup" for the Medical Center in light of her international reputation and sterling record of scholarship in the nursing profession. During the 1960s, she chaired the Department of Nursing Education at Teachers College, Columbia University, and directed the Division of Health Services, Sciences, and Education. In addition to holding office in several national organizations, she was a consultant to foundations, governmental agencies, and academic institutions. Lambertsen was also a member of several committees and commissions that dealt with important timely educational and social issues.

Her interests extended into the political realm as it affected nursing and health care, and early in the decade she campaigned for the re-election of Governor Nelson Rockefeller. As chairman of "Nurses for Rockefeller in New York City," she supported his promotion of state legislation to increase funding to $24,000,000 to expand nursing enrollment. "We must make an intensive effort on our part to urge our colleagues, families, and friends to return the experienced team to Albany in November," she stated (59). Her legislative activities to advance nursing education and involvement in organizations enhanced her prominence in the profession, and in 1970 she was nominated for the presidency of the American Nurses Association (60).

Toward the end of her tenure as dean, Muriel Carbery succeeded in securing a retirement annuity for the faculty with the awarding of TIAA-CREF coverage (61). In accordance with University policy, eligible faculty members included assistant professors and those of higher rank. The program was initiated on July 1, 1970, when Eleanor Lambertsen began her official duties at the School. Some months earlier, Carbery had written to her, suggesting that they have dinner together some evening. "I'm also asking Mr. Palmer Baker to invite you to the next meeting of the Committee on Nursing on May 22. And I look forward to seeing you again" (62). At the time, Lambertsen already knew some of the faculty, who had studied at Teachers College or were taking courses there.

The timing of the new dean's arrival at the School coincided with a variety of complex health problems confronting the nation as it began to initiate new patterns of health care delivery. Some experts characterized the health field as "rapidly becoming the largest industry in the United States" (63). A trend that became markedly apparent at the outset of the decade was the rise in health care costs in all components of the system, with cost containment becoming the watchword. This development, along with the uneven quality of health care and inaccessibility of health services, became a source of public and governmental concern.

Reporting to the Governors, David Thompson, director of The New York Hospital, portrayed health care as "a right and not a privilege" (64). "Yet the cost of such care is far beyond personal means," he asserted (65). Although it was not known what kinds of mechanisms were to be developed, he seemed convinced that some form of insurance would be made available to all citizens. "Finding a means of providing health care of uniform quality will take medico-social engineering of a high order to solve the problem in the coming decade" (66).

According to Kenneth Hannan, president of the Board of Governors, operating costs continued to be a great concern, with an increase to $62,000,000 in 1970 from $32,000,000 five years earlier (67). Further, the salary of nurses had doubled over that same period of time, reaching the annual figure of $9,420. Hannon stated that salaries accounted for 70% of the Hospital's costs (68).

At the beginning of the 1970s, a national trend gaining some momentum was the evolving Women's Liberation Movement. The nursing profession had a great stake in the issue since the majority of its members were women. Although early leaders such as Lillian Wald, Irene Sutliffe, and Annie Goodrich had been committed to equal opportunities for women, nurses as a whole, as well as other women, remained passive or indifferent to the cause. But it became a stimulus to progressive nurses who saw a parallel between the struggle for women's rights and the struggle of nursing to become an autonomous profession.

Around this time, a new type of worker appeared known as the physician's assistant, an individual whose role had yet to be defined

(69). While programs for physician's assistants developed, nurses applied their expertise in instituting creative patterns of patient care. In the middle 1960s at the University of Colorado, Loretta Ford, a nurse educator, and Henry Silver, a physician colleague, launched the first demonstration project in the country for the preparation of nurse practitioners (70). The five-year experiment aimed in the beginning to improve the health care of children in ambulatory settings by expanding the scope of practice of the registered nurse without altering the nature of nursing, and to explore the implications of this change for program development in collegiate schools of nursing (71). As the concept of the nurse practitioner expanded, the movement rapidly gained some prominence, as nurses assumed responsibility for the primary care of patients in other settings.

In November 1971, the federal government issued a report, *Extending the Scope of Nursing Practice*, which represented the combined efforts of nursing, medicine, hospital administration, and health disciplines, to define problems in health care and recommend methods for enlarging the scope of nursing practice. The report categorized nursing practice in three broad areas: primary care, acute care, and long-term care. Primary care encompassed the individual's initial contact in any given episode of illness with the health care system leading to decisive action, and the responsibility for continuation of care, including health maintenance, evaluation, and management of symptoms and referrals (72).

Another development was the introduction of health maintenance organizations (HMOs), which were created through Congressional legislation to replace the regional medical programs of the late 1960s. Under HMOs, comprehensive services were offered for a per capita fee. Organized nursing supported the HMO plan, which included such services as primary care, emergency care, acute inpatient and outpatient care, and rehabilitation for chronic and disabling conditions (73).

In the nursing profession, a corps of clinical specialists demonstrated skills far beyond the reach of the average nurse. New clinical specialty organizations proliferated quickly and tended to fragment nursing care even further (74). Another group consisting of a small number of deans and directors of college and university nursing schools banded together after breaking away from the NLN Council of

Baccalaureate and Higher Degree Programs. They established their own organization on May 26, 1969, later called the American Association of Colleges of Nursing (75). The following month, Ruth Kelly shared this news with the faculty after attending a meeting of NLN's Council of Baccalaureate and Higher Degree Programs in Nursing (76).

The 1970s proved to be a fertile time in the nursing education arena. In academia, the growing number of health professions and increasing enrollments stimulated a trend toward the clustering of pre-professional and professional programs in health science centers within universities. On the organizational front, the NLN intensified its interest in health care legislation and in 1971 the Council of Baccalaureate and Higher Degree Programs prepared a position paper on national health insurance. Earlier, the NLN had adopted a statement endorsing the "open curriculum" in nursing education, a new concept that took into account the different purposes of the various types of nursing program but recognized common areas of achievement. The system permitted student mobility according to ability, and changing career goals and aspirations (77).

In the fall of 1971, the Government Relations Department of the American Nurses Association announced that appropriations expected under the forthcoming Nurse Training Act would fall far below the budget requested—disturbing news to nursing school deans (78). Whereas $78,000,000 had been proposed in the original request for nursing capitation grants, only $31,500,000 was appropriated (79). After reviewing copies of the Act, Dean Eleanor Lambertsen highlighted its provisions and shared them with Hugh Luckey (80). She explained with some dismay that the funds were earmarked for a three-year period, but it was not possible to know the nature of federal support for undergraduate programs.

Lambertsen's concern was predictable, having been fully apprised of the School's financial status prior to accepting the deanship. At the time, the Board of Governors assured her of the program's economic viability under the joint agreement with Cornell University and the existing pattern of cost containment (81). Nevertheless, she found the arrangement with the Hospital troubling. "We are the only collegiate program in the country totally financed through this mechanism and tuition and other fees from students," she told the Governors (82).

Early in her administration, Lambertson began to examine critically the nature and structural relationship of the School of Nursing within the complex administrative organization of a private university and voluntary hospital (83). In addition to the major problem of how the School related directly or indirectly to the financial bases of support, she was greatly disturbed by the social and professional isolation of the faculty as well as the inadequacy of educational resources and facilities (84).

Eleanor Lambertsen was introduced to students in the School of Nursing at the senior convocation in 1970 when she spoke on the extended role of nurses. In her view, there were two distinct groups of nursing personnel, with clearly defined areas of practice for the future. She referred to nurses capable of developing innovative patterns of patient care while others practiced within the framework of the existing structure (85).

At a meeting with the faculty in September of that year, she shared information about the School's enrollment. Among the 270 students there were 259 females and 11 males, with 53% from New York State. The group included 11 African American and two Asian students (86).

From the outset, Lambertsen discovered that the majority of the faculty did not understand the existing organizational relationships, and at their request she eventually prepared a comprehensive statement on the governance of the School of Nursing (87). She began her review with historical background, highlighting the 1927 agreement between Cornell University and The New York Hospital, and the establishment of the Joint Administrative Board to conduct the therapeutic and educational work of the two institutions under the title of The New York Hospital-Cornell Medical Center (88). She described the roles and titles of the various administrative officials of the Medical Center, including Dr. Hugh Luckey, president and chief executive. He also served as vice president of medical and nursing affairs and vice president for medical affairs of Cornell University. In the late 1960s, the complexity of the task had led to the appointment of Dr. Robert Buchanan, dean of the Medical College, as assistant vice president of the Medical Center (89).

While defining her philosophy and assumptions about academic governance, Lambertsen stated that the combined position of dean and professor represented a blend of administration and scholarship. She perceived the dean's role to be one of curriculum leadership, responsible for long-range planning as well as safeguarding the quality of the educational program (90). "The primary aim of the dean must rest with the school in its entirety rather than with one particular phase of the program or institution or with isolated groups of faculty or students," she asserted (91). As for the faculty, she explained that their primary responsibility was in curriculum development, subject matter and method of instruction, research, faculty status, and those aspects of student life relating to the education process (92). Student participation, she noted, had to be ensured within a framework of attainable effectiveness.

In concluding her statement on governance, Lamberten shared with the faculty her reasons for accepting the position of dean. "It was largely the milieu conducive to the study of the potential of nursing practice in the multidisciplinary health service and science setting. I have had positive evidence of this in all of my associations since being appointed" (93). She added that her interest lay in exploring mechanisms that fostered the continuing development of a center for education, experimentation, and research in nursing (94).

During her first year, the Executive Faculty Committee was disbanded and replaced by an Administrative Advisory Committee to the dean "to receive, devise, conduct, discuss, and recommend proposals for the administrative conduct of the school" (95). Another change suggested by the faculty was that all standing committees include nursing students elected or appointed by the Student Senate. The members also proposed releasing course chairmen from their clinical supervision of students, but Lambertsen pointed out that this would not be possible because of budgetary restrictions (96).

When Luckey addressed the nursing faculty on November 23, 1970, he presented the long-range plan for the Medical Center and cited housing for nursing and medical personnel as being high on the list of priorities (97). It would take four years to complete construction of a new student residence, the Jacob S. Lasdon House on 430 East 70th Street (98).

Lasdon was a well-known industrialist and supporter of the arts and sciences. His generous gift had special meaning for the School of Nursing dating back to 1967 when The New York Hospital submitted a proposal to the Lasdon Foundation requesting a contribution to support the expansion of the nursing program (99). At the time, Jacob Lasdon and his brother William had been involved in firming up their plans for philanthropy, and indicated an interest in nursing with the possibility of a $5,000,000 gift to the endowment (100). Expectations loomed high among the nursing community, but for whatever reason or influences, the School's hopes soon dissipated when the Lasdons turned their sights toward other needs of the Medical Center.

In recent years, the nursing students had been living in deteriorating quarters, while complaints for improvement echoed widely. An accompanying problem was the inadequate space for operating the School, located in the same facility. A residence committee was formed to explore the matter along with an architectural survey, which concluded that renovation would be impractical and unable to meet modern standards. The solution appeared to lie in constructing a new building for the students to be separate from the educational plant. In April 1970, Patricia Long, chairman of the residence committee, informed Jeffrey Hill, president of the Student Senate, about the results of an opinion poll about the housing needs of the nursing students. It revealed that the majority favored an apartment-like residence (101).

On July 31, 1974, the dedication of the Jacob S. Lasdon House took place with a host of dignitaries present to celebrate the occasion. The speakers included the mayor of New York City and officials of Cornell University and The New York Hospital-Cornell Medical Center. Lambertsen participated in the observances along with the Hospital director and deans of the Medical College and the Graduate School of Medical Sciences (102).

The project cost nearly $11,000,000 for the building and almost $4,000,000 for the land. The 15-story tower contained 236 furnished apartments ranging from studios to two bedrooms (103). Accommodations were available to married students and couples with children, who had become an increasing visible segment of the student population (104). For the first time at the Medical Center, students from the various disciplines were going to be housed under the same roof, generating a promise of hope that the new arrangement would encourage more informal interchange and broaden the educational experience.

CHAPTER 13

The 1970s: The Decisive Years

In December 1970, Eleanor Lambertsen informed the faculty about a critical report of the Joseph Musio case that appeared in the winter issue of the *AAUP Bulletin* (1). The seriousness of the matter was reopened and intensified when Dorothy Ozimek, secretary of the NLN Board of Review of Baccalaureate and Higher Degree programs, wrote to the dean that the article had attracted the attention of League staff and a number of concerned nursing educators. She pointed out that if the allegations were accurate, then the School could be in violation of certain accreditation criteria (2). In response, Lambertsen sent Ozimek background materials relative to the case while refuting the AAUP's charges. She claimed that it could not be determined whether the decision to terminate Musio's services had been based on "considerations violative of his academic freedom," and elaborated as follows:

> The Faculty and Administration of the School of Nursing are assuming that the Board [NLN] is concerned with policies and procedures rather than upon attempting to reconstruct conflicting evidence in the chronology of events of interpretation of the circumstances of the termination of Professor Musio's services (3).

Aware that the next accreditation visit would be coming up in another year, Lambertsen clarified the issue in subsequent discussions. She had no desire to jeopardize the status of the School. Work had already begun on revising the grievance appeal procedure by adapting the Cornell University model (4). At a meeting on June 30, 1972, the

189

Faculty Council approved the statement, describing a grievance as "an injustice or harm arising from a specific situation involving an act or acts of unfairness. A grievance concerns only matters which have actually occurred" (5). A few months later, the members concurred with the dean on developing a method to handle faculty grievances and outlined an appeals procedure to be used in cases of individual grievances (6). They requested that advice be sought from officials at the University regarding the appropriate process (7).

In her letter of April 11, 1975, to Martin Lapidus, AAUP director and secretary, Eleanor Lambertsen reported the progress of the faculty committee in revising the grievance procedure (8). She assured him that in the event of terminating a faculty member with more than seven years of service, the School would conform to the principles espoused by the University (9). Furthermore, the information would be included in the School's annually revised *Educational and Administration Policy Manual*. According to a policy enunciated by the AAUP, a faculty member must be notified one year in advance of the decision not to reappoint (10).

Early in her administration, Lambertsen had expectations of developing continuing education programs in primary care, a concept that she passionately supported. Her hopes were realized when a tripartite contract was awarded to the School of Nursing, Cornell Medical College, and the Visiting Nurse Service of New York (11). In 1971, the PRIMEX Program was launched with Doris Schwartz, associate professor of nursing, and Frederic Kirkhein, M.D. as codirectors. Funded by the Health Services and Mental Health Administration, U.S. Department of Health, Education, and Welfare, the project aimed to train registered professional nurses as family nurse practitioners (FNPs), to complement the care given by physicians in ambulatory clinics and community settings (12). The FNPs would be expected to assume the principal responsibility for the primary health care of individuals and families, as well as supportive care for the elderly and those with chronic health problems (13).

The program required one semester or 18 weeks of intensive theory and clinical practice followed by seven and a half months of supervised work or internship in the employing agency, and a certificate awarded on completion (14). In December 1971, Lambertsen notified Muriel Carbery, whom she recently appointed the associate dean of continuing education, that the course was scheduled to begin the following February (15). In her report for the 1971–1972 academic year, she hailed the establishment of the Division of Continuing Education at the Medical Center as "a model of collaborative and collegial relationships of personnel with the three constituent units" (16).

The School of Nursing, the Medical College, and The New York Hospital initiated another program on primary care in 1972. A grant from the Health Services Administration provided for the training of registered professional nurses as pediatric nurse associates (PNAs) to serve in child health stations operated by New York City and the U.S. Public Health Service. "Ours was the first pediatric nurse program in a big city and the first to be a joint enterprise between a medical center and a public health agency," declared Dean Lambertsen (17). The project required public health nurses to spend four months in classes, followed by an eight-month internship in the stations or clinics before receiving their certificate. In May 1972, the first graduating class of 15 PNAs completed the program (18).

With her extensive experience in nursing service as well as in education, Lambertsen encouraged collaborative relationships in the practice setting with the medical community. In addition to the continuing education programs on primary care, several offerings evolved jointly among the School of Nursing, the Medical College, and the Hospital. Unless supported by grants, the programs became self-supporting through tuition fees from the participants. The Premature Institute Program continued to function well under the direction of a physician and Alice DonDero, head of the pediatric department and professor of clinical practice (19).

Another interdisciplinary undertaking was the Coronary Care Nurse Training Program coordinated by Muriel Carbery and a physician colleague, and assisted by Professor Nina Argondizzo from the School of Nursing. The Graduate Nurse and Technician Training Program for Hemodialysis, cosponsored with the nursing service staff of the Department of Surgery, was also instituted (20).

Lambertsen held strong convictions about the importance of continuing education for nurses. In her view, the department heads in nursing service should be faculty members with responsibility for program development and evaluation. "The primary function is the education of the *practicing nurse*," she asserted in a comprehensive document for the Board of Governors on long-range planning for the School (21). In the section on continuing education, she stated that it was an area in which department heads and clinical specialists could make a distinctive contribution. Also, the full-time faculty should have the option of teaching selected continuing education courses.

Lambertsen's position on the future of a graduate program in nursing became apparent in the early stages of her tenure. She believed that the purpose of master's degree education was to prepare graduate nurses for specialization in a particular field of nursing. The baccalaureate program, she emphasized, aimed to educate the nurse for beginning professional practice as a generalist (22). Although this view was widely held by most deans in collegiate programs, some nursing educators began to consider other patterns. For example, in 1962 the New York Medical College introduced an extremely innovative nursing program with Frances Reiter as the dean. Her vision involved the recruitment of non-nursing graduates of liberal arts colleges to prepare for a two-year master's degree program in nursing without being required to earn another baccalaureate (23).

Planning was also in progress at Yale University for another entry-level master's program designed for college graduates with a non-nursing major. Expected to open in 1973, the program was designed to prepare nursing students to become clinical specialists or nurse practitioners by the end of three years without offering a bachelor's degree. Both schools of nursing at the New York Medical College and Yale initiated a second master's program in clinical specialization for registered nurses with previous baccalaureate preparation (24).

With her knowledge and contacts, Eleanor Lambertsen surely must have been familiar with these nontraditional programs, but there were no indications as to whether she had considered moving in that direction in the near future, especially since the School of Nursing was already operating a baccalaureate program for college graduates. The possibility of changing the focus of this group to a generic master's program seemed unlikely since she believed that generalist preparation culminated in a baccalaureate degree (25). Although greatly interested in developing a graduate nursing program for clinical specialists, she pointed out the impracticality of pursuing such an undertaking at that time without proper resources. Planning would have to be delayed until faculty with doctorates were recruited and financial support assured (26).

At a meeting on October 10, 1972, the faculty concluded that the Faculty Council had not served them effectively and should be dissolved (27). They pointed out that the grievance procedure replaced any duties previously described and a 15-minute open discussion period during a faculty meeting could replace the Council's function as a forum (28). An ad hoc committee was formed with Jean Kijek as chairman, to explore methods of communication among and between the faculty-at-large (29).

During their deliberations, the new group cited the importance of finding a mechanism for dealing with small problems difficult to resolve but not requiring consultation with the grievance committee. Before disbanding, the committee recommended that the nursing faculty (1) examine their role outside the School, which would include dialogue and sharing with the Medical College on a formal level; (2) establish a regular in-service program to further growth and development; and (3) schedule a faculty meeting in January 1973 to discuss the curriculum and plans underway for the spring semester (30).

Following a successful site visit in the fall of 1971, the NLN Board of Review granted continuing accreditation to the baccalaureate programs of the School of Nursing (31). Presiding at the November 21 meeting, Louise Hazeltine, the new associate dean, shared with members the preliminary report of the accreditation visitors, including their recommendations. Among the strengths identified were the number and qualifications of the faculty, the excellent library resources, the potential for interdisciplinary experiences, and the effective use of clinical agencies (32). The following January, Hazeltine informed the faculty that Cornell's President Dale Corson had received NLN's approval and recommendations of the Board of Review:

- continue support of faculty and students in efforts toward full participation in matters which effect progress in meeting the School's objectives;
- continue joint planning of faculty with students and peers to develop a systematic approach to evaluation of teaching effectiveness;
- suggest faculty continue to clarify and develop the philosophy, purposes, objectives, and conceptual framework, and the revised statement in the curriculum design; and
- suggest faculty further delineate expected behavioral objec-

tives which differentiate between levels of achievement
during the program, and utilize these as part of an overall
plan to systematically evaluate the effectiveness of the curriculum in relation to students as graduates (33).

To follow through on some of the areas cited, Lambertsen
appointed a committee of faculty and students to develop, adapt, or
accept an instrument for faculty evaluation by students (34). During
the next few years, work was completed on tools for self and peer evaluation and for course chairmen to evaluate the performance of faculty
(35). Another undertaking involved independent study to be initiated
as a pilot project with 20 students. The dean also announced that a
joint committee of faculty and students in the School of Nursing and
their counterparts from the Department of Public Health of the
Medical College, would be appointed in the near future to develop a
proposal for interdisciplinary study and practice in the area of community health (36).

Despite ongoing efforts and those projected for the future,
Lambertsen experienced an uneasiness about the nursing program's
financial support. In his annual report to the Governors, David
Thompson commented on the persisting financial difficulties. "This
war of attrition against the viability of The New York Hospital comes
from many sources—from legislative actions, third party insurers, and
from well meaning but short sighted community groups," he soberly
recounted (37). Although Eleanor Lambertsen became increasingly
concerned about the Hospital director's observations, the Board of
Governors continued to reassure her about the School of Nursing's economic viability. Nevertheless, she viewed the situation to be a major
problem and stated that "it can be predicted that there will be a change
in policy and the practice of reimbursement by third party payers for
the educational costs of the School" (38).

On June 20, 1973, David Thompson presented a proposal to the
Executive Committee of the Board of Governors that would have a
marked impact on the future direction of nursing at the Medical
Center. He believed that organization changes indicated a realignment
of administrative responsibilities. "The Nursing Service leadership will

need to be more intimately involved in the practice and teaching of nursing," he explained and called for a parallel relationship of nursing and medical practice and a more compatible framework for medical and nursing services (39).

Thompson urged greater participation in staff education as well as the enhancement of the medical-nursing dyad in specialty practice occurring in both disciplines. His impression of Eleanor Lambertsen's harmonious relationship with the medical staff, and the effective educational programs developed for staff nurses had prompted him to recommend her for the appointment of associate director of The New York Hospital for Nursing Service (40).

The announcement meant a return to the dual administrative pattern, which would be accompanied by increased responsibilities in program planning and budgetary matters (41). In September 1973, the Governors enthusiastically endorsed her expanded position to begin the following July, and stated that in the new arrangement she would report to the Medical Board on all nursing policies affecting the treatment of patients (42).

The changing administration of the Division of Nursing at The New York Hospital coincided with the retirement of Muriel Carbery, who had spent 40 years in the service of the institution. Addressing the Governors, Thompson characterized her as a person who "won the esteem of all at the Hospital for her advancement of nursing as a career, and for the expertise and personal warmth which she brought to the practice of the profession" (43). Until the time she retired at the end of the year, Carbery agreed to assume the task of collecting and updating the School's archival material. In the spring of 1974, the Alumnae Association selected her to be the first recipient of the distinguished alumnus award, citing her "outstanding leadership and achievement at the local, national, and international level" (44).

Lambertsen's perception of the dual administrative role represented an interface of nursing service and academic programs within the Medical Center. "Its value is constantly reflected in responsive programs of education and research," she asserted. "More significantly, nursing faculty and students are constantly exposed to problems of health care delivery and the social and economic environment of health care" (45). She stressed that her work required building a strong and energetic support staff capable of horizontal as well as vertical problem solving. "Delegation must be perceived as a practical force rather than abdication of responsibility by the chief administrative officer for nursing to others in the hierarchy" (46).

By the mid-1970s, the dean had acquired the new title of senior hospital director, and an administrative team in nursing service consisting of Joanna Foster as executive assistant director of nursing, Edna Danielson, assistant director of staff education, seven clinical department heads, and a director of the psychiatric nursing administrative division (47). In the School of Nursing, the dean's management team included Louise Hazeltine as her associate, Gloria Wilson, the assistant dean, and two administrative assistants (48). Among the 51 faculty members, all were nurses except for three that included psychologist, Dr. Lee Salk, who conducted a seminar on the humanistic approach to life (49).

With her added responsibilities as senior hospital director, Lambertsen devoted considerable time to reorganizing the Hospital's nursing services. She merited high praise from Stanley de J. Osborne, president of the Board of Governors, who stated that she had brought "a whole new standard of managerial excellence to our institution" (50). In redefining the role of the clinical department heads, she was determined to change their focus from an institutional service orientation to a patient care service orientation (51). Under her leadership, a nursing council and a head nurse advisory committee were formed during 1975 (52). As a decision-making body in the Division of Nursing, the nursing council coordinated the activities and general policies of the various clinical departments as well as with other constituent units and departments of the Medical Center. In addition to proposing objectives and programs, it acted for the staff as a whole and monitored the reports and activities of the Division's committees. Consisting of assistant directors of nursing service and clinical nursing department heads, the nursing council met weekly with Lambertsen as chairman (53).

The dean also met bimonthly with the Head Nurse Advisory Committee, which operated as an official channel of communication within the Division. Each clinical nursing department elected two representatives to serve as members, who discussed policies relating to the provision of patient-care services. The committee was also responsible for developing a program of continuing education for head nurses (54).

Lambertsen encouraged the instructional staff and staff nurses to present papers and publish them, attend meetings and conventions of nursing organizations, and participate in a variety of other professional activities (55). As a relentless advocate of doctoral education, her hopes met with some success when several of her master's-prepared faculty pursued more formal study, mostly on a part-time basis. The number increased from three with earned doctorates during the 1972–1973 academic year to six in 1974 (56). When invited to a Medical College Retreat, she asked Nina Argondizzo, who recently became assistant dean, to accompany her (57).

In 1976, Lambertsen supported the appointment of faculty member Jeanne Dorie to a subcommittee to develop examinations for the newly established New York State Regents External Degree Program (58). A nontraditional approach to nursing education, the program was designed for graduates of associate degree and hospital diploma programs who wanted to earn a baccalaureate in nursing. Characterized as a university without walls, a growing concept in education, the instruction was self-paced by the individual and did not take place in the classroom (59).

The School of Nursing claimed a cadre of faculty with impressive backgrounds. Among them was Eleanor Herrmann who not only had taught at the Universities of Wyoming, Syracuse, and Colorado, but also had considerable international experience. Before joining the Cornell faculty, the same year that Lambertsen began her deanship, Herrmann had served as a consultant for Project Hope in Ecuador and for the Pan American Health Organization in Belize, and spent two years in Guatemala working with the Behrhorst Clinic in Chimaltenango, which cared for hundreds of Mayan Indians (60).

When a major earthquake struck Guatemala on February 4, 1976, Herrmann and her husband, an attorney and former field program director for the Pan American Development Foundation, initiated a major fund-raising project to secure supplies, medicine, food, and equipment for the devastated population (61). "The terror is mounting," Eleanor wrote to her colleagues at the School and graphically described the plight of the survivors (62). A videotaped interview about the catastrophe was shown on the television program "Straight Talk." The dean and faculty members expressed their sentiments with donations for the victims (63). Through a sustained international fund-raising effort, the Herrmanns continued their support of the rebuilding efforts as members of the Board of Directors of the Behrhorst Clinic Foundation (64).

During Lambertsen's administration, the relocation of the school became a prime concern after the students were settled in their new living quarters at the Lasdon House. In June 1974, the Medical Center's Development Committee presented a progress report on their efforts to explore space requirements and site operations (65). The following March, the Governors announced that arrangements were underway to renovate the "S" Building on East 71st Street between York Avenue and the East River (66). By the end of the summer, occupancy was anticipated along with the admission of students for the fall semester.

The first two floors of the air-conditioned building were designed for learning activities and contained a multimedia laboratory and convertible classrooms, which could be subdivided by sound-proof screens to create three rooms to accommodate 20 students each. A six-bed laboratory enabled the students to practice nursing skills and simulated hospital facilities. The 10th floor had been reconstructed to house administrative and faculty offices (67).

For some time, Lambertsen considered introducing a baccalaureate program for graduate nurses with associate degrees and diplomas from hospital schools. The idea had been brewing since the late 1960s when the School unsuccessfully sought grant funding from the Division of Nursing, U.S. Public Health Service. With the increasing number of inquiries reaching the dean, she was eager to move ahead in launching the registered nurse-baccalaureate program. In 1973, Eleanor Herrmann, secretary of the faculty, reported that at the June meeting the question of admitting RN nursing students was thoroughly discussed. Although some adverse reaction occurred, most of the faculty decided to support the completion program and endorsed the principle of offering advanced standing at the undergraduate level by use of college proficiency examinations (68).

While plans proceeded with the RN-baccalaureate program, enrollment in the other two undergraduate programs continued to grow, reaching 121 and representing the highest number to date (69). On August 28, 1973, the faculty suggested that a questionnaire be distributed to graduate nurses employed by the Hospital's Division of

Nursing to elicit their interest in enrolling in the upcoming program to acquire a baccalaureate degree (70). It seemed reasonable to open admissions to qualified nurse employees at the Medical Center and enroll them in courses offered to the other students.

As a work-study program, the graduate nurse student could continue as a staff nurse part time and be eligible for tuition benefits and fringe benefits (71). One important aspect of the new undertaking was the effect on clinical nurse specialists and the increasing number of dual appointments required. They would be expected to apportion their time to guide the clinical study of the seasoned graduate nurse student with a highly individualized approach (72).

In the fall of 1974, representatives of the New York State Education Department visited the School to clarify and supplement materials submitted for the re-registration of the program for college graduates as well as approval of the RN-BSN Program (73). Program I, which had enrolled students with 60 complete credits of general education, admitted its last class and would be phased out in two years (74). During their site visit, the evaluators conferred with Lambertsen, Hazeltine, and Hospital and University officials. They also met with nursing faculty and observed the clinical experience of the third- and fourth-year students (75).

In individual interviews with students who were college graduates, a number of critical issues surfaced that revealed a general lack of satisfaction with classroom instruction in the nursing courses (76). The major problem areas included a lack of the faculty's ability in classroom teaching, and inadequate information about the master's degree program for those who wanted to pursue graduate study. In contrast, the students expressed positive feelings about the biological courses and faculty instruction (77).

Following the visit, the report prepared by Mildred Schmidt, executive secretary of the New York State Board of Nurse Examiners, was shared in June 1975 with Lambertsen, Dr. Luckey, and President Corson (78). Directed toward the faculty, the main recommendations included: (1) institute an in-service plan to improve teaching methods and skills to be implemented; (2) establish a mechanism to promote informal exchange of views with students so that potential conflicts can be determined and resolved; and (3) critically evaluate the structure of the curriculum to delineate the concepts, subconcepts, and theoretical formulation contained in the philosophy and implemented in the courses (79).

The observations of the site visitors created some consternation when Lambertsen distributed the report to the faculty. She requested specific information from them to be used in her rebuttal (80). Although disappointed in some of the comments expressed by the visitors, she welcomed their support of the re-registration of the program for college graduates, and the granting of interim registration to the proposed baccalaureate program for registered nurses, scheduled to begin in September (81).

In the spring of 1975, David Thompson reported that The New York Hospital, like other teaching hospitals, was faced with a freeze on reimbursement rates from Blue Cross and Medicare, which together provided half of the institution's income. "The freeze reduced our projected income for 1976 by over five million dollars," he explained. "Not only will we be restricted in what we can build but what services we can provide" (82). Earlier in the year, Lambertsen had apprised the faculty of the deteriorating financial situation and noted that it was "a time of holding action" at the School. She urged them to use resources in new and different ways and to demonstrate their creative skills. "Our school must be one of scholarly professionals" (83).

The changes in Medicare and Blue Cross regulations affecting hospital reimbursement for educational purposes had serious repercussions for the School of Nursing. When a provider furnished financial support to an approved nursing program that was not the legal operation, its contribution could not be included in the hospital's allowable costs for Medicare reimbursement purposes (84).

Despite the financial crisis that appeared to be building, the Governors expressed a guarded optimism during 1976 about conditions at the Hospital, which President Osborne attributed to the cooperation of all professional and administrative units, and the heads of the clinical departments and disease centers (85). He also acknowledged the income derived from endowments and generous donors as well as the annual contributions of devoted friends (86).

In June 1976, a perinatal center opened in the new neonatal intensive-care unit, followed by the establishment of a comprehensive burn center that would become one of the most famous in the nation (87). A $510,000 award from the National Institutes of Health (NIH) to the Medical Center's Division of Infectious Diseases provided for the study of bacterial organisms related to sexually transmitted diseases (88). Another NIH grant, totaling $8,500,000 and earmarked for the Clinical Research program, aimed to maintain research beds for the study of patients with various health problems such as diabetes, hypertension, Parkinson's disease, and endocrine disorders (89).

When Thompson asked Lambertsen in May 1976 to review the steps taken by the School regarding its financial problems, she informed him that the faculty was aware of the situation (90). She further stressed the commitment to honor faculty contracts and student admissions through the 1978 academic year (91). On October 10, she notified the Governors that the School was exercising every precaution to maintain continuing eligibility for reimbursement and "we must give serious thought to finding ways to assure the future financial integrity of the School of Nursing" (92).

According to the dean, it was necessary to reduce the number of students seeking admission to the School. Of the 243 qualified candidates, a total of 119 college graduates and 15 registered nurses students were accepted in the 1976 fall class (93). Lambertsen pointed out that requests for financial aid had increased markedly, but assistance remained uncertain in light of the withdrawal of governmental and foundation monies due to cost containment. On the brighter side, Lambertsen announced that for the first time, eight nursing students were nominated and appointed to membership in *Who's Who in American Universities and Colleges* (94).

On May 11, 1976, when President Corson addressed the Executive Committee of the Board of Trustees, he expressed his concern about the precarious financial status of the nursing program. "There is the possibility that new regulatory guidelines issued by HEW will preclude The New York Hospital from including costs of the School of Nursing in the Hospital's expense budget, which is the basis for third party reimbursement" (95). Corson pointed out that the annual operating budget for the School amounted to approximately $1,300,000 and that the faculty had been notified of a one-year appointment through June 30, 1977 (96).

In the coming months, the financial condition of the Medical Center began to show signs of worsening, with many programs in jeopardy. The Hospital suffered significant deficits created by unsatisfactory reimbursement policies of third-party agencies, further compounded by rigid controls, inadequate repayment, and other factors (97). At the national and state levels, problems intensified, with the withdrawal of funds for research, federal wage and price controls, inadequate staffing needed to handle new and complex medical and surgical treatments, and the absence of a national health program (98).

On May 26, 1976, the Medical Center introduced a new initiative when it launched a fund-raising campaign known as the Third Century Fund, co-chaired by Hugh Luckey and Mrs. Vincent de Roulet, vice president of the Board of Governors. Setting a goal of $260,000,000 to be reached over the next 10 years, the drive was designed to acquire funds targeted to programs for expanding and improving patient-care research, and medical and nursing education (99).

From the beginning, the Third Century Fund received wide visibility, boosted by coverage in *The New York Times* that described the undertaking as "an outstanding demonstration of the role volunteerism can play in breathing new life and vigor into New York City" (100). The campaign took off in a spirit of great cooperation with $27,000,000 already received toward the first phase of the program. Within the provisions of the Fund, a total of $5,000,000 was to be allocated toward program support and a $15,000,000 endowment for the School of Nursing (101).

Outside of the annual giving fund of the School's Alumni Association, which produced modest contributions, the Endowment Fund, initiated almost 20 years earlier, seemed to have reached a plateau at $330,774.29 with minimal change occurring since the summer of 1970 (102). Thus, the present need for achieving the goal seemed more critical than ever. The time was approaching for decisions at the highest level of Cornell University, that would have a serious impact on the future of the School of Nursing.

CHAPTER 14

A Noble Ending: Hail and Farewell

In the spring of 1977, hundreds of congratulatory letters and telegrams poured into the office of Dean Eleanor Lambertsen, honoring the 100th Anniversary of the founding of the School of Nursing that proclaimed the theme, "A Century of Excellence in Nursing Education." Stanley de J. Osborne, president of the Society of The New York Hospital, presented a resolution stating that the Governors saluted the achievements of present and past faculties and staff, students, and alumni practicing throughout the medical world (1).

In his address given at the Church of the Epiphany in New York City, President Dale Corson expressed the pride of Cornell University's Trustees in the educational and service accomplishments of the School of Nursing (2). He quoted from a letter written in 1867 by Ezra Cornell to his young granddaughter, in which the founder shared his vision of making university education available to women on a basis equal to men. Cornell had stated his hope that she would attend the university (to open a year later) and lead the life of service that he visualized for all the graduates (3). To preserve the memorabilia of the Centennial, the Medical College Alumni Association contributed a gift of $500 (4).

Writing from St. Petersburg, Florida, Anna Wolf, former director of the School, expressed her regrets for not being able to attend the festivities and "join colleagues in manifesting their just pride and deep satisfaction in the prestigious accomplishments of the School to the many services of its graduates" (5). Another letter, sent to the Alumni Association, came from Virginia Dunbar, who expected to be in Switzerland at the time of the celebration. Although several years had passed since she spearheaded the Endowment Fund, Dunbar continued to follow its progress. "We need to speak up for the nursing school without the least feeling of begging," she wrote, "Tell the story and keep on telling it because we are rendering a wonderful service" (6). In closing, she added that the nursing school was very much on her mind and in her heart.

Prior to the annual meeting on May 7, the Alumni Association paid tribute to Muriel Carbery, professor emerita, in a brief ceremony unveiling her portrait. The painting would be added to the display of former directors and deans of the School (7). Among the 600 people attending the Centennial, over 350 had graduated from the School. Lambertsen spoke at the Convocation, highlighting the future of health care and the challenges for nurses. She noted that the most significant advances had occurred as a result of the efforts of nurses to define knowledge, judgment, values, and skills required for safe, efficient, and therapeutically effective nursing care services (8). During the celebration, alumni and guests attended programs on national health policy, health care, and nursing education, toured the Medical Center, and visited exhibits in the library.

The event concluded with a gala evening at the St. Regis Hotel that began with a toast by Ezra Cornell III, Cornell trustee, followed by a message sent from President Jimmy Carter praising the School's 100-year commitment to the highest standard of nursing education in our country. Featured as dinner speaker was Dr. Eileen Jacobi, dean of the School of Nursing, University of Texas at El Paso and former executive director of the American Nurses Association. She addressed the topic, "Health Care-Nursing Care: Patients and Challenge" (9).

A spirit of marked optimism accompanied the nostalgia of the Centennial with its focus on the School's achievements over the decades. If there were doubts about the future of the nursing programs, they were muted, avoided, or discussed privately. The School's financial picture could not have been a surprise to the faculty and students because they had been apprised earlier of the situation. Like the dean, they remained hopeful of a favorable outcome.

On May 23, 1977, a few days before her visit to Ithaca where she anticipated a successful meeting with the Board of Trustees, Lambertsen shared with the faculty the findings of a study commissioned by Corson to explore the feasibility of alternative programs for the School of Nursing. Three options emerged from the study committee's findings: (1) continue the present program, (2) terminate the program, or (3) consider the possibility of a graduate program (10).

The committee had concluded that priority should be placed on the third option, and recommended a "three-year degree program for college graduates leading to the preparation of primary nurse practitioners for ambulatory care settings and clinical specialists for acute and long-term care in institutional settings" (11). During an ensuing faculty meeting, the dean discussed her proposal for a master's program, developed as a continuum of education from beginning or general preparation in nursing to specialized education at the graduate level. She pointed out that the clinical and educational milieu of The New York Hospital, and the availability of other health care resources from an urban social environment would provide unusual opportunities for the study of nursing practice roles.

When Lambertsen met with Cornell's Board of Trustees on May 29, 1977, her hopes were crushed by their unexpected announcement to terminate the School of Nursing on June 30, 1979 (12). Although they based their rationale largely on financial considerations, the Trustees believed that there were many other sound baccalaureate nursing programs operating in public institutions in New York State. Furthermore, undergraduate nursing education was not a high-priority program at a leading university like Cornell, which favored nursing preparation at an advanced level (13). The Trustees suggested that faculty, students, and staff of the School, as well students admitted to the September class, be informed of the Board's action before June 30. They indicated their support for maintaining and expanding continuing education programs in nursing (14).

When Lambertsen presented the Trustees with her proposal for a three-year master's program based on the recent deliberations of Corson's committee, they endorsed the concept but could not make a commitment in light of existing financial pressures (15). The members added, however, that because of the obvious high quality of the proposed graduate program, it would be prudent to permit Cornell's incoming president, Frank Rhodes, to evaluate the University's academic priority in relation to the many needs and limited funds (16).

Despite previous warnings of the School's possible closing, the faculty expressed anger and resentment on hearing the news (17). When Corson met with them on June 7, he stated that the Trustees had recommended that a master's program be considered in the future if funding could be assured. He also lauded Lambertsen, "who had conducted herself with remarkable fine dignity during this most distressing time for so many people" (18). During the next few weeks, Lambertsen was busy sending letters to faculty, returning and incoming students, and regulatory agencies, notifying them of the School's status.

At a meeting on June 24, the faculty elected an ad hoc committee to serve as a channel of communication with the dean for the purpose of securing benefits for them and developing strategies "to save our school" (19). The action demonstrated a strong resistance to accepting the decision of the Trustees to terminate the baccalaureate programs. Some faculty suggested contacting the New York State Nurses Association, but Lambertsen cautioned that any attempt to initiate collective bargaining would be inappropriate (20). She informed faculty members who had signed up for the 1977–1978 school year that prior to their vacation they could expect contracts to be offered for the academic period through June 1979. She also pointed out that 13 highly qualified faculty had requested to be released from their present contracts. Student admissions for the 1977 fall term, however, seemed to be holding up, with 100 applicants accepted (21).

In a letter sent later that month to the alumni about the School's pending dissolution, she stated that student admissions for college graduates would be discontinued after September 1977. Also, the following September was set as the final date to enter registered nurse students (22). When mentioning her proposal for a master's degree program, she declared that graduate education had been one of the School's planning goals since 1970 (23).

The dean's letter stunned many of the alumni who were not cognizant of the School's deteriorating financial situation. Some of the graduates seemed to know very little about the baccalaureate programs, or that The New York Hospital had been funding the School since its inception in 1877 (24). On July 1, 1977, Jeanne Dorie, president of the Alumni Association, sent identical letters to President Osborne and Robert Purcell, chairman of Cornell's Board of Trustees, in which she expressed the concern of members:

> The Alumni must consider making an effort to save the School.... We believe that to do less would be a betrayal of all who have gone before us in our illustrious one hundred year his-

tory.... Would you support an organized effort of the alumni to seek an endowment? (25)

Osborne responded by alluding to the Third Century Fund in progress and the proposed endowment. "We will of course continue to support the fund raising efforts for the School of Nursing if the decision is made to establish the master's program" (26). Purcell's letter of August 5 noted the following: "Personally, I am very unhappy about the school of nursing situation and will be overjoyed if an endowment fund were suddenly to appear. Before committing to a drive, we would like to be confident that it will have a reasonable chance of success" (27).

When writing to the nursing alumni earlier that summer, Dorie emphasized the need to participate in a campaign for the endowment. She urged their support for what would require "an enormous effort requiring energy and time" (28). Lambertsen subsequently reported on the numerous comments received from alumni as well as faculty, students, medical staff, and other interested individuals. "Their attempts," she pointed out, "are directed primarily toward securing an expression of intent of priority of effort in fundraising for an endowment for the School of Nursing for immediate sources of funds" (29).

News about the pending termination of the School spread rapidly throughout the Medical Center. The dean informed the faculty of an article to appear in a forthcoming issue of *The Cornell Alumni News* that presented an historical review of the nursing program and the events leading up to its closing (30). She also mentioned her intention to invite junior nursing students to attend the September 6 meeting as observers when Frank Rhodes, the new president of Cornell, was expected to address the faculty. After distributing copies of the proposal for a master's program, she was encouraged when hearing a number of favorable comments (31).

Reporting to the Board of Governors in the summer of 1977, President Osborne characterized the closing of the undergraduate nursing program as "one of the unhappiest duties of the Hospital and Cornell University. . . . Every avenue was explored in seeking a solution that might have obviated the decision to end the 100-year program" (32). He added that Frank Rhodes was planning to appoint an ad hoc committee to study the matter. In an exchange of correspondence with Rhodes, Lambertsen suggested that he consider inviting Dr. Mary K.

Mullane, a distinguished nursing leader, to serve on the committee (33).

Toward the end of August, Lambertsen requested a commitment from the faculty to the proposed master's program. "This is not the time to vacillate and ask for a return to the baccalaureate program. The faculty must be unified," she asserted (34). She noted that both the New York State Education Department and the National League for Nursing (NLN) had been apprised of the decision to terminate the programs. The NLN accreditation visit scheduled for the fall would be cancelled, but approval of the continuing education program was granted through 1979 (35).

When the faculty met with Rhodes, they raised several questions about the future of the School (36). He stated that plans were in progress to appoint an ad hoc committee to review the feasibility of developing a master's level program in nursing (37). In late September, the committee was formed with Dr. Alison Casarett, associate dean of the graduate school of Cornell University, serving as chairperson. Other members included Dr. Carolyn Davis, a nurse and associate vice president for academic affairs, University of Michigan; Dr. Mary K. Mullane, executive director, American Association of Colleges of Nursing; and Dr. Raymond Handlin, director of development, Cornell University. Associate Dean Louise Hazeltine of the School and Associate Dean James Curtis of the Medical College served as executive liaison to the committee (38).

At the outset, Rhodes defined the charge to the group and set forth three requirements for a master's program to be acceptable: "(1) There must be a clearly demonstrated need for graduates of this program; (2) it must be a program of professional and intellectual distinction that can be validated, and demonstrated that Cornell can offer a distinguished program; and (3) the program must be self-supporting. New funds must be found to cover the existing expenses" (39).

On November 11, 1977, Eleanor Lambertsen wrote to Dr. Dorothy Ozimek, director of the Department of Baccalaureate and Higher Degree Programs at the NLN, updating her on developments at the School (40). She pointed out that by the following March the faculty would have to indicate whether they intended to leave or retain their appointments. Louise Hazeltine had announced her willingness to remain for an additional two years or longer (41). On December 15, associate professors Marjorie Miller, Deanna Pearlmutter, Reva Rubenstein, and Doris Schwartz issued a statement to the ad hoc committee expressing strong support for a program offering a master's degree in nursing to students with a baccalaureate degree in another discipline. They urged that closer ties be established on the University's Ithaca campus, stating the following:

> We should consider the possibility of nursing students studying in Ithaca for a semester of class work, and that of faculty from Ithaca lecturing in New York City. Conversely, the use of nursing and medical faculty should be considered for special classes, conferences, and seminars on the Ithaca campus (42).

While the ad hoc committee proceeded with its task, the Society of The New York Hospital and Cornell University amended the historic agreement of 1927 that led to the establishment of the Joint Administrative Board (43). During 1977, a five-member committee consisting of Cornell's Trustees and the Hospital's Governors conducted an in-depth study to evaluate the relationship of the Medical College to its two-parent organization involving activities, costs, and needs (44). As a result, the function of the Joint Board was shifted from an administrative body to an advisory and coordinating capacity. In the new arrangement, formalized in October, the Joint Board of The New York Hospital-Cornell Medical Center consisted of four representatives each of the Governors and Trustees, charged to promote the development of the enterprise and public affairs (45).

In March 1978, Eleanor Lambertsen notified the faculty that she had conferred with Margaret Walsh, general director of the NLN, about job opportunities for them in baccalaureate programs. Walsh had offered assistance in locating positions and suggested that the instructional staff meet with Dorothy Ozimek (46). In addition to her frequent communications to NLN officials, the dean mentioned that she intended to write to selective collegiate nursing program and incorporate summary statements with biographical information supplied by the faculty (47).

At a meeting on April 17, Lambertsen announced that Dr. William Herbster, senior vice president of Cornell University, indicated

interest in receiving the curriculum vitae of the faculty if they wanted
to be considered for other academic appointments when the undergraduate program closed (48). She also shared the good news that for
the first time 100% of the 1977 graduating class had passed the state
board examination (49).

Later that month, Chairperson Alison Casarett wrote to
Lambertsen, informing her that the ad hoc committee had completed
its work and the report would be distributed shortly (50). In the meantime, she enclosed a summary of the committee's recommendations:

- An academically sound innovative master's level program
  can be established at Cornell University to provide individuals who have bachelor's degrees in nursing with additional skills and orientation needed for them to serve efficient-
  ly as primary care practitioners in rural or inner-city communities.
- Such a program can be accomplished best on the Ithaca
  campus based in the College of Human Ecology.
- The program should include campus-based education for
  approximately three semesters and a one-semester
  practicum at appropriate off-campus clinical sites. Total
  program time should be two academic years with a summer. About 20 students would be accepted each year.
- On-campus education should include a core curriculum of
  graduate nursing courses to be taught and/or coordinated
  by a core nursing staff. A thesis based on research at the
  clinical site would lead to a master of science degree.
- Funding for program planning and development should
  be requested from the U.S. Department of Health,
  Education, and Welfare under the Nurse Training Act,
  foundations, and individual donors. The State University
  of New York and Budget Office of the State of New York
  should be asked to provide "core" support. The program is
  particularly appropriate in view of the land-grant mission
  of Cornell University (51).

During their exploration, members of the ad hoc committee met
individually and collectively with various experts in education and
health care. They believed that basing the proposed program on the
Ithaca campus was an appropriate setting for the study of primary care

in a rural environment (52). Also, the high quality and diversity of graduate courses and other educational opportunities, as well as a flexible philosophy of graduate education, tended to encourage individual initiative and the intellectual growth of students. Another advantage was the variety of primary care services in New York's Tompkins County (53).

The ad hoc committee urged that a special effort be undertaken to attract many students from metropolitan areas who were concerned with inner-city community health problems. The New York Hospital-Cornell Medical Center represented a potential site although it focused more on tertiary care. In pursuing the possibility of a graduate nursing program, the committee estimated that a period of 18 months to two years would be needed for the initial planning phase, fund raising, and discussions with officials of the New York State Department of Education before firming up a decision to move forward (54).

On May 22, 1978, when Lambertsen distributed copies of the ad hoc committee's report to the faculty, several members raised questions about areas requiring clarification. It was obvious that a dramatic change had occurred in the original proposal from a three-year entry-level master's program for non-nursing college graduates to a two-year program designed for registered nurses with a baccalaureate degree. The concerns of the faculty included the proposed program's organizational relationship to the College of Human Ecology; the core curriculum; the rationale for reducing the length to two years and the practicum to only one semester; and a perceived limited definition of primary care and the nurse practitioner (55).

In early June at the Medical Center, the faculty shared with President Rhodes and Dr. Casarett a series of questions prepared in advance (56). Later that month when Dean Lambertsen asked for an endorsement of the revised proposal for a master's program in the College of Human Ecology, only one faculty member dissented (57).

During the summer, Dr. Evelyn Gioiella, president of the School's Alumni Association, wrote to Rhodes expressing the organization's support of the graduate nursing program. "We are eager to assist the efforts being made to move into a new period for nursing at Cornell. We are willing to serve as a resource of people" (58). In his response to her, Rhodes appeared delighted, but noted that it might be a while before any formal reply would be forthcoming because of the arrival of Dr. Jerome Ziegler, the new dean of the College of Human Ecology (59). It was not until late October that Rhodes informed Lambertsen that he intended to ask Casarett to arrange a meeting with Ziegler and faculty representatives from the School of Nursing (60).

While discussions were in progress regarding the master's degree program, nursing students at the School were preoccupied with planning for what would be the last graduating class. They indicated a desire to close on a positive note by featuring some type of program in the period between examinations and graduation (61). The Alumni Association's Board of Directors readily supported the students and invited them to participate in Alumni Day activities. They suggested a two-day program to be planned by a steering committee that would involve faculty participation (62).

Accompanied by a few faculty members, Lambertsen went to Ithaca on February 12, 1979, to meet with Rhodes and representatives from the College of Human Ecology (63). The session was apparently productive because a month later Rhodes asked Ziegler to form a special committee to consider the role of the College in the health field (64). Under the direction of Phil Schoggen, chairman of Health Programs, Human and Family Studies, the committee members made some compelling observations. They emphasized that it was essential to conceive of the health field in broad terms that extended beyond traditional medical and nursing practice that focused on pathology (65).

In the view of the Special Health Programs Committee, the growth of the concept of holistic health had made more central the roles of nutritional, environmental, social, and behavioral sciences in the definition of the health services. The limited role of the College of Human Ecology was also pointed out . The members called upon the College to consider exploring the possibility of developing a Master of Public Health Program, particularly since Columbia University offered the only other such program in the State (66). They supported the recommendations of the Casarett committee and suggested that the University immediately appoint a task force, headed by a staff professional, to conduct a study to determine the feasibility of a high-quality nurse practitioner program within the College of Human Ecology. Curriculum, cost, funding source, and the availability and location of clinical sites would all have to be investigated (67).

When Lambertsen met with the Executive Committee of the Board of Governors in April, she spoke of the approaching closure of the nursing program, and the responsibility of the Hospital to continue to participate in affiliations with other schools of nursing. She believed that the recruitment of nurses graduating from these programs had to be considered for future staffing of the clinical departments. Lambertsen reminded the Governors that after June 30, a major source of graduates of the Cornell University-New York Hospital School of Nursing would be lost (68).

That same month she received encouraging news that Rhodes had authorized the sum of $45,000 to conduct the proposed feasibility study and college-wide planning to be undertaken by a task force chaired by Betty Lewis, associate dean for research and graduate education in the College of Human Ecology (69). In a follow-up letter to Ziegler, Rhodes asked him to keep Lambertsen informed of the latest developments (70). Ziegler had already pointed out that a well-developed plan would require about a year of work before presenting it for faculty approval. He cautioned that unless funding could be assured, it was doubtful that the mood of the faculty would permit them to vote positively for a new program on health (71). "At the same time, there was considerable support within the faculty for new initiatives," Ziegler declared. "While it is certainly too early to predict, I am reasonably confident of a favorable outcome" (72).

As far back as January 1942, the Joint Administrative Board of The New York Hospital-Cornell Medical Center stipulated that if the time ever came when a surplus of funds existed in the School of Nursing, the monies should revert to the general funds of the Society (73). In 1977, the disposition of the funds became an extremely relevant issue with the pending termination of the School. On July 6 of that year, Eleanor Lambertsen sent a statement to William Herbster that listed the names of donors and the amount contributed to the Endowment Fund as well as funds targeted for special purposes (74). Over the decades, the official records had been maintained by staff in the Hospital's financial office. The dean mentioned that David Thompson, director of the Hospital, had requested a review of the documents by the secretary of the Society and Thomas Martin of the law firm Kelley, Drye, and Warren (75).

On March 27, 1979, Lambertsen wrote to Martin concerning his progress on the matter. "We need to come to some conclusion," she asserted while raising important questions: "Are the funds designated for scholarships for students applicable to the proposed master's program of Cornell University on the Ithaca campus? If we were to organize as a New York Hospital School of Continuing Education, could the endowment funds be diverted? And how are these funds invested?" (76).

In April, she received an extensive fact sheet prepared by Gregory S. Meredith, explaining that the funds had always been received, administered, and invested by the Hospital, which turned over the income from the investment directly to the School (77). The document noted that the monies were separated into two groups consisting of (1) the Endowment Fund, donated for the purpose of operating the School, and (2) the Scholarship Fund for nursing students. Of the $650,192 principal amount, $385,737 fell into the Endowment Fund category and $265,055 was allotted for scholarships (78).

As to the ownership of the funds, Meredith's fact sheet concluded that The New York Hospital and not Cornell University was the corporation that fit the description cited in Section 513 of the New York Not-for-Profit Law. He emphasized that the Board of Governors had established the School's Endowment Fund, with all gifts made to the Hospital. It seemed probable, therefore, that the Endowment monies would be absorbed by the institution's general funds (79). Also to be resolved was the issue concerning the disbursement of gifts to the Scholarship Fund sponsored by the Alumni Association. For years, the members had campaigned to secure financial aid for the education of nursing students (80).

With the weeks drawing closer to graduation on May 23, the School of Nursing presented a symposium early in the month organized by the students (81). Addressing the large assembly, President Rhodes expressed high hopes of having a master's degree program for training nurse practitioners to take place within a proposed program on health education in the College of Human Ecology (82). At the faculty meeting on May 14, Lambertsen announced that Louise Hazeltine and the assistant administrator agreed to remain on staff for two years to work on students' loans and records, as well as those of the faculty (83). She also mentioned the upcoming visit of Dean Ziegler to the Medical Center to confer with her and Hazeltine, Dean Theodore

Cooper of the Medical College, and Dr. George Reader, head of the Department of Public Health (84).

It turned out to be a bittersweet occasion when the School of Nursing graduated its 103rd class in a combined commencement with Cornell University Medical College, held at the Alice Tully Hall in Lincoln Center. A total of 104 nurses received their baccalaureate degree, which brought the total number of graduates to 4,377 since the first commencement exercises of The New York Hospital Training School for Nurses in 1878 (85). In addition to the keynote address by Dr. Joseph Lederberg of Rockefeller University, words of high praise for the School came from many dignitaries, including Governor Hugh Carey of New York and President Jimmy Carter (86). Commenting on her long tenure as dean, Lambertsen spoke of the "great sadness that today's commencement marked the ending of the School" (87). The trend in the future, she noted, would be for nurses to seek higher levels of education to prepare themselves to meet society's health demands. In an attempt to assuage some of the existing resentment, President Frank Rhodes urged the graduates to let the School's proud role live on through them (88).

A month following the graduation, Lambertsen received a letter from Rhodes that lifted her spirits. "I have been especially proud of the way you have continued to provide magnificent leadership during the two troubled and difficult years," he wrote. "I count it a privilege to have worked with you and I shall look forward to staying in close touch" (89). Rhodes added that he intended to seek her advice in moving forward on the proposed master's program in the College of Human Ecology. After June 30, she would no longer hold the title of dean, but her position as senior associate director of the Hospital and head of the Division of Nursing seemed secure. Lambertsen also was accorded the rank of professor of nursing in the Department of Medicine, Cornell University Medical College, and professor emerita of Cornell University (90).

In the fall of 1979, Lambertsen requested approval from President Rhodes to establish a school of continuing education for nurses (91). She explained that the school would become a constituent of The New York Hospital's Division of Nursing, and as such, the institution would assume full financial support (92). As the chief administrator, her status would be comparable to that of the clinical nursing heads of the individual departments, while management of the day-to-day operations would be delegated to Louise Hazeltine (93). Within a few months, The New York Hospital-Cornell Medical Center School of Continuing Education in Nursing became a reality when approved by the Society's Board of Governors (94). The action proved beneficial to the Alumni Association when a ruling by the Attorney General of New York State authorized the transfer of the monies in the Scholarship Fund for Annual Giving to the new school of continuing education (95).

During the early stages of developing continuing education policies and procedures, another major effort had been underway for some months. In October 1979, Rhodes commissioned a study "to further assess the possibility of a master's degree program in nursing in the College of Human Ecology" (96). Three previous investigations had supported the concept of such a program, but certain areas required more in-depth exploration before proceeding with the implementation phase. Facilitated through Betty Lewis, the new feasibility study was conducted by Fran A'Hern Smith, a doctorally prepared nurse as project consultant (97).

During three intensive months of research, Smith investigated the nature of other nursing programs in Ithaca and surrounding areas, evaluated the availability of local agencies and institutions as resources for clinical experiences, obtained data on potential funding, and identified legislation that affected nursing (98). In her survey of registered nurses in the region, she found that the highest priority was given to a master's degree program with a rural health specialization that had a provision for a nurse practitioner option (99).

The study also explored the question of funding for a new graduate program and yielded some sobering observations. With the expiration of federal health legislation anticipated on September 30, 1980, no clear indication existed about the allocation of funds. When conferring with Dr. A. Norman Haffner, associate chancellor for health sciences, State University of New York (SUNY), Smith learned that there would be no funding for new programs that year because of recent cutbacks in the State University's budget (100).

From the information collected for the feasibility study, the focus of the proposed graduate program shifted entirely to rural health nursing with an option for functional roles in administration, teaching, or nurse practitioner certification (101). In recommending this approach, Smith explained that only one other program of this nature existed in the country and that Cornell's interdisciplinary resources and strengths would allow for the development of a truly innovative program. She believed that educating nurses to work in sparsely populated areas would generate contributions to the theory of nursing practice and rural health delivery systems (102).

The study's recommendations soon became moot. Continuing to support a master's degree nursing program at the College, Dean Ziegler presented the case before officials of the State Education Department and SUNY's budget office in Albany (103). His efforts to seek funding, however, proved unsuccessful because available monies had already been targeted to several other nursing education programs operating under the SUNY system. Another setback was the lack of start-up funds through the Nurse Training Act without assurance of continuing support from the State (104).

The news shattered the hopes of the nursing community of The New York Hospital and Cornell University, which had endured a troubling decade and the closing of a school of nursing with a glorious history. Despite that fateful happening, hopes had remained reasonably high for the establishment of a new program on the Ithaca campus. Although deeply affected by the loss of the School and the outcome of the proposed graduate program, Lambertsen set her sights for the next few years on strengthening nursing services. To carry on that goal, Helen Van Shea succeeded her on January 11, 1982, as senior associate director for nursing at the Hospital (105). A former vice president for nursing at St. Luke's-Roosevelt Hospital Center, Shea assumed the responsibility of directing a staff of 1600 and administering the continuing education program and seven clinical nursing departments.

Until her retirement in 1983, Lambertsen served as special assistant to Dr. David Thompson, director of The New York Hospital. During that period, she was lauded for her contributions at a number of receptions at the Medical Center. On January 5, 1982, the Division of Nursing hosted an open house for nursing personnel and friends. Two days later at a formal event, the Board of Governors and Medical Board presented her with a "captain's chair" as a token of their appreciation (106). On the occasion of her retirement, June 23, 1983, a symposium was held, in which Dale Corson, president emeritus of Cornell University, offered some telling comments:

> The decision to close the school was not Eleanor's doing, and she had no responsibility whatever for that decision. . . . However that made life difficult for her particularly in her relationship with faculty. She organized the closing of the school effectively, protected the interests of the students, and to the best of her ability, she protected the interests of the faculty and she did it all with dignity (107).

Commentary: The Legacy Lives

A century of excellence in nursing education remains the pervasive theme in the history of the Cornell University-New York Hospital School of Nursing. Before the end of the 19th century, training schools for nurses in America were founded in an era when modern nursing practice had its origins in reform movements for the improvement of the care of the sick and disabled in hospitals. The Society of The New York Hospital had a long record of service and prominent physicians who recognized the need to establish a school of nursing with a corps of young women superior to those usually employed in public institutions.

From the outset, the Board of Governors indicated their desire to select a limited number of candidates meeting a high standard of education and eager to devote themselves to the specialty of nursing with proper preparation. The Governors had no problem meeting their goal, but they admitted to the first class only a small number of the caliber they were seeking. The pupil nurses represented a homogenous group, having grown up in affluent homes, attended schools beyond secondary education, and worked as teachers or in some other responsible employment capacity. Most of them entered the nursing program in their twenties and showed some level of maturity as well as certainty about the career they chose to pursue.

Unquestionably, there must have been a uniqueness about these young women of privilege who decided to become nurses at a time when other attractive opportunities began to open up for women in colleges and universities. Whether or not prospective students were aware of the regimented, restrictive lifestyle awaiting them, the major-

219

ity completed the program. Despite the hardships, the experience fostered a spirit of camaraderie and collegiality that often lasted for years.

During the School's nascent period, the letters of candidates clearly revealed their motivations for entering the nursing program. In most cases, there appeared to be a universal desire to serve humanity, accompanied by a need for self-fulfillment. The drive toward economic independence was also a strong factor. As daughters of physicians with exposure to certain aspects of the medical world, some of the women had opted for a career in medicine as their first choice but reconsidered and turned to nursing. Years later, Julia Stimson, a 1908 graduate, declared that she had intended to become a doctor but changed her mind and never regretted it. Mentored as a student by the great Annie Goodrich, Stimson herself emerged in time as one of the profession's outstanding leaders.

While expressing a genuine interest in caring for patients, some of the pupil nurses may have harbored a desire, consciously or otherwise, to meet and eventually marry a doctor. Apparently, such an expectation was not unrealistic because a third of the Training School's graduates followed this pattern, settled into married life, and no longer practiced nursing. It was significant that an unusually large number of future leaders, who strove valiantly to advance the profession and participated in efforts relating to the health concerns of the larger society, had never married.

From the School's inception, many of the graduates were in the forefront of the modern nursing movement and nurtured its development in the ensuing years. Irene Sutliffe, class of 1880, deserved much credit for her role, not only as the fifth directress of the program but also for her involvement in the work of the alumni association and the newly founded national nursing organizations. Her classmate, Clara Weeks, was appointed the first superintendent of nurses at New Jersey's Paterson General Hospital, and a few years later was the first nurse to write a nursing textbook in America. Another alumna, Nora Livingston, class of 1889, opened the first training school for nurses in the province of Québec at Montreal General Hospital. An 1890 graduate, Katherine Sanborn, received high honors for her 40 years of service as superintendent of nurses at St. Vincent's Hospital in New York.

After graduating in 1893, Anna Duncan accepted a post as the first nurse employed in a department store. Her work was followed by the first textbook on industrial nursing written by Lydia E. Anderson, class of 1897, an excellent teacher and a wise and understanding faculty member. Although a number of the School's alumni journeyed to different parts of the country to establish schools of nursing, others took the overseas route to set up and administer new nursing programs. In 1922, Caroline Robinson, a 1908 graduate, organized a training school in Albania under the auspices of the American Red Cross. That same year, Marion Doane, class of 1913, established a nursing school in Port au Prince, Haiti, where she was honored with that nation's medal of honor.

The nursing program had prepared an illustrious group of nurses who shared their expertise, nationwide and internationally, to raise education standards and enrich the quality of people's lives through improved patient-care services. In the annals of American nursing, graduates Annie Warburton Goodrich and Lillian Wald became legendary. As contemporaries and close colleagues, they had practiced nursing, taught students, and administered programs while becoming prime movers in stimulating the collective action of nurses in professional activities. Charismatic, cultured, and independent, Annie Goodrich, class of 1892, was the foremost leader of her time in nursing education, in which she introduced many reforms. Her appointment as the first dean of the Yale University School of Nursing in 1923 probably represented the zenith of her distinguished career.

As the founder of public health nursing, Lillian Wald, an 1891 graduate, established a corps of dedicated Henry Street nurses whose work evolved into the Visiting Nurse Service of New York. Through her influence, the The New York Hospital Training School for Nurses introduced the first course on public health nursing and employed the first public health nursing instructor. A dynamic, caring person, Wald was concerned with many of the social ills affecting people as well as their need for better health care, and she participated in progressive movements to improve conditions.

The heads of the Training School, whose administrative style set the climate for the nursing program, were undoubtedly an important influence in the development of the pupil nurses. Irene Sutliffe assumed her post as directress in 1886 and began a 16-year tenure that profoundly affected the future direction of the school. Like her predecessors, she was also responsible for nursing services in the Hospital.

Sutliffe continued the tradition of recruiting highly desirable candidates and became an exemplary role model to them. Beloved by the pupil nurses, colleagues, and the alumni, she was greatly respected by the Hospital hierarchy. The poignancy of letters from graduates of the School, postmarked from countries around the world, reflected their enduring admiration of Sutliffe and the impact that she had on their lives.

Early on, Sutliffe recognized the need to strengthen and extend the length of the nursing course, and successfully challenged the medical staff who wanted to increase the service experience of the pupil nurses in lieu of more theoretical content. Although the doctors encouraged the long hours in the patient-care setting, they empathized with the rest deprivation of the students as well as their cramped living quarters. In addition to authorizing a new residence for the nurses, the Governors often acceded to Sutliffe's wishes, recognizing her ability to enhance the reputation of the School. Furthermore, her loyalty and long devotion to the Hospital could never be doubted, as demonstrated by her various activities even after retiring.

When Annie Warburton Goodrich took over the administrative reins in 1902 with the title of superintendent, she had every expectation of gaining the support of the Hospital's officials. Although markedly different in temperament from Sutliffe, she shared similar values and convictions and quickly won over the pupil nurses with her vibrant personality, wit, and passion to enforce high standards. It was a new century of scientific discovery and a changing health care scene, which required innovations in nursing education and patient care. Goodrich brought an international perspective to the program that emanated from her childhood schooling in Europe as well as her contacts abroad. It wasn't surprising that from 1912 to 1915 she served as president of the International Council of Nurses.

At the beginning of her tenure at The New York Hospital, Goodrich succeeded in instituting a series of changes until she sensed a gradual undermining of her authority by the Medical Board. As an astute observer, she recognized the futility of convincing them to continue forward-looking policies to strengthen the School. In 1907, she resigned but not before accepting a position as the general superintendent of the training school at Bellevue and Allied Hospitals. Although many of her reforms were abolished soon after leaving The New York Hospital, she left her mark, and, in the view of the students whom she mentored, Annie Goodrich "had made it a school."

Many of the women who graduated from the School of Nursing could point to their wartime military service as their finest hour. The heroic efforts of such nurses as Anne Williamson in the Spanish-American War, Julia Stimson in World War I, and Marie Troup in World War II come to life in their diaries, correspondence, and other forms of communication. When the United States declared war on Spain on April 25, 1898, Williamson was one of the first to report to the Red Cross Auxiliary along with 40 other volunteers from The New York Hospital who offered their services in Cuba, Puerto Rico, and the Philippines.

Williamson was one of the pioneers in army nursing. During World War I, she worked to maintain an adequate nursing supply at home while organizing nursing service units in the army and navy. In her seventies at the onset of World War II, she never lost her patriotic fervor and maintained it by assisting nurses in preparing for emergency services in her community. From 1908 to 1925, she served as director of the California Hospital in Los Angeles, followed by 30 more years as director of social service.

When World War I seemed imminent, The New York Hospital mobilized a contingent of physicians and nurses in preparation for pending service. Four months after the United States entered the war on April 7, 1917, medical officers, nurses, a chaplain, and enlisted personnel set sail for France. From St. Louis where she held a dual administrative position, Julia Stimson accepted the formidable task of directing nursing services overseas, functioning as a liaison officer between the Army Nurse Corps and the Red Cross. Endowed with superb executive ability and a strong commitment to action, she successfully supervised nursing services provided by more than 10,000 nurses.

Stimson's humanity became evident in the numerous letters to her mother in which she shared her feelings about the conduct of the war and the courage shown by the young men sent to the front. She provided a fascinating account, interspersed with a touch of humor, of her resourcefulness in arranging the transfer of her wounded brother Phillip, a medical officer, from a hospital in Flanders to her headquarters in Rouen where she could look after him.

By the end of the war, Stimson had received several citations and awards for her outstanding military service that were followed by other honors in the years to come. In 1920, when an Act of Congress granted relative rank to the Army Nurse Corps, she became the first woman accorded the title of major by virtue of her position as superintendent of the corps. Twenty-seven years later, army nurses achieved full commissioned rank. From 1919 to 1933, Julia Stimson succeeded Annie Goodrich as the second dean of the Army School of Nursing.

In the decade following World War I, a cultural revolution erupted that affected all aspects of American life. Minnie Jordan, the nursing directress of The New York Hospital Training School for Nurses, commented on the changing behavioral characteristics of the student population, who seemed more outspoken and eager for professional advancement. The Hospital was in the forefront of medical and scientific innovation, introducing such dramatic discoveries as the test for early detection of cervical cancer by Dr. George Papanicolaou, and the work of Dr. Harold Wolff, the father of psychoanalytic medicine and the first full-time academic neurologist in the country.

In the patient-care environment, graduate nurses were employed in the private pavilion to add to the needed complement of staff, while the less seasoned students worked in the wards on an eight-hour-a-day or -night schedule. The affiliations of pupil nurses increased at other institutions, including the Henry Street Visiting Nurse Service, the Manhattan Maternity and Dispensary, and the Maternity Center Association. Conversely, Julia Stimson arranged to have a number of her students in the Army School of Nursing affiliate at The New York Hospital.

The establishment of The New York Hospital-Cornell Medical Center in 1927 represented a pivotal time for the School of Nursing because the seeds were planted in the joint agreement for forming a new and different type of educational program. In a few years, the term "training" would disappear from the School's name and the School would shed many of the trappings of the traditional hospital program. The reality of a collegiate program, however, would be long in coming, partly due to the inability to obtain an endowment during the years of the Great Depression. Despite the disturbing economic picture, it did not stop the Medical Center from forging ahead with ambitious programs that involved mergers or cooperative relationships with other hospitals.

In 1931 when Chairman Mary Beard and the Committee on Nursing Organization recommended Anna Dryden Wolf to be the first director of the School of Nursing and nursing services at the new Medical Center, they selected the right person at the right time in the right place. Born in India of Lutheran missionary parents, Wolf acquired a *Weltanschauung* early in life that defined her as a caring and brilliant leader. From the beginning of her appointment, she had a clear vision of how nursing could fit into the changing system.

A graduate of Goucher College in Baltimore before entering the nursing program at Johns Hopkins, Wolf held strong views about liberal arts education for nursing students and ensured that such values were incorporated into the curriculum. She encouraged the development of a democratic student organization and initiated separate student exchange arrangements with Temple University and Cornell University. Because of her stature in the nursing profession, as well as the reputation of the School of Nursing, she had no problem attracting an exceptionally able faculty. Despite a severe nursing shortage during the Depression years, she strengthened nursing services by coordinating the activities of all clinical departments in the Hospital.

Wolf's knowledge and diplomatic skills merited her considerable admiration from the hospital and university community. She formed excellent working relationships with Canby Robinson, director of the Joint Administrative Board, the Board of Governors, and Presidents Farrand and Day of Cornell, who supported her expectations of placing the School on a collegiate basis within the University system. Movement toward this goal proved to be tedious and discouraging because of opposition from the executive faculty of the Medical College. By the time the physicians relented and endorsed the baccalaureate program in nursing, Wolf had resigned her position after nine years to return to Hopkins to administer its school of nursing and nursing services. Her efforts, however, had laid the groundwork for the establishment of the Cornell University-New York Hospital School of Nursing in the summer of 1942.

When America's entry into World War II was declared in December 1941, The New York Hospital had already released a large number of medical and nursing personnel for military service. Members of the Ninth General Hospital Base Unit had prepared for this eventuality and geared up for active duty. Marie Troup, the chief nurse, and her unit were shipped to the South Pacific in the summer of 1943. In correspondence with Bessie Parker, interim director of the School, as well as with some of the Governors, Troup, a 1926 graduate, described the Spartan conditions faced by the unit. On the home front, the Hospital had assumed the lead in developing emergency measures as the District Hospital Control Center in Manhattan to promote stability and maintain a safe and protective environment for the patients. The Governors put a system in place that involved the use of emergency field units and evacuation plans.

Soon after the war ended, the Committee on Deanship, following a lengthy search, announced its success in finding a highly desirable candidate. When Virginia Matthews Dunbar accepted the appointment, her administration began a new era in the history of the School of Nursing. She had traveled in many of the same professional circles as her friend Anna Wolf, and like her predecessor studied nursing at the Johns Hopkins Hospital after graduating from Mount Holyoke College. A year after assuming the position, she began an extremely productive working relationship with Dr. Stanhope Bayne-Jones, the director of the Joint Administrative Board. During the next few years, the collegiality that they shared made it possible for Dunbar to initiate many of her forward-looking ideas.

An internationalist, educator, and recent director of the American Red Cross Nursing Services, she began her new role by implementing the directive of Cornell's President Day to admit only students with two years of previous college preparation. Dunbar promoted closer relationships between faculty and students, involved the entire faculty in policy-making decisions, and encouraged faculty and student involvement in research. In addition to meeting with other deans on the Ithaca campus, she spoke before Cornell women's groups and encouraged the annual visits of the nursing students to the University.

During her tenure, some of the faculty began experimenting with dual appointments, but in the early 1950s as her own work intensified, Dunbar agreed with Bayne-Jones that it would be more advantageous to relinquish her post as director of nursing service to Muriel Carbery. As a result, she became the School's first full-time dean, an action that seemed to please the students and faculty. Mary Millar, a student at the time, shared a poignant recollection:

Miss Dunbar inspired awe. . . . She was lofty, by which I mean
that she seemed to be someone you did not approach with triv-
ial matters. She was always kind, and I believe had a genuine
affection for students. She had a quiet confidence, a conviction
that nurses had a great contribution to make.

Virginia Dunbar's passion to seek funding for the School never
waned because she recognized that the survival of the program
depended on it becoming independent. At that time, the Hospital continued to finance the total cost of the nursing program. In 1952, with
the support of the Alumnae Association and Bayne-Jones, she spearheaded an Endowment Fund with the goal of $8,000,000, which grew
to $138,000 in six years. When she retired in 1958, Dunbar had con-
verted the School into one of true university status.

When Muriel Carbery succeeded her as dean, it proved to be a
difficult act to follow. Carbery came to her new position at a time when
the School was at a high point, with excellent faculty, bright young students with college preparation, and a Medical Center with ongoing
innovations in the clinical environment. Her decision to return to the
dual position was not surprising because Carbery's main interest and
top priority had always been nursing service. Although opposed by the
faculty, she believed that nursing students should spend more time in
the clinical area for the purpose of giving service beyond the planned
learning experience.

Carbery's administrative skills in the patient-care setting could
not be matched as attested to by the Governors and the nursing and
medical nursing staff. She strengthened the nursing departments by
employing clinical nurse specialists and supporting their efforts in creating new patterns of patient care. Carbery was well liked by the staff
nurses, who appreciated her frequent evening rounds on the units to
confer with them and visit the patients. In light of her strong commitment to nursing service, she delegated the daily operations of the
School to Veronica Lyons, who continued in her role as associate dean
and was given a fair amount of authority in dealing with education
concerns. To what extent the dean shared with her associate the financial arrangement with the Hospital is not known, but Carbery was well
informed of the School's status because she attended all the meetings

of hospital administration on budgetary matters. She also tended to zealously guard the nursing education budget.

Most of the School's progress was made by the faculty, particularly in areas of curriculum revision and evaluation, and in introducing an experimental baccalaureate program for non-nursing college graduates, a truly notable achievement at the time. As industrious as the faculty were, however, they lacked the direction of a strong, visible leader. Dissension in the ranks was already apparent when Ruth Kelly became associate dean on the retirement of Lyons.

Many of the faculty expressed frustration when the dual role in nursing service was discontinued after 1964. There was also dissatisfaction with the lack of uniformity in academic appointments. Another issue related to the complaints of nursing department heads that their involvement with nursing students was being undermined by the action of course chairmen to assume total responsibility for clinical assignments. With Kelly as her ally, Carbery tried to pacify the faculty and resolve the situation but her attempts proved ineffective. Despite her experience and expertise in the educational arena, Kelly was a polarizing figure whose abrasive, autocratic manner alienated the faculty further.

During the 1960s, two unique opportunities arose that held promise for ensuring the longevity of the School of Nursing. An endowment fund and the momentum needed to sustain it through whatever means were available had been established. The passage of the federal Nurse Training Act of 1964 and the Fund for Medical Progress of the Society of The New York Hospital seemed to hold the key to a stable future for the nursing program. Whether the School could meet the challenge that lay ahead would depend largely upon the vision and ingenuity of an energized leadership.

The Nurse Training Act authorized $283 million over a five-year period to fund nursing schools, traineeships to graduate nurses, student loans, and construction grants. When Carbery shared the provisions of the legislation with the faculty, she encouraged them to suggest projects that would enhance the quality of the nursing program. With the availability of federal traineeships, it seemed reasonable to assume that the master's prepared faculty would take advantage of the opportunity for full-time doctoral study to increase their knowledge and maintain the excellent image of the nursing program.

As to whether the School followed through on applications for government project grants under the Nurse Training Act, the evidence appeared to be sparse. Did this mean that no proposals were prepared or submitted? Or were they submitted and rejected? Was there a lack of faculty interest, inertia, or a preoccupation with too heavy a workload and other activities? Was it possible that the faculty, or even the dean, could not see the long-term benefit of securing grants for creative undertakings that would increase the School's visibility and make it more attractive to seek funds from other sources? Certainly, the development of exciting new projects would have highlighted the value of the nursing program and served as a stepping-stone to obtaining a substantial endowment from a prospective donor.

Another issue was related to the reluctance of the faculty to apply for federal traineeships. There was no record of individuals taking leaves of absence to advance their credentials, while faculty from other schools flocked to institutions of higher education under the traineeship program. The situation began to change when Dr. Eleanor Lambertsen became dean in 1970 because of her determination to increase the complement of faculty with earned doctorates.

In 1961, the Society of The New York Hospital initiated the Fund for Medical Progress and earmarked a $10,000,000 goal for the School's endowment. President Perkins of Cornell University and some of the Governors presented opportunities to Carbery to meet with interested donors, but in a number of cases she either failed to submit acceptable proposals or pursue requests for further information. A conference with a representative of the Kellogg Foundation looked promising, but the dean's inordinate delay in responding and then submitting a limited presentation ended any possibility of funding from that source. In another case, when an endowed professorship seemed possible, she did not prepare the requested proposal.

It is difficult to understand Carbery's response, or lack thereof, to the opportunities provided to her in pursuing an endowment. Perhaps she simply did not have the knowledge or conceptual ability to frame an appropriate appeal. Or, she may not have realized the urgency of the matter since the Governors reassured her of the Society's continuing financial support. Another factor was her relationship to the Hospital as the consummate insider, who had come up the ranks and in a sense became a favorite of the hierarchy.

It was possible that Carbery may have been too inbred in the system, which gave her a limited perspective as well as a certain amount of comfort in maintaining the status quo. In any case, the School's endowment did not assume the highest priority. It was an unfortunate miscalculation because the fund-raising campaigns of the University and the Society of The New York Hospital yielded little support to the School of Nursing.

By the time Eleanor Lambertsen came to the School in July 1970, some of the best opportunities for securing a desperately needed endowment may have come and gone. How informed she was on her predecessor's involvement in the fund-raising efforts and the ensuing failures is not known. On resuming the role of a full-time dean for the next few years, she asked Carbery to continue in nursing service and appointed Louise Hazeltine as assistant to the dean. An able and loyal colleague, Hazeltine worked well with Lambertsen and was greatly respected by the faculty.

After examining the structural and organizational relationships of the School within the Medical Center complex, Lambertsen established an ambitious agenda for the nursing program. From the outset, she identified her goals as promoting nursing research by the faculty, urging them to pursue doctoral education, strengthening joint continuing education offerings with the Medical College, and introducing a baccalaureate program for registered nurses. As a long-term aim, she envisioned the development of a graduate program for clinical specialization.

At the time of Lambertsen's appointment, a climate of optimism permeated the academic community because of her sterling reputation in the health professions and vast experience in both nursing education and organized nursing service. Before long, however, faculty tensions began to surface, created by the new dean's rather blunt, doctrinaire manner and an attitude that sometimes bordered on the dismissive. A common complaint was that when developing a plan and policies for the program, she did not elicit the faculty's ideas or reactions in advance, and thus the faculty began to distrust her. Another problem was the aura of secretiveness surrounding the administration because the dean only shared selectively.

Prior to accepting the position, Lambertsen was fully apprised of the School's financial situation. Expressing her concern about it, she continued to be reassured by the Governors and Hospital Director of the program's economic viability despite clear evidence of rising health care cost. In 1975, the financial crisis came to a head when contributions to the School of Nursing from the Hospital could no longer be included in reimbursements from third-party payers. The implications of the information were startling, but Lambertsen's hopes rose when the Governors announced the Third Century Fund with a goal of $260,000,000 to begin the following year. It may have been wishful thinking on her part, because she already had a plan in the works to initiate a master's degree program in clinical specialization that would build on the present baccalaureate program for non-nursing college graduates.

Lambertsen's overconfidence may have been her Achilles' heel. In May 1977, when she met with the University's Board of Trustees in Ithaca to present her plan for the School, it never entered her mind that a decision would be made to terminate the baccalaureate programs. Louise Hazeltine remembered vividly the despair of the dean on her return to New York, and the pain she must have experienced when explaining the Trustees' action to an angry faculty.

It would be unfair to hold Lambertsen largely responsible for the demise of the School of Nursing, but she must assume some accountability for the furor that followed the decision. Why was the faculty so stunned? Were they so uninformed about the School's financial situation? Did they and the alumni not understand the significance, even the urgency, of having an endowment and the implication of not obtaining one?

Although the lack of ongoing funding could be cited as the main reason why the School closed, it was not the only factor that contributed to or even accelerated its failure to survive. In 1942 when the Cornell University-New York Hospital School of Nursing was established, the joint agreement had defined the arrangement with the Hospital to assume the financing of the nursing program until other appropriate sources could be found. With that understanding, the

School was vulnerable from the outset, and perhaps the final outcome was inevitable. Realistically, however, it was more than probable that lacking the Hospital's financial commitment, university affiliation would not have materialized, at least at that time.

A major factor relevant to the continuing operation of the School was the leadership of the deans during the years of seeking an endowment. An inspirational leader, Virginia Dunbar announced the Fund at the 75th Anniversary in 1952 so that alumni could participate from the beginning. During her administration, the endowment effort claimed a modicum of success. In her commitment to education and her stature in the nursing profession, as well as contacts with foundations, Dunbar was an articulate spokesperson for the School when approaching prospective donors.

In contrast, her successor did not follow a similar course. Throughout her tenure, Muriel Carbery placed nursing service needs before those of the educational program. She lacked standing in the academic community and failed to follow through on opportunities that may have helped to secure an endowment. When Eleanor Lambertsen arrived on the scene, it may have been too late to activate the endowment campaign. The opportune conditions of the preceding decade no longer existed, and funding possibilities were diminished.

On reflection, one can only speculate that if an individual with the leadership capabilities of Anna Wolf or Virginia Dunbar had been in command during the critical 1960s, the chances of obtaining an endowment might have been more likely and a positive outcome assured. In light of that observation and the foregoing compelling evidence, could the demise of the School of Nursing have been prevented? Perhaps the only fair response to such a searching question must be a guarded "yes."

––––––––––––––––––

Although 1979 marked the end of the 100-year journey of one of the nation's most prestigious schools of nursing, its magnificent heritage endures. As trailblazers at the beginning of modern nursing, the graduates spread their mission around the world to raise education standards and improve the quality of patient-care services. These legendary figures laid the foundation for professional nursing, and those that followed became leaders in the forefront of inevitable change to improve the conditions of health in peace and war.

Many of the nurses who graduated from the School after it affiliated with Cornell University continued to demonstrate their skills in a variety of positions, such as deans and professors of nursing, vice presidents for nursing, and consultants to national and international organizations. Others remained closer to The New York Hospital, serving as staff nurses or as clinical specialists and nurse practitioners. One of the School's outstanding graduates and a former president of the Alumnae Association was Doris Glick, class of 1966, who administered nursing service in the 1990s and became vice president for patient-care services until her retirement in 2004.

Throughout the years, nursing students were exposed to a rich laboratory in an institution that evolved into a famous academic medical center, dedicated to innovation and scientific discovery. In January 1998, The New York Hospital merged with the Presbyterian Hospital of New York City. It represented a move that combined two institutions with long and illustrious histories.

Almost 30 years have passed since the Cornell University-New York Hospital School of Nursing was terminated, but its legacy continues to shine. It will live on in remembrance because of the distinguished graduates, the passionate pioneers who made nursing a profession!

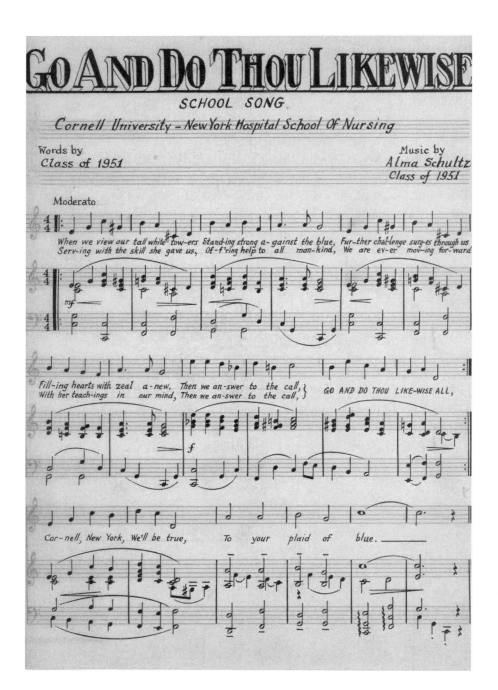

GO AND DO THOU LIKEWISE

SCHOOL SONG

Cornell University - New York Hospital School Of Nursing

Words by
Class of 1951

Music by
Alma Schultz
Class of 1951

Moderato

When we view our tall white tow-ers Stand-ing strong a-gainst the blue, Fur-ther chal-lenge surg-es through us
Serv-ing with the skill she gave us, Of-f'ring help to all man-kind, We are ev-er mov-ing for-ward

Fill-ing hearts with zeal a-new, Then we an-swer to the call,}
With her teach-ings in our mind, Then we an-swer to the call,} GO AND DO THOU LIKE-WISE ALL,

Cor-nell, New York, We'll be true, To your plaid of blue.

Appendices

A. Bylaws of The New York Hospital, adopted by Board of Governors, July 2, 1878

1. There shall be a Training School for the instruction of Female Nurses, in which the course shall extend over a period of eighteen months, divided into three terms of six months each.

2. The School shall consist of twenty four pupils, divided into two classes of eight, who shall serve respectively the first six months as Junior Assistants, the second six months as Senior Assistants, the third six months as Head Nurses, but the Visiting Committee may vary the number at their discretion.

3. Applicants for tuition in the Training School must be between twenty-five and thirty-five years of age, and possess a good common school education. They must produce certificates of good character, good health and physical capacities for the duties of nurses, satisfactory to the Conference Committee, and must make their applications to the Principal of the School not later than the twentieth of June or the twentieth of December.

4. If admitted, they will be expected to serve one month on probation, during which time they will receive board and lodging, but no compensation unless accepted as pupils, when they must sign an agreement to remain in the School and subject themselves to the rules of the Hospital for the full period of eighteen months, unless failing of promotion.

5. At the end of each term there shall be an examination of the graduating class, conducted under the supervision and in the

presence of the Conference Committee, which, being creditably passed, shall entitle its members to a diploma under the seal of the Hospital. The promotions from lower classes shall also be under the direction and control of the Conference Committee.

6. The Principal of the School shall exercise the functions of her office subject to the general authority of the Superintendent. With this reservation the School shall be under her direct supervision and control, and her authority shall extend over all that pertains to the duties and discipline of the nurses in the wards, as well as to the details of their instruction in the School. All the servants and orderlies shall be responsible to her in the performance of such duties as relate to the nursing of the patients.

7. In case of misconduct or insubordination, the Principal may suspend members of the classes from duty, and refer the case to the Visiting Committee for final decision.

8. Instruction shall be given by all the medical officers of the Hospital, by the Principal of the School, and by the Head Nurses of the wards.

B. Policies of The New York Hospital School of Nursing and Nursing Service, approved by Board of Governors, 1932

1. The curriculum of the School would provide a longer pre-clinical period of study. This would allow more complex and thorough courses to be given in the psychological and sociological aspects of nursing, and in the fundamental biological sciences and chemistry. It would also permit more careful supervision of elementary nursing at the bedside.

2. The clinical curriculum would provide for the inclusion of more varied types of clinical and public health courses for which the students would have proper facilities for study.

3. All courses would be of collegiate grade as to content and instruction.

4. All students would be admitted to the School once instead of twice a year. If possible, those students should have more than high school education and be over the age of twenty.

5.   Student schedules, including class and practice, would not exceed forty-four hours a week.
6.   The faculty members would be selected because of their special preparation and success in various fields of study.
7.   The clinical nursing departments would be organized with responsible heads who would direct all nursing activities and instruction in their respective departments.
8.   The size of the student body would be limited to the number of students who could be offered proper experience in the smallest clinical department. The School would be enlarged in numbers through the admission of graduate and affiliated students.
9.   A graduate staff would be maintained because of the rapid turnover of students in a given clinical department, so as not to jeopardize patient care.
10. Health education would be stressed and staff and student health be emphasized.

C. Cornell University-New York Hospital School of Nursing. Recommendations approved by Board of Governors, The New York Hospital, and Board of Trustees, Cornell University, January 1942

1.   That the name of the affiliated school include both the name of Cornell University and The New York Hospital School of Nursing.
2.   That the affiliation become effective with the opening of the next term, in which first year students in the School begin work.
3.   That the School have as its administrative head a dean or director who should also be director of the nursing service of The New York Hospital.
4.   That the basic requirement for admission to the School of Nursing be two years of college work acceptable to Cornell University. (It may be well to provide, however, that in exceptional cases, applicants with less than two years of completed college work but showing unusual ability and promise be admitted to the School with the approval of the dean or director).

5. That the proposed curriculum of the School of Nursing be presented in tentative form at this time and be so developed as to require not less than two and a half years (thirty months) exclusive of vacations.

6. That the faculty of the School of Nursing include the heads of the several departments of the Cornell University Medical College.

7. That the faculty of the School of Nursing be responsible for the curriculum and for the maintenance of instruction of college grade meeting the academic standards of the other colleges of the University.

8. That, upon satisfactory completion of the required course of study in the School of Nursing, candidates be eligible for an appropriate degree from Cornell University and for a diploma in nursing from the Society of The New York Hospital. It should be provided that in the exceptional cases cited in #4, the diploma from the Hospital be awarded although the degree from the University is not conveyed.

9. That the Society of The New York Hospital assume full financial responsibility for the School of Nursing, including any increase in the costs of operating the present School, which may be made necessary through the formal affiliation with the University.

10. That the University appoint the Society of The New York Hospital as fiscal agent for the University for handling all funds employed in connection with the School of Nursing. (As such fiscal agent, the Society of The New York Hospital would be required to render an account to Cornell University in such form as to meet the requirements of the University auditors. It is also understood that additional periodic reports from the fiscal agent would be rendered as requested by the University).

11. That any increase of income resulting from an increase in student fees be applied toward increased costs of the School of Nursing, or with the approval of the Joint Administrative Board, held in reserve by the Society of The New York Hospital, against any deficits in the operation of the School, or applied to current deficits.

12. That any increase in fees introduced in connection with the affiliation of the School shall not apply to students now enrolled in The New York Hospital School. However, such students who

meet the requirements of the University and are permitted to apply for the degree may be required when admitted to candidacy for the degree to make additional payments designed to meet the expenses incurred by the University in connection with the granting of the degree.

D. Nurse Administrators, Cornell University-New York Hospital School of Nursing: 1877–1979

Juliet E. Marchant	Principal	1877–1878
Jane A. Sangster	Principal	1878
Eliza Watson Brown	Principal	1879–1882
Zilpha E. Whitaker	Principal	1882–1886
Irene H. Sutliffe	Directress	1886–1902
Ida Nudel	Acting Directress	1902
Annie W. Goodrich	Superintendent	1902–1907
Lottie Bushnell	Acting Superintendent	1907
Adeline Henderson	Superintendent	1907–1915
Bertha H. Lehmkuhl	Acting Superintendent	1915–1916
Minnie H. Jordan	Directress	1916–1931
Sarah E. Moore	Acting Directress	1932
Anna D. Wolf	Director	1931–1940
Bessie A. R. Parker	Director	1940–1942
Bessie A. R. Parker	Acting Director/Dean	1942–1946
Virginia M. Dunbar	Dean	1946–1958
Muriel R. Carbery	Dean	1959–1970
Eleanor C. Lambertsen	Dean	1970–1979

E. Distinguished Alumnus Award

The Distinguished Alumnus Award was established in 1973 by the Board of Directors of the Cornell University-New York Hospital School of Nursing Alumni Association to recognize graduates who made significant contributions to nursing.

The Board established the following nomination criteria:

1. A record of achievement in one or more of the following fields of nursing:
   a. Clinical practice
   b. Administration
   c. Education
   d. Research
2. Significant professional contributions in one or more of the following ways:
   a. Publishing.
   b. Lecturing, program participation, and community service beyond that of the usual job requirements.
   d. Original research (this may be based on doctoral dissertation).
   e. Clinical studies which lead to the improvement of patient care.

In addition to a nominating letter, the Board requested:

1. Curriculum Vita completed within the preceding 12 months
2. A minimum of two letters of support—one from an alumnus; one from a non-alumnus
3. A maximum of three sample publications if available

On the next page is a list of award recipients.

Distinguished Alumnus Award Recipients

1974	Muriel R. Carbery '37
1975	No award given
1976	Barbara McKinley Resnick '50
1977	No award given
1978	Jean E. Steel '60
1979	Louise S. Hazeltine '49
1980	No award given
1981	No award given
1982	Evelyn Ruth Hayes '65
1983	Dorothy W. Smith '47S
1984	Josephine Kelly Craytor '38
1985	G. Maureen Turecan Chaisson-Stewart '62
1986	No award given
1987	Evelynn Clark Gioiella '59
1988	Jane Van Sickle Feil '46S
1989	Alma Schelle Woolley '54
1990	Dorothy McMullen Pisani '35
1991	Lynn Gates Keegan '66
1992	Frances M. Farthing '42 and Marie Kurihara '50
1993	Doris Troth Sommerfield Lippmann '65
1994	Ruth Blatt Merkatz '61 and Virginia Burggraf '64
1995	Carol Noll Hoskins '55 and Gladys Balbus Lipkin '47F
1996	Gail B. Malloy '56 and Nancy R. Adams '68
1997	Mary Beth Zimmerman Mathews '65 and Anne H. Sheetz '66
1998	Janet R. Sawyer '46S
1999	Barbara Geesey Valanis '65 and Mary Woods Byrne '66
2000	Lois White Lowry '55 and Joyce Edgar Schickler '57
2001	Sandra Roberts Byers '60 and Jeanette Dontzow Johnson '47S
2002	Gloria Richards Gelmann '57
2003	Margaret Wines '58 and Ruth Fischbach (no data)
2004	Kathleen Wheeler '76
2005	Doris M. Glick '66
2006	Doris Dickerson Coward '60

Notes

Abbreviations used in the notes:

ACSN   Association of Collegiate Schools of Nursing
ANA   American Nurses Association
CUMC   Cornell University Medical Center
CU-NYHSN   Cornell University-New York Hospital School of
              Nursing
JAB, NYH-CMC Joint Administrative Board, New York Hospital-
              Cornell Medical Center
NLN   National League for Nursing
NLNE   National League of Nursing Education
NOPHN   National Organization for Public Health Nursing
NYH   The New York Hospital
NYWCMCA   New York Weill Cornell Medical Center Archives

CHAPTER 1

1. Sandra Opdycke, *No One Was Turned Away – The Role of the Public Hospital in New York City since 1900* (New York: Oxford, 1999), 38. In private or voluntary hospitals, a governing board was standard practice. In contrast, public hospitals generally had commissioners or salaried officials operating the facility at the pleasure of the mayor. By the early 1900s, however, the status of Bellevue and Allied Hospitals changed when granted a semi-autonomous board. In this respect, Bellevue paralleled the nature of The New York Hospital with dedicated, public-spirited citizens.

2. Eric Larrabee, *The Benevolent and Necessary Institution—The New York Hospital, 1771–1971* (New York: Doubleday, 1971), 212. After Dr. Morton patented the procedure, he found himself embroiled in a bitter dispute over the discovery of the anesthetic. The controversy brought him near poverty and destroyed his prac-

tice. See also G.C. Sanchez, "William T.G. Morton," in *Dictionary of American Medical Biography*, Vol. 2, Martin Kaufman, Stuart Galishofff, Todd L. Savitt, edit. (Westport, Connecticut: Greenwood Press, 1984), 540.

3. Dickens' satire portrayed Sairey Gamp as an unsympathetic, incompetent, uncouth, and tipsy woman who contributed to human suffering. The origin of the expression "a regular Gamp" stemmed from Sairey, who was characterized as a low-class, uneducated maternity nurse.

4. Dr. William Van Buren to Board of Governors, New York Hospital (NYH), report of Surgical Division, October–November 1859; box 3, folder 5; Records of Secretary-Treasurer, NYH: 1811–1933; New York Weill Cornell Medical Center Archives (NYWCMCA); Helene Jamieson Jordan, *Cornell University-New York Hospital School of Nursing, 1877–1952* (New York: The Society of the New York Hospital, 1952), 10, 12–15.

5. Florence Nightingale, *Notes on Nursing, What It Is and What It Is Not* (London: Harrison and Sons, 1960, reprint of 1860 first edition).

6. Jessie M. Keyes, "Present Day Opportunities," extracted from a speech given to Dubuque County registered nurses, as reproduced in *American Journal of Nursing* 11 (February 1911), 46.

7. Majority and Minority Reports of a Special Committee of the Board of Governors, NYH, 17 April 1866, 6–8,12; NYWCMCA; Jordan, *Cornell University-New York Hospital*, 9.

8. Ibid.; Jordan, *Cornell University-New York Hospital*, 8.

9. Ibid.

10. James A. Harrar, *Story of the Lying-In Hospital* (New York: The Society of the Lying-In Hospital, 1930), 21–22. On February 3, 1801, a committee of the Board of Governors of NYH proposed a union with Lying-In Hospital, in which a lying-in ward would operate under the direction of the Governors. The arrangement appeared to be the first of its kind in the United States where male medical students were permitted to witness deliveries in a maternity ward.

11. Larrabee, *The Benevolent*, 155–156. The name "Bloomingdale" was derived from the Dutch *Bloomendael* meaning "Vale of Flowers," given to Manhattan's upper west side by the early settlers. Surrounded by 70 acres of landscaped grounds, the building was designed to avoid any impression of being a prison or a place of punishment.

12. Ibid., 271.

13. "History of the Bloomingdale Training School, 1897–1934," one sheet typescript; NYWCMCA.

14. Larrabee, *The Benevolent*, 271.

15. Joellen W. Hawkins, "Dorothea Lynde Dix," in *Dictionary of American Nursing Biography*, Martin T. Kaufman, edit. (Westport, Connecticut: Greenwood Press, 1988), 97.

16. Larrabee, *The Benevolent*, 262–263.

17. Edith Abbott, *Some American Pioneers in Social Reform: Selected Documents with Editorial Note* (Chicago: University of Chicago Press, 1937), n.p.

18. See "Florence Nightingale" at http://en.wikipedia.org/wiki/Florence_Nightingale (accessed 9/30/2005). The Union Army approached Nightingale for advice on organizing field medicine. The United States Sanitary Commission was inspired by her ideas, as well as those of Dorothea Dix, Clara Barton, and other women who volunteered their services during the Civil War.

19. Jane E. Mottus, "The New York Nightingales; The Emergence of a Profession at Bellevue and New York Hospitals, 1850–1920" (Ph.D. diss., New York University: 1980), 54, 57. (University Microfilms International, Catalog Number 8017582.)

20. Ibid.

21. Jill K. Conway, *The Female Experience in Eighteenth and Nineteenth Century America – A Guide to the History of Women* (New York: Garland, 1982), 82.

22. Kate Cumming, *The Journal of a Confederate Nurse*, Richard Barksdale Harwell, edit. (Baton Rouge, Louisiana: State Press, 1959). Cumming was a volunteer nurse from Mobile, Alabama, who worked as a matron, cared for the ill and wounded, and took charge of all domestic activities. Published after the war, her journal provided poignant recollections of the lives of the soldiers, doctors, and nurses.

23. Hawkins, "Clarissa Harlan Barton," in *Dictionary of American Nursing*, 17–20.

24. Ibid. Clara Barton became the first president of the American Red Cross in 1881 and served in that office until May 14, 1904.

25. C. L. Meigs, *The Invincible Louisa* (Boston: Little Brown, 1968), 104.

26. Hawkins, "Louisa May Alcott," in *Dictionary of American Nursing*, 3–4.

27. Larrabee, *The Benevolent*, 203.

28. Jordan, *Cornell University-New York Hospital*, 23; Mottus, *New York Nightingales*, 3. The proportion of women in the professional category doubled from 25 to 47.4%. This marked growth could be attributed to the feminization of the teaching and librarian fields, as well as the increase and inclusion of the traditional women's occupations like nursing and social work.

29. Morris Bishop, *A History of Cornell University* (Ithaca: Cornell University Press, 1962), 20.

30. Ibid., 613. See also Carol Kammen, *Cornell—Glorious to View* (Ithaca: Cornell University Library, 2003), xi.

31. Kammen, *Cornell—Glorious to View*, 27.

32. Ibid., 42–43. See also "The Cornell Women's Handbook—History of Women at Cornell" at http://www.rso.cornell.edu/cwh/historyn.html (accessed 9/30/2005).

33. Kammen, *Cornell—Glorious to View*, 44–46. Although Jennie Spencer successfully passed her tests and was highly regarded, she decided to leave after the first week. In 1873, Emma Sheffield Eastman became the first woman to graduate, and by 1998 women made up almost half of the student body.

34. Charles Rosenberg, "The Practice of Medicine in New York a Century Ago" in *Readings in the History of Medicine and Public Health*, Judith Leavitt and Ronald Numbers, edit. (Madison, Wisconsin: 61 QWI Press, 1978), 64.

35. Ibid.

36. Larrabee, *The Benevolent*, 235.

37. Majority and Minority Reports of a Special Committee of the Board of Governors, NYH, 17 April 1866, 6–8,12; NYWCMCA. Until 1877, when NYH relocated to its new site on West 16th Street, it remained an imposing edifice for decades facing Broadway in lower Manhattan. The building was opposite Pearl Street and surrounded on the west side by Church, on the south by Duane, and on the north by Worth Streets.

38. Ibid.

39. Ibid.

40. "Remonstrance Against Removal of The New York Hospital," *The New York Times* (4 January 1869); box 5, folder 2; Records of Secretary-Treasurer, NYH:

1811–1933; NYWCMCA.

41. Report, Investigating Committee to Board of Governors, NYH, 1871; Annual Report, NYH, 1872, 9; NYWCMCA.

42. Minutes, Board of Governors, NYH, 3 February 1920; NYWCMCA. From 1875 to 1894, NYH maintained the House of Relief at No. 160 Chambers Street, where it was widely known as Chambers Street Hospital. It was the only hospital in that part of the city.

43. Annual Report, NYH, 1893, 11; NYWCMCA. In the early 1890s, the Governors purchased a plot of land with the intent to erect a new House of Relief. By 1894, the building was ready for occupancy.

44. Mottus, *New York Nightingales*, 99–100.

45. Ibid.

46. Opdycke, *No One Was Turned Away*, 38.

47. Minutes, Board of Governors, NYH, 6 January 1874; NYWCMCA.

48. Mottus, *New York Nightingales*, 102.

49. Ibid., 116.

50. Opdycke, *No One Was Turned Away*, 39.

51. W. H. Van Buren, M.D., "An Address Delivered on the Occasion of the Inauguration of the New Building of The New York Hospital," 16 March 1877, 22; NYWCMCA.

52. "Hospital Life in New York," *Harper's New Monthly Magazine*, Vol. LVII, No. 338 (July 1878).

53. Larrabee, *The Benevolent*, 242.

54. "The New York Hospital," *Harper's Weekly* (7 April 1877); NYWCMCA.

55. Annual Report, NYH, 1877, 10; NYWCMCA.

56. Report, Committee on a Village of Cottage Hospitals, 24 February 1876; W. H. Van Buren, M.D., "An Address Delivered on the Occasion of the Inauguration of the New Building of The New York Hospital," 16 March 1877, 20; NYWCMCA.

57. Annual Report, NYH, 1877, 10; NYWCMCA. On 3 May 1877, *The New York Times* featured an article titled "A New Training School for Nurses" that announced the opening of the School in July.

58. Mottus, *New York Nightingales*, 123.

59. Bylaws and Regulations, NYH, 1878, chapter xxii; NYWCMCA.

60. Bylaws and Regulations, NYH, 1878, chapter xv; NYWCMCA.

61. Bylaws and Regulations, NYH, 1878, chapter iv; NYWCMCA.

62. Juliet Marchant to Visiting Committee, letter, 8 October 1877; box 8, folder 8; Records of Secretary-Treasurer, NYH: 1811–1933; NYWCMCA. See also George Plunkett Red, *The Medicine Man in Texas* (Houston, Texas: Standard Printing Company, 1930). No archival documents could be located regarding Marchant's qualifications and credentials before she accepted the position as principal. After leaving the Training School, the career of Juliet Marchant took a unique turn when she obtained a license to practice medicine in Oneida County, Rome, New York. She moved to LaPorte, Texas, in 1893 and remained there the rest of her life. Marchant's neighbors related how she walked many miles to see patients and that her services were a blessing. She died in LaPorte on 24 April 1929, at the age of 84.

63. Jane Sangster to Visiting Committee, report, 19 August 1878; box 9, folder 9;

Records of Secretary-Treasurer, NYH: 1811–1933; NYWCMCA.

64. Minutes, Conference Committee, NYH, 1 May 1880; NYWCMCA.
65. Minutes, Conference Committee, NYH, 25 September 1878; NYWCMCA.
66. Minutes, Conference Committee, NYH, 10 January 1879; NYWCMCA.
67. Minutes, Visiting Committee, NYH, 11 August 1879; NYWCMCA.
68. Minutes, Visiting Committee, NYH, 23 June 1879; NYWCMCA.
69. Minutes, Conference Committee, NYH, 9 October 1879; NYWCMCA.
70. Ibid.
71. Minutes, Conference Committee, NYH, 5 December 1881; NYWCMCA.
72. Minutes, Conference Committee, NYH, 2 October 1882; NYWCMCA.
73. Minutes, Conference Committee, NYH, 30 December 1882; NYWCMCA.
74. Minutes, Conference Committee, NYH, 6 November 1882; NYWCMCA.
75. Jordan, *Cornell University-New York Hospital*, 78–79.
76. Minutes, Conference Committee, NYH, 5 March 1883; NYWCMCA.
77. Annual Report, Conference Committee, NYH, 1883, 4; NYWCMCA.
78. Ibid.
79. Minutes, Conference Committee, NYH, 6 October 1884; NYWCMCA.
80. Minutes, Conference Committee, NYH, 18 May 1885; NYWCMCA.
81. Annual Report, Conference Committee, NYH, 1885, 3; NYWCMCA.
82. Minutes, Conference Committee, NYH, 7 November 1885; NYWCMCA.
83. Zilpha Whitaker to Conference Committee, NYH, letter, 2 January 1886; box 15, folder 10; Records of Secretary-Treasurer, NYH: 1811–1933; NYWCMCA.
84. Minutes, Conference Committee, NYH, 1 February 1886; NYWCMCA.
85. Annual Report, Conference Committee, NYH, 1885, 4; NYWCMCA.
86. Ibid. See also Minutes, Conference Committee, NYH, 23 November 1885; NYWCMCA.
87. Annual Report, NYH, 1886, 11; NYWCMCA.

CHAPTER 2

1. Record of Services, NYH Training School for Nurses: 1877–1897; NYWCMCA.
2. Ibid.
3. Class Records, NYH Training School for Nurses: 1878–1920; NYWCMCA.
4. Ibid.
5. Ibid. See also Mottus, *New York Nightingales*, 199–200. Widowed and divorced women tended to be older. The School later decided not to accept divorced women, a policy that stayed in effect for several years.
6. Class Records, NYH Training School for Nurses: 1878–1920; NYWCMCA.
7. Hawkins, "Annie Warburton Goodrich," in *Dictionary of American Nursing*, 154.
8. Beatrice Siegel, *Lillian Wald of Henry Street* (New York: Macmillan, 1983), 19.
9. Hawkins, "Jane Elizabeth Hitchcock," in *Dictionary of American Nursing*, 193.
10. Mottus, *New York Nightingales*, 216.
11. Clipping, *The New York Sun* (12 May 1937); box 7, folder 4; Julia Stimson Papers: 1875–1949; NYWCMCA.
12. Lillian Wald, letter of application; box 2; Class Records, NYH Training School for Nurses: 1878–1920; NYWCMCA. See also Siegel, *Lillian Wald*, 15–16.
13. Class Records, NYH Training School for Nurses: 1878–1920; NYWCMCA.

14. Anne A. Williamson, *50 Years in Starch* (Culver City, Calif.: Murray and Gee, 1948), 21–22.
15. Class Records, NYH Training School for Nurses: 1878–1920; NYWCMCA.
16. *Announcements*, NYH Training School for Nurses, 1907–1908; NYWCMCA.
17. Williamson, 50 Years, 66.
18. Lillian Wald, *House on Henry Street* (New York: Henry Holt, 1915), 1; Siegel, *Lillian Wald*, 17.
19. Esther A. Werminghaus, *Annie Goodrich—Her Journey to Yale* (New York: Macmillan, 1950), 23.
20. Minutes, Executive Committee, NYH, 2 May 1887; NYWCMCA.
21. Minutes, Executive Committee, NYH, 1 April 1895; NYWCMCA.
22. Report, Conference Committee, NYH, 9 March 1885; Minutes, Conference Committee, NYH, 6 April 1885; NYWCMCA.
23. Report, Conference Committee, 30 April 1886; NYWCMCA.
24. Siegel, *Lillian Wald*, 16.
25. Williamson, *50 Years*, 63.
26. Anonymous, biography of Irene Sutliffe, n.d.; box 1, folder 1; Irene Sutliffe Papers: 1878–1940; NYWCMA.
27. Minutes, Executive Committee, NYH, 1 November 1886; NYWCMCA.
28. Minutes, Executive Committee, NYH, 31 January 1887; NYWCMCA. Includes Dr. Hoppin's report of 3 November 1886.
29. Ibid.
30. Ibid.
31. Ibid. Clara Weeks' text, *Nursing for the Use of Training Schools, Families, and Private Students*, sold more than 100,000 copies in the ensuing years and underwent 58 printings. See Jordan, *Cornell University-New York Hospital*, 30. It was of interest that as a speaker at the graduation exercises of the Training School in 1911, Dr. Peabody apparently changed his attitude about the theoretical instruction of pupil nurses when he stated the following: "It would not be possible to say how much or exactly what has been contributed by nurses to advance in clinical knowledge which has of late been so rapid for my part. I wish to accord you your full share." Jordan, *Cornell University-New York Hospital*, 44.
32. Minutes, Executive Committee, NYH, 31 January 1887; NYWCMCA.
33. Ibid.
34. Minutes, Conference Committee, NYH, 5 December 1887; NYWCMCA.
35. Minutes, Conference Committee, NYH, 30 April 1886; NYWCMCA; Jordan, *Cornell-University-New York Hospital*, 27.
36. Minutes, Conference Committee, NYH, 25 September 1886; NYWCMCA.
37. Minutes, Executive Committee, NYH, 28 September 1886; NYWCMCA.
38. Minutes, Executive Committee, NYH, 4 February 1888; NYWCMCA.
39. Ibid.
40. Ibid.
41. Ibid.
42. Ibid.
43. Minutes, Board of Governors, NYH, 5 February 1888; NYWCMCA.
44. Annual Report, NYH, 1891, 11; NYWCMCA.
45. Jordan, *Cornell University-New York Hospital*, 30.
46. Minutes, Executive Committee, NYH, 28 June 1892; NYWCMCA.
47. Mottus, *New York Nightingales*, 203–207.

48. Helen Fraser to NYH Training School for Nurses, letter, 16 October 1896; box 3 (Narusa); Class Records, NYH Training School for Nurses: 1878–1920; NYWCM-CA. The student, Shidzu Narusa, was a graduate of the Class of 1900.

49. Joseph Hirsch and Beka Doherty, *The First Hundred Years of the Mount Sinai Hospital of New York: 1852–1952* (New York: Random House, 1952), 68.

50. Mottus, *New York Nightingales*, 199, 222.

51. Ibid., 295.

52. George Peabody, commencement address, 2 March 1911, 7; box 1, folder 1; Commencements, CU-NYHSN: 1884–1979; NYWCMCA.

53. Jurgen Thorwald, *The Century of the Surgeon* (New York: Pantheon, 1956).

54. Ibid. William Stewart Halsted, first professor of surgery at Hopkins, was renowned for his numerous contributions to the field.

55. Nurses Registry: Assignment Records, Alumni Association, CU-NYHSN, ca. 1898–1946; box 1, folder 2; NYWCMCA.

56. Ibid.

57. Minutes, Executive Committee, NYH, 27 August 1919; NYWCMCA. In the early period, the more common violations committed by graduates of the School can be found in the Executive Committee Minutes of 5 November 1888, 1 January 1891, and 4 April 1892.

58. Mottus, *New York Nightingales*, 289–290.

59. Class Records, NYH Training School for Nurses: 1878–1920; NYWCMCA.

60. Ibid.

CHAPTER 3

1. Annie Goodrich, President's Address, Twelfth Annual Convention of the Superintendents' Society, New York, 1906, in *Legacy of Leadership*, Nettie Birnbach and Sandra Lewenson, edit. (New York: National League for Nursing Press, 1993), 63.

2. Opdycke, *No One Was Turned Away*, 23.

3. Annual Report, NYH, 1891, 11; NYWCMCA.

4. Susan Bastable, "Recruitment of Students into Basic Nursing Education Programs in the United States, 1893–1940: An Historical Survey," (Ed.D. diss., Teachers College, Columbia University, 1979). (University Microfilms International, Catalog Number 80066988.)

5. Nettie Birnbach and Sandra Lewenson, *First Words: Selected Addresses from the National League for Nursing, 1894–1933* (New York: National League for Nursing Press, 1993), prologue, xxii.

6. Richard Olding Beard, "Hospital Economics of the Nursing Situation," *Modern Hospital* 21 (October 1923), 394.

7. Teresa E. Christy, "Nurses in American History: The Fateful Decade, 1890–1900," *American Journal of Nursing* 75 (February 1975), 163.

8. Loretta Higgins, "Irene H. Sutliffe," in *Dictionary of American Nursing*, 361. Irene Sutliffe believed in the value of organization as shown by her support of an Alumnae Association for the School, and later The New York Hospital's Nurses' Club.

9. Lyndia Flanagan, *One Strong Voice—The Story of the American Nurses Association* (Kansas City, Missouri: American Nurses Association, 1976), 29–31.

10. Lystra Gretter, President's Address, Ninth Annual Convention of the

Superintendents' Society, Detroit, Michigan, 1902, in *Legacy of Leadership*, Nettie Birnbach and Sandra Lewenson, edit. (New York: National League for Nursing Press, 1993), 45.

11. Higgins, "Irene H. Sutliffe," in *Dictionary of American Nursing*, 361.

12. Minutes, Executive Committee, NYH, 5 May 1893; NYWCMCA.

13. Minutes, Executive Committee, NYH, 4 April 1892; NYWCMCA.

14. Historical Scrapbook, Alumnae Association, NYH Training School for Nurses, 1893–1932; NYWCMCA. See also CU-NYHSN *Alumni Newsletter* (Summer 2001), Mary Belmont, edit.

15. Agnes S. Brennan, "Comparative Value of Theory and Practice on Training Nurses," 1897, in *First Words: Selected Addresses from the National League for Nursing*, 23.

16. M. Elizabeth Carnegie, *The Path We Tread* (New York: National League for Nursing Press, 1995, 3rd edition), 74.

17. *Circular Information*, NYH Training School for Nurses, 1907–1908; NYWCMCA.

18. Carnegie, *The Path We Tread*, 17–25. By 1965, 71 of the 91 black hospital schools had closed; after 1982, none remained.

19. Flanagan, *One Strong Voice*, 29, 611. In 1901, the Nurses Associated Alumnae was incorporated under the laws of the State of New York, making it necessary to remove the reference to Canada in the title.

20. Jordan, *Cornell University-New York Hospital*, 32.

21. Annual Reports & Minutes, Alumnae Association, NYH Training School for Nurses: 1893–1902; NYWCMCA. See also Historical Scrapbook, Alumnae Association, NYH Training School for Nurses: 1893–1932; NYWCMCA. The original title of the organization was the Alumnae Association of the School for Nurses of The New York Hospital. References for changes in the title in 1945 and 1974 appear in the minutes of the Association during those years.

22. Ibid.

23. Jordan, *Cornell-University-New York Hospital*, 31.

24. Ibid.

25. Ibid., 36.

26. *The Alumnae News*, Vol. 1, No. IV (May 1907), 7; NYWCMCA.

27. Jordan, *Cornell University-New York Hospital*, 41.

28. Ibid.

29. The first copy of *The Alumnae News* was introduced in 1896 and listed the officers as well as members of the Association's executive committee and the Fund for Sick Nurses. For several years, the newsletter format was that of a pamphlet until it became a Quarterly. In 1916, Clara Weeks Shaw assumed the editorship.

30. Siegel, *Lillian Wald*, 49–50.

31. Ibid., 27–28.

32. Jordan, *Cornell-New York Hospital*, 42

33. Karen Buheler-Williamson, "The Call to the Nurse," in *Healing at Home* (New York: Visiting Nurse Service of New York, 1993), 9–15.

34. Siegel, *Lillian Wald*, 50, 87–88.

35. Hawkins, in *Dictionary of American Nursing*, 193–195. Jane Hitchcock enjoyed an illustrious career, including her appointment as the first secretary of The New York State Board of Nurse Examiners in 1903. She served in that post for the next

16 years. Hitchcock was responsible for the questions on public health nursing that appeared in the state licensing examination.

36. Annual Report, NYH, 1907, 36; NYWCMCA.

37. Jordan, *Cornell University-New York Hospital*, 42–43.

38. Ibid., 43. In 1913, Irene Sutliffe organized a similar social service department at the House of Relief.

39. Ibid.

40. Minutes, Executive Committee, NYH, 29 October 1912; NYWCMCA. Hannah Josephi had specialized in social service nursing and gave lectures on the relationship between the social service department of a hospital and patient care. She frequently spoke to medical students at Cornell University Medical College and the College of Physicians and Surgeons, Columbia University.

41. Minutes, Executive Committee, NYH, 15 April 1896; NYWCMCA.

42. Ibid.

43. Minutes, Executive Committee, NYH, 4 October 1897; NYWCMCA. In the fall of 1908, the Training School resumed its association with Sloane Maternity Hospital, which operated under new management. See also Minutes, Executive Committee, NYH, 24 February 1909; NYWCMCA.

44. Report of Special Committee in Minutes, Executive Committee, NYH, 5 April 1897; NYWCMCA. The library of NYH was considered one of the best medical repositories in the United States. Although the pupil nurses had their own small library, it was not likely that they had access to the Hospital library.

45. Ibid. On March 5, 1898, a Committee on the Library of the New York Academy of Medicine accepted the offer and decided to feature a plaque identifying the donation. At the time, the Academy was located at 1721 West 43 Street. (The Academy moved in 1905 to its present site at 1216 Fifth Avenue and 103 Street.) The committee decided to accept the entire collection before arranging for the handling of duplicates and cataloging. Subsequently, bookmarks were made for the number of holdings to be housed in the Academy's rare book collection. All of the books were integrated into the card catalog, but no information has been presently found about the disposition of the original plaque, if it existed. Arlene Shaner, Reference Librarian, Historical Collection, New York Academy of Medicine to Shirley H. Fondiller, e-mail communication, 11 January 2005; NYWCMCA.

46. "Oliver H. Payne Gives $1,500,000 to Found a Medical College," *The New York Herald* (1 September 1898); NYWCMCA.

47. Bishop, *History of Cornell*, 320; Larrabee, *The Benevolent*, 288–289. The founding of the Medical College stemmed initially from a disagreement involving faculty members of New York University and Bellevue Medical College. The dissenters were distinguished men who resigned and decided to establish their own medical college. They acquired the support of Oliver Payne as a generous benefactor.

48. Larrabee, *The Benevolent*, 288–291. Dr. Stimson was an uncle of Julia Stimson and her younger brother, Philip Stimson, a graduate of Cornell University Medical College.

49. *The New York Herald* (1 September 1898); NYWCMCA.

50. Larrabee, *The Benevolent*, 293; Robinson, *Adventures*, 193.

51. Bishop, *History of Cornell*, 320.

52. Robinson, *Adventures*, 195.
53. Ibid.
54. Ibid., 197.
55. Jordan, *Cornell University-The New York Hospital*, 45.
56. Ibid.
57. Christy, *Cornerstone*, 17–19. The course was a remarkable innovation because no one could foresee that it would eventually evolve into the Division of Nursing Education, making Teachers College, Columbia University, the premier institution for educating graduate nurses throughout the world for many decades. This was a significant event because it placed nursing within the system of higher education and represented a giant step toward advancing the profession.
58. Ibid.
59. Minutes, Executive Committee, NYH, 20 July 1900; NYWCMCA.
60. Christy, *Cornerstone*, 9.
61. Ibid.
62. Ibid.
63. Ibid.
64. Siegel, *Lillian Wald*, 99.
65. "1898–1998: Centennial of Spanish-American War": http://www.zpub.com/cpp/saw.html (accessed 9/30/2005).
66. Jordan, *Cornell University-New York Hospital*, 34–35.
67. Williamson, *50 Years*, 116.
68. Ibid.
69. "Women Were There": http://userpages.aug.com/captbarb/femvets3.html (accessed 9/30/2005). At the outset of the war, Congress authorized the U.S. Army to procure female nurses without military status. Recruited as civilians, over a thousand women served under contract.
70. Hawkins, "Dita Hopkins Kinney," in *Dictionary of American Nursing*, 218–220.
71. Minutes, Board of Governors, NYH, 4 December 1928; NYWCMCA. For her years of devotion to NYH, "Belle" Walton was honored at a festive reception with a large turnout from the medical and nursing community.
72. Williamson, *50 Years*, 117.
73. Ibid.
74. Ibid.
75. Ibid., 23.
76. Ibid., 121.
77. Ibid.
78. "The World of 1898: The Spanish-American War": http://www.loc.gov/rr/hispanic/1898/intro.html (accessed 9/30/2005).
79. Jordan, *Cornell-New York Hospital*, 34–35.
80. Mary Roberts, *American Nursing: History and Interpretation* (New York: Macmillan, 1959, 3rd printing), 144–145. The war years and the aftermath generated an increased demand for military and civilian nursing services.
81. Jordan, *Cornell University-New York Hospital*, 35. Irene Sutliffe served on the executive committee of the Nurses Associated Alumnae.
82. Ibid., 36.
83. Ibid. In 1922, the Spanish-contract nurses were granted a pension. On July 2, 1925, Public Law 448 granted the contract nurses full military status in the Army Nurse Corps. See Philip A. Kalisch, "Heroes of '98: Female Army Nurses in the Spanish-American War," *Nursing Research* 24 (November–December, 1975),

410–425.

CHAPTER 4

1. "Early 1900s in N. America": http://www.cyberessays.com/History/12.htm (accessed 9/30/2005).
2. Lystra E. Gretter, President's Address at Ninth Annual Convention of ASSTSN, in Birnbach and Lewenson, *Legacy of Leadership*, 45.
3. Ibid.
4. Annual Report, NYH, 1905, 86; NYCMCA.
5. Annual Report, NYH, 1900, 13; NYWCMCA.
6. Minutes, Training School Committee, NYH, 7 January 1907; NYWCMCA.
7. Ibid.
8. Jordan, *Cornell University-New York Hospital*, 38.
9. Annual Report, NYH, 1900, 13; NYWCMCA.
10. Siegel, *Lillian Wald*, 19.
11. Hawkins, "Annie W. Goodrich," in *Dictionary of American Nursing*, 155.
12. Ibid.
13. Minutes, Executive Committee, NYH, 4 April 1902; NYWCMCA.
14. Minutes, Training School Committee, NYH, 10 June 1902; NYWCMCA.
15. Ibid.
16. Minutes, Training School Committee, NYH, 22 March 1904; NYWCMCA.
17. Ibid.
18. Ibid.
19. Minutes, Board of Governors, NYH, 5 April 1904; NYWCMCA.
20. Ibid.
21. Minutes, Training School Committee, NYH, 28 March 1905; NYWCMCA.
22. Minutes, Training School Committee, NYH, 2 January 1906; NYWCMCA.
23. Ibid.
24. Minutes, Training School Committee, NYH, 26 September 1906; NYWCMCA.
25. Ibid. Goodrich's letter of 22 August 1906 to Dr. Hoppin evoked intense discussion at the meeting.
26. Minutes, Training School Committee, NYH, 28 November 1906; NYWCMCA.
27. Ibid.
28. Minutes, Training School Committee, NYH, 11 December 1906; NYWCMCA.
29. Minutes, Board of Governors, NYH, 5 February 1907; NYWCMCA.
30. Minutes, Training School Committee, NYH, 4 February 1907; NYWCMCA.
31. Alumnae Association, letter, 1907; box 40, folder 5; Records of Secretary-Treasurer, NYH, 1811–1933; NYWCMCA.
32. Werminghaus, *Annie Goodrich*, 23. Goodrich's impact on her students had an enduring effect that sustained them throughout their professional career. Many of the nurses became famous in their own right, devoting their lives to social reforms and strengthening the nursing profession. As an example, Mary Beard was recognized throughout the world for her advocacy of public health and preventive health services.
33. Helen V. Connors, *Laws Regulating the Practice of Nursing* (Lexington, Kentucky: State Governments, 1967).
34. Joseph Hill, *Women in General Occupations*, 1870–1920 (Washington, DC: Government Printing Office, 1929), 4.
35. Winifred Hector, *The Work of Mrs. Bedford Fenwick and the Rise of Professional*

Nursing (London: The Royal College of Nursing and National Council of Nurses of the United Kingdom, 1970), 48. A younger contemporary of Florence Nightingale, Fenwick challenged her on many issues, including the registration of nurses, which Nightingale vehemently opposed. Nightingale believed that the educational program should be of such quality that it would not be necessary for the individual to acquire approval from the government.

36. Ibid., 61.
37. Flanagan, *One Strong Voice*, 41–42, 611. See Nettie Birnbach, "The Genesis of the Nurse Registration Movement in the United States, 1893–1903" (Ed.D. diss., Teachers College, Columbia University, 1982). (University Microfilms International, Catalog Number 8313393.) Since the State laws stipulated that nurses be licensed to practice, the term *licensure* became widely accepted. At the time of the early statutes, however, *registration* was the term universally accepted.
38. M. L. Shannon, "Our First Four Licensure Laws," *American Journal of Nursing* 75 (August 1975), 1329.
39. Bernice Anderson, *The Facilitation of the Interstate Movement of Registered Nurses* (Philadelphia: J.B. Lippincott, 1959), 4.
40. Minutes, Training School Committee, NYH, 28 February 1906; NYWCMCA; Jordan, *Cornell University-New York Hospital*, 39.
41. Minutes, Medical Board, NYH, 5 February 1913; NYWCMCA.
42. Ibid.
43. Ibid.
44. Minutes, Executive Committee, NYH, 6 May 1913; NYWCMCA.
45. Ibid.
46. Anderson, *Facilitation of Interstate Movement*, 36.
47. Minutes, Training School Committee, NYH, 27 February 1907; NYWCMCA.
48. Minutes, Training School Committee, NYH, 29 May 1907, 105; NYWCMCA.
49. Minutes, Training School Committee, NYH, 26 January 1910, and 10 November 1910; NYWCMCA.
50. Minutes, Training School Committee, NYH, 26 May 1909; NYWCMCA.
51. Minutes, Training School Committee, NYH, 27 October 1909; NYWCMCA.
52. Minutes, Training School Committee, NYH, 30 November 1910; NYWCMCA.
53. Opdycke, *No One Was Turned Away*, 45.
54. Ibid., 56.
55. Minutes, Executive Committee, NYH, 16 March 1915; NYWCMCA.
56. Robinson, *Adventures*, 57.
57. Ibid., 60.
58. Ibid., 60–61.
59. Ibid., 61. In the United States, the decline in the number of four-year medical schools was striking, showing a decrease from 155 in 1910 to 76 in 1956. The schools were approved by the American Medical Association and the Council on Medical Education and became an integral part of universities. Cornell University Medical College required a bachelor's degree beginning in 1908 for admission to the school.
60. Richard Olding Beard, "The University Education of the Nurse," paper presented at the Fifteenth Annual Convention of the American Society of Superintendents of Training Schools for Nurses, 1909.
61. Christy, *Cornerstone*, 55–56.
62. M. Adelaide Nutting, "A Report of the Committee on Education, 1911," in *First Words: Selected Addresses from the National League for Nursing, 1894–1933*, Nettie

Birnbach and Sandra Lewenson, edit. (New York: National League for Nursing Press, 1991), 30–34.

63. National League of Nursing Education, *Standard Curriculum for Schools of Nursing, A Report Prepared by the Committee on Education* (Baltimore: Waverly Press, 1917).

64. M. Louise Fitzpatrick, *The National Organization for Public Health Nursing, 1912–1952: Development of a Practice Field* (New York: National League for Nursing, 1975), 30.

65. Ibid., 35

66. Annual Report, NYH, 1914, 100; NYWCMCA.

67. Ibid.

68. Ibid. Anna Reutinger had resigned in 1912 as assistant superintendent to accept the position of chief nurse and matron at Lying-In Hospital.

69. Annual Report, Alumnae Association, 1915; NYWCMCA.

70. Jordan, *Cornell University-New York Hospital*, 46–47.

71. Minutes, Board of Governors, NYH, 1 August 1916; NYWCMCA.

72. Ibid.

73. Raymond Shiland Brown, *The New York Hospital in France: Base Hospital Number Nine, A.E.F.: A History of the Work of The New York Hospital Unit during Two Years of Active Service* (New York: n.p., 1920), 30; NYWCMCA.

74. Minutes, Board of Governors, NYH, 5 September 1916; NYWCMCA.

75. Minutes, Board of Governors, NYH, 8 November 1916; NYWCMCA.

76. Annual Report, NYH, 1917, 42–43; NYWCMCA.

77. Ibid.

78. Brown, *Hospital in France*, 10–11.

79. Ibid.

80. Report, Alumnae Association, in *The Alumnae News* (April 1918), 66–67; NYWCMCA.

81. Annual Report, NYH, 1917, 42; NYWCMCA.

82. Brown, *Hospital in France*, 27–29; NYWCMCA.

83. Ibid., 43.

84. Ibid., 55.

85. Ibid., 73.

86. Finding aid; Julia C. Stimson Papers: 1875–1849; NYWCMCA. Stimson reported that her original group consisted of 65 American nurses, who were assisted by English volunteer aides. Eventually, 30 more nurses joined the unit.

87. Alice H. Friedman, "Julia Catherine Stimson," in *Dictionary of American Nursing*, 350–352. One of the most prominent nurses in the first half of the 20th century, Julia Stimson was known for her dynamic personality and extraordinary leadership style, which became legendary during World War I.

88. Robinson, *Adventures*, 123.

89. Julia Stimson, *Finding Themselves—The Letters of an American Army Chief Nurse in a British Hospital in France* (New York: Macmillan, 1920). Several Stimson letters to her mother have been reprinted in this small anthology. Some of the original handwritten correspondence has been maintained at NYWCMCA along with other letters written to her family, which do not appear in the book.

90. Ibid., 112.

91. Ibid., 113.

92. Ibid., 117.

93. Ibid., 220.
94. Ibid., 231.
95. Report, Alumnae Association, April 1920, 9; NYWCMC; See Friedman, "Julia C. Stimson," in *Dictionary of American Nursing*, 352.
96. Anna Reutinger to Irene Sutliffe, letter, 10 November 1918; box 1; Irene Sutliffe Papers: 1878–1940; NYWCMCA.
97. Minutes, Board of Governors, NYH, 4 March 1918; NYWCMCA.
98. Ibid.
99. Ibid.
100. Minutes, Board of Governors, NYH, 15 March 1918; NYWCMCA.
101. Ibid.
102. Minutes, Board of Governors, NYH, 3 February 1920; NYWCMCA.
103. Annie Goodrich, "Contributions of the Army School of Nursing," *Proceedings of the Twenty Fifth Annual Convention of the National League of Nursing Education*, Chicago, 24–28 June 1919, 47–48; NLNE Archive.

CHAPTER 5

1. "Immigration Restrictions in the 1920s": http://www.msu.edu/course/mc/112/1920s/Immigration/index.html (accessed 9/30/2005). People emigrated from other countries to seek better economic conditions in America, but they were often exposed to strong feelings of prejudice and nationalism. Many immigrants became victims of discrimination in the work place in addition to facing a host of other problems. They represented various ethnic groups and within large cities, like New York, herded together forming their own groups in discrete communities.
2. E. Poole, *Nurses on Horseback* (New York: Macmillan, 1932), 1–3, 16.
3. Hawkins, "Mary Breckinridge," in *Dictionary of American Nursing*, 41.
4. Hawkins, "Margaret Louise Sanger," in *Dictionary of American Nursing*, 322–325.
5. Ibid., 324.
6. Susan Reverby, "The Search for the Hospital Yardstick: Nursing and the Rationalization of Hospital Work," in *Health Care in American Life: Essays in Social History*, Susan Reverby and David Rosner, edit. (Philadelphia: Temple University Press: 1979), 213.
7. Nightingale often cited "character" as the quintessential attribute of the pupil nurse. "Character, character, character, all the influences of the training and the organization must be to form or develop her character," she stated. "God, decency, no overcrowding interest for her leisure moment. . . discipline, obedience to order, all that tends to form character." Nightingale Papers, Vol. CLXIV, British Museum.
8. Annual Report, NYH, 1921, 52; NYWCMCA.
9. Minutes, Executive Committee, NYH, 30 December 1919; NYWCMCA
10. Reverby, "The Search for the Hospital Yardstick," 206.
11. Ibid.
12. Annual Report, NYH, 1921, 51; NYWCMCA.
13. Annual Report, NYH, 1922, 56; NYWCMCA.
14. Annual Report, NYH, 1920, 51; NYWCMCA.
15. Annual Report, NYH, 1925, 44; NYWCMCA. In 1924, 36 affiliate students from

other schools sought theoretical and practical instruction in the various services. A total of 40 students from the Training School went on affiliation to outside institutions in addition to the 25 obtaining obstetrical training.

16. *Nursing and Nursing Education in the United States: Report of the Committee for the Study of Nursing Education* (New York: Macmillan, 1923). The report was named after Josephine Goldmark, a sociologist and the principal investigator of the study.
17. Christy, *Cornerstone*, 67.
18. Werminghaus, *Annie Goodrich*, 79.
19. Hawkins, "Annie Warburton Goodrich," in *Dictionary of American Nursing*, 155.
20. Ibid.
21. Ibid.
22. Higgins, "Mary Beard," in *Dictionary of American Nursing*, 22.
23. Christy, *Cornerstone*, 82–83.
24. Robert Piemonte, "A History of the National League of Nursing Education: Great Awakening in Nursing Education, 1912–1932" (Ed.D. diss., Teachers College, Columbia University, 1976). (University Microfilms International, Catalog Number 7617291.)
25. Ibid.
26. Christy, *Cornerstone*, 62.
27. Piemonte, "History of National League."
28. Minutes, Executive Committee, NYH, 5 April 1927; NYWCMCA.
29. *Commemorative Exercises of the School of Nursing of the New York Hospital, Fiftieth Anniversary, 1877–1927* (New York: The Society of the New York Hospital, 1927); NYWCMCA.
30. Ibid.
31. Ibid.
32. Ibid., 44.
33. Annual Report, NYH, 1927, 45; NYWCMCA.
34. Minutes, Board of Governors, NYH, 14 June 1927; NYWCMCA.
35. Minutes, Board of Governors, NYH, 2 March 1920; NYWCMCA.
36. Minutes, Board of Governors, NYH, 2 January 1923; NYWCMCA.
37. Minutes, Board of Governors, NYH, 2 October 1923; NYWCMCA.
38. Minutes, Board of Governors, NYH, 6 May 1924; NYWCMCA.
39. Minutes, Board of Governors, NYH, 25 May 1927; NYWCMCA.
40. Minutes, Board of Governors, NYH, 7 December 1926; NYWCMCA.
41. Ibid.
42. Larrabee, *The Benevolent*, 314.
43. Minutes, Board of Governors, NYH, 1 November 1927; NYWCMCA.
44. Robinson, *Adventures*, 198.
45. Ibid., 199.
46. Annual Report, NYH, 1927, 45; NYWCMCA.
47. Ibid.
48. Annual Report, NYH, 1928, 24–25; NYWCMCA.
49. Ibid, 44.
50. Bishop, *History of Cornell*, 515. Robinson was also appointed director of the Medical College but he did not hold the official title of dean.
51. Robinson, *Adventures*, 184.

52. Ibid., 201.
53. Ibid., 184.
54. Bishop, *History of Cornell*, 516. "Black Friday" occurred during the fateful October of 1929. In the days that followed, the resources of NYH were greatly reduced.
55. Robinson, *Adventures*, 199.
56. Ibid.
57. Larrabee, *The Benevolent*, 319.
58. Robinson, *Adventures*, 184.
59. Minutes, Board of Governors, NYH, 2 April 1929; NYWCMCA.
60. Ibid. See Jordan, *Cornell University-New York Hospital*, 54–55.
61. Jordan, *Cornell University-New York Hospital*, 55.
62. Robinson, *Adventures*, 218.
63. Jordan, *Cornell University-New York Hospital*, 60.
64. Minutes, Board of Governors, NYH, 1 July 1930; NYWCMCA.
65. Ibid.
66. Robinson, *Adventures*, 216.
67. Jordan, *Cornell University-New York Hospital*, 60–61.
68. Minutes, Board of Governors, NYH, 2 June 1931; NYWCMCA. Before Mary Beard approached Anna Wolf, the Committee on Nursing Organization approved Canby Robinson's request to ascertain Julia Stimson's interest in the position of director. At a meeting in Washington, DC, Stimson told Robinson that she preferred to continue in her present position as dean of the Army School of Nursing. Minutes, Joint Administrative Board, NYH-CMC, 20 November 1930; NYWCMCA.
69. Hawkins, "Anna Dryden Wolf," in *Dictionary of American Nursing*, 406.
70. Mary Roberts, *Nursing: History and Interpretation*, 223.
71. Hawkins, "Anna Dryden Wolf," in *Dictionary of American Nursing*, 406.
72. Ibid.
73. Transcript of Doris Schwartz interview with Anna Wolf at Wesley Palms, San Diego, California, 1970; NYWCMCA. A long time faculty member, nurse researcher, and innovator, Schwartz made important contributions to nursing and health care at CU-NYHSN as well as to the nursing profession.
74. Minutes, Board of Governors, NYH, 7 July 1931; NYWCMCA. Following Minnie Jordan's retirement, the Alumnae Association established a scholarship fund in her name.
75. Minutes, Board of Governors, NYH, 2 February 1932; NYWCMCA.
76. Ibid.
77. Annual Report, NYH, 1938, 20–21; NYWCMCA.
78. Transcript of Doris Schwartz interview with Anna Wolf, 1970; NYWCMCA.
79. Ibid.
80. Transcript of Doris Schwartz interview with Margery T. Overholzer, 21 July 1970; NYWCMCA. Margery Oberholzer held three different positions during her tenure of 28 years at NYH. Following an earlier interest in maternal nursing, she eventually turned to public health nursing and became the head of the department. She also held the academic title of associate professor of public health nursing.
81. Transcript of Doris Schwartz interview with Anna Wolf, 1970; NYWCMCA.
82. Ibid.
83. Ibid.

84. Anna Wolf to Dr. G. Howard Wise, letter, 23 May 1932; box 1, folder 1; Records of Council, CU-NYHSN, 1931–1939; NYWCMCA.

85. Ibid.

86. Minutes, Board of Governors, NYH, 31 May 1932; NYWCMCA.

87. Minutes, Executive Committee, NYH, 2 August 1932; NYWCMCA.

88. Larrabee, *The Benevolent*, 316. The architecture of the building was modeled after the Palace of the Popes in Avignon, France, "with its rugged mass, Gothic grandeur, tall pointed windows." Bishop, *A History of Cornell University*, 516.

89. Jordan, *Cornell University-New York Hospital*, 59.

90. Annual Report, NYH, 1932, 27; NYWCMCA.

91. Ibid.

92. Minutes, Board of Governors, NYH, 7 June 1932; NYWCMCA.

93. Annual Report, NYH, 1932, 33; NYWCMCA.

94. Transcript of Doris Schwartz interview with Bessie A.R. Parker, 24 July 1981, NYWCMCA. In 1932, Parker joined the staff of NYH as evening administrative assistant, and four years later was appointed assistant director of nursing and head of the department of medical and surgical nursing. After Anna Wolf resigned in 1940, she became director of nursing service and acting dean of the new university school of nursing.

95. Ibid.

96. Ibid.

97. *The Architectural Forum* (February 1933), 108; NYWCMCA.

98. Jordan, *Cornell University-New York Hospital*, 62.

99. Minutes, Board of Directors, NYH, 2 August 1932; NYWCMCA.

100. Anna Wolf's letter appeared in the *Student Handbook*, 1933–1934, published by the Student Organization. In 1935, the School's name was officially changed to The New York Hospital School of Nursing. Minutes, Executive Committee, NYH, 12 November 1935; NYWCMCA.

101. Annual Report, NYH, 1932, 27; NYWCMCA.

102. Ibid., 27,30.

103. Annual Report, NYH, 1933, 31; NYWCMCA.

104. Ibid.

105. Annual Report, NYH, 1932, 31; NYWCMCA.

106. *Proceedings of a Conference of the Proposed Association of Collegiate Schools of Nursing*, Teachers College, Columbia University, 20–21 January 1933, typescript (New York: Sophia F. Palmer Library, American Journal of Nursing Company).

107. Ibid.

108. Nellie Hawkinson, President's Address, Proceedings of the Forty-third Annual Convention of the NLNE, Boston, Massachusetts, 1937, in Birnbach and Lewenson, *Legacy of Leadership*, 306.

109. Friedman, "Euphemia Jane Taylor," in *Dictionary of American Nursing*, 362–364. A graduate of the Johns Hopkins School of Nursing, Effie Taylor followed Annie Goodrich as the second nursing dean at Yale. At the time of the founding of the ACSN, she was president of the National League of Nursing Education.

110. Jordan, *Cornell University-New York Hospital*, 64.

111. Minutes, Board of Governors, NYH, 8 April 1932; NYWCMCA.

112. Ibid.

113. Minutes, Executive Committee, NYH, 9 October 1934; NYWCMCA.

114. Opdycke, *No One Was Turned Away*, 88.
115. Annual Report, NYH, 1935, 20; NYWCMCA.
116. Minutes, Council, CU-NYHSN, 31 January 1934; NYWCMCA.
117. Ibid.
118. Ibid.
119. Bishop, *History of Cornell*, 516.
120. Robinson, *Adventures*, 221.
121. Ibid.
122. Ibid.

CHAPTER 6

1. "The Social Security Act and the Nurse," *American Journal of Nursing* 36, No. 12 (February 1936), 153–155.
2. Ibid. See also Philip Kalisch and Beatrice Kalisch, *The Advance of American Nursing* (Boston: Little, Brown and Company, 1978), 432.
3. "Analysis of Roosevelt's New Deal": http://cyberessays.com/History/84.htm (accessed 9/30/2005).
4. "Livingston Farrand": http://www.cornell.edu/president/history_bio_farrand.cfm (accessed 9/30/2005).
5. Kammen, *Cornell - Glorious to View*, 105.
6. Ibid., 125. Dr. Day became the fifth president of Cornell University.
7. Kalisch and Kalisch, *The Advance of American Nursing*, 498, 501.
8. Address of President Nellie Hawkinson, *Proceedings of the Forty-third Annual Convention of the National League of Nursing Education*, Boston, Massachusetts, 1937, in Birnbach and Lewenson, *Legacy of Leadership*, 306.
9. Christy, *Cornerstone*, 86.
10. Ibid.
11. Report, Executive Secretary, *A Curriculum Guide for Schools of Nursing*, 1937; NLNE Archive, microfilm #3.
12. Minutes, Council, NYH School of Nursing, 14 April 1938; NYWCMCA.
13. Address of President Nellie Hawkinson, *Proceedings of the Forty-fifth Annual Convention of the National League of Nursing Education*, New Orleans, Louisiana, 1939, in Birnbach and Lewenson, *Legacy of Leadership*, 324–325.
14. Annual Report, Department of Measurement and Guidance, National League of Nursing Education, 1951; NLNE Archive, microfilm #5. See Minutes, Board of Directors, NLNE, January 1952, 21–25; NLNE Archive.
15. Ibid.
16. Transcript of Doris Schwartz interview with Margery Overholzer, 21 July 1970; NYWCMCA.
17. Minutes, Council, NYH School of Nursing, 11 April 1940; NYWCMCA.
18. Annual Report, NYH, 1935, 47; NYWCMCA.
19. Transcript of Doris Schwartz interview with Anna Wolf, 1970; NYWCMCA.
20. Hawkins, "Anna Dryden Wolf," in *Dictionary of American Nursing*, 406–407.
21. Transcript of Doris Schwartz interview with Anna Wolf, 1970; NYWCMCA.
22. Minutes, Council, NYH School of Nursing, 18 November 1937; NYWCMCA.
23. Ibid.
24. Ibid.

25. Annual Report, NYH, 1935, 25; NYWCMCA.
26. Ibid.
27. Ibid., 48.
28. Annual Report, NYH, 1938, 102; NYWCMCA.
29. Annual Report, NYH, 1937, 72; NYWCMCA.
30. Ibid., 72–73.
31. Annual Report, NYH, 1938, 87; NYWCMCA.
32. Annual Report, NYH, 1937, 74; NYWCMCA.
33. Ibid., 58.
34. Ibid., 23.
35. Ibid., 67.
36. Lillian Wald to Alumnae Association, NYH School of Nursing, 4 June 1937; box 3, folder 17; Records of Office of the Dean, CU-NYHSN: 1920–1970; NYWCM-CA.
37. Ibid.
38. Minutes, Council, NYH School of Nursing, 18 November 1937; NYWCMCA. Included is Anna Wolf's report of the 60th anniversary of the School.
39. Livingston Farrand had a long time interest in public health concerns. Prior to World War I, he served as director of the International Anti-Tuberculosis Commission under the International Health Provisions of the Rockefeller Foundation. His success in that effort led to an appointment after the war as chairman of the Central Committee of the American Red Cross.
40. Annual Report, NYH, 1937, 67; NYWCMCA. As requested in her will, Irene Sutliffe was buried next to Laura York, the abandoned baby girl that she grew to love and care for when directress of the Training School in the 1890s.
41. Transcript of Doris Schwartz interview with Anna Wolf, 1970; NYWCMCA.
42. Anna Wolf to Edmund Day, letter, 26 October 1937; box 1, folder 1; Records of Council, CU-NYHSN: 1931–1939; NYWCMCA.
43. Minutes, Council, NYH School of Nursing, 10 November 1938; NYWCMCA.
44. Minutes, Council, NYH School of Nursing, 23 January 1939; NYWCMCA.
45. Minutes, Council, NYH School of Nursing, 1 April 1939; NYWCMCA.
46. Minutes, Council, NYH School of Nursing, 29 May 1939; NYWCMCA.
47. Minutes, Executive Committee, NYH, 6 June 1939; NYWCMCA.
48. Minutes, Board of Governors, NYH, 6 June 1939; NYWCMCA.
49. Minutes, Board of Governors, NYH, 8 November 1939; NYWCMCA.
50. Ibid.
51. Minutes, Board of Governors, NYH, 4 November 1939; Minutes, Joint Administrative Board, NYH-CMC, 31 December 1939; NYWCMCA. Farrand had served on the JAB from its inception until he retired in July 1937. Excerpts from *The New York Times* obituary were reproduced in the *Cornell Daily Sun* (4 October 1963); NYWCMCA.
52. Minutes, Faculty, NYH School of Nursing, 12 December 1939; NYWCMCA. Margaret Farrand to Margaret Wyatt, letter, 31 May 1940; Livingston Farrand biographical folder; NYWCMCA. Veronica Lyons later succeeded Margaret Wyatt, Assistant Director of the School.
53. Annual Report, NYH, 1939, 34–35; NYWCMCA.
54. Ibid., 22.
55. Ibid. On 16 March 1938, an arrangement took place between NYH and the New

York City Board of Health to open the Kips Bay-Yorkville Health and Teaching Center. The facility aimed to provide services and improve health conditions of low-income residents in the community. Annual Report, NYH, 1938, 20; NYW-CMCA.

56. Annual Report, NYH, 1939, 19; NYWCMCA. In 1947, Manhattan Maternity Hospital and Nursery and Child's Hospital merged with Long Island Hospital of the City of New York.

57. Minutes, Council, NYH School of Nursing, 1 November 1939; NYWCMCA. Dr. George Heuer had been a disciple of Dr. William Halsted at Johns Hopkins when Canby Robinson recruited him earlier in the decade to NYH-CMC.

58. Minutes, Executive Faculty, Cornell University Medical College (CUMC), 15 December 1939; NYWCMCA.

59. Ibid.

60. Minutes, JAB, NYH-CMC, 21 December 1939; NYWCMCA.

61. Ibid.

62. Transcript of Judith Allen interview with Margery Overholzer, August 1980; NYWCMCA.

63. The Alumnae News, Vol. 13, No. 2 (April 1940), 2; NYWCMCA. Julia Stimson was outgoing president of the Alumnae Association at the time.

64. Transcript of Doris Schwartz interview with Anna Wolf, 1970; NYWCMCA.

65. Eugene Dubois to Executive Faculty, CUMC, memorandum concerning "The Question of Establishing a New York Hospital Training School for Nurses on a Collegiate Basis"; Minutes, Executive Faculty, CUMC, 14 May 1940; NYWCMCA.

66. Ibid.

67. Ibid.

68. Ibid. Anna Wolf greatly admired Eugene Dubois and viewed his concept of care and education as remarkable. In an interview with Doris Schwartz (1970), she reiterated Dr. Dubois' comment: "You can face the trouble when you have something constructive to work on. That's the thing to look for in leadership."

69. The Alumnae News, Vol. 13, No. 3 (July 1940), 5; NYWCMCA. During President Henry's administration, Mrs. Charles S. Payson was elected to the Board of Governors, NYH. She was the first female member to serve on the Board.

70. Minutes, Council, NYH School of Nursing, March 1940; NYWCMCA. At the meeting, Wolf shared her view of what had been accomplished during her eight and a half years as director of the School. She stated her purpose in accepting the position was to care for patients and to teach students; "We tried to set up a professional school and we selected personnel carefully. An attempt was made to establish a nursing service and practices that met the best standards of nursing."

71. Hawkins, "Anna Dryden Wolf," in Dictionary of American Nursing, 407.

72. Minutes, Board of Directors, American Nurses Association, 22 January 1939; Archive of the American Nurses Association (ANA Archive).

73. Ibid., 10. The action of the ANA Board stemmed from a recommendation of the Oregon State Nurses Association that requested the parent organization to consider further study and consolidate ANA, NLNE, and NOPHN.

74. Minutes, Board of Governors, NYH, 4 June 1940; NYWCMCA.

75. The Alumnae News, Vol. 13, No. 2 (April 1940), 4; NYWCMCA.

76. Transcript of Doris Schwartz interview with Bessie Parker, 24 July 1970; NYW-CMCA.

77. Transcript of Doris Schwartz interview with Henderika Rynbergen, November 1970; NYWCMCA. A non-nurse and professor of science at the School from 1934 to 1961, Rynbergen taught chemistry, nutrition, and physiology.
78. Transcript of Judith Allen interview with Marjory Overholzer, August 1980; NYWCMCA.
79. Minutes, JAB, NYH-CMC, 18 April 1940; NYWCMCA.
80. Minutes, Executive Committee, NYH, 4 June 1940; NYWCMCA.
81. Minutes, Executive Committee, NYH, 15 October 1940; NYWCMCA.
82. Minutes, Executive Committee, NYH, 20 August 1940; NYWCMCA.
83. Minutes, Council, NYH School of Nursing, 28 May 1940; NYWCMCA.
84. Annual Report, NYH, 1940, 86; NYWCMCA.
85. Minutes, Council, NYH School of Nursing, 28 May 1940; NYWCMCA.
86. Annual Report, NYH, 1940, 86; NYWCMCA.
87. *The Alumnae News*, Vol. 14, No. 1 (1941), 17, NYWCMCA.
88. Minutes, Executive Faculty, CUMC, 4 June 1941; NYWCMCA.
89. Minutes, Executive Faculty, CUMC, 18 December 1941; NYWCMCA.
90. JAB, NYH-CMC to Nursing Council, memorandum, 6 January 1942; box 1, folder 2; Records of Council, NYH School of Nursing: 1940–1942; NYWCMCA. Includes plan of the New York Hospital-Cornell University School of Nursing.
91. Minutes, Council, NYH School of Nursing, 9 January 1942; NYWCMCA.
92. Ibid.
93. Ibid.
94. William Jackson to Edmond Day, letter, 15 January 1942; box 1, folder 1; Records of Office of the Dean, CU-NYHSN: 1942–1983; NYWCMCA.
95. Proceedings, Board of Trustees, CU, 24 January 1942; NYWCMCA.
96. Ibid.
97. Minutes, Executive Committee, NYH, 17 February 1942; NYWCMCA.
98. Minutes, JAB, NYH-CMC, 26 February 1942; NYWCMCA.
99. Minutes, Council, NYH School of Nursing, 19 May 1942; NYWCMCA.
100. Ibid.
101. Annual Report, NYH, 1942, 54; NYWCMCA.
102. Bishop, *History of Cornell*, 549.
103. Report of the President, CU, 1942–1943, 11; NYWCMCA.

CHAPTER 7

1. Flanagan, *One Strong Voice*, 113–114.
2. Ibid., 114. See Friedman, "Julia Catherine Stimson," in *Dictionary of American Nursing*, 350–352. Stimson served as President of the ANA from 1938 to 1944. On October 4, 1942, she was a violin soloist at a benefit in New York for the Nursing Council for National Defense. *The Alumnae News*, Vol. 13, No. 4 (October 1942), 2; NYWCMCA.
3. "A Date Which Will Live in Infamy," draft of President Roosevelt's speech, 8 December 1941: http://www.archives.gov/education/lessons/day-of-infamy/ (accessed 9/30/2005).
4. Report of the President, CU, 1941–1942, 5; NYWCMCA.
5. Minutes, Board of Directors, NLNE, 22–24 October 1945; NLNE Archive, microfilm #5. Voting members of the National Council included the ACSN, ANA,

NLNE, National Association of Colored Graduate Nurses, NOPHN, and the American Red Cross Nursing Service. In 1942, the American Association of Industrial Nurses became a member.

6. Hawkins, "Anna Dryden Wolf," in *Dictionary of American Nursing*, 407.

7. "Ninth General Hospital Unit Report for Duty," *The Pulse*, Vol. IV (July 1942); NYWCMCA. *The Pulse* was the official house organ of NYH-CMC employees. Marie Troup Papers: 1927–1982; box 1, folder 6; NYWCMCA.

8. Ibid. Marie Troup Papers. Troup was director of the Nursing Bureau of Westchester, NY, from 1936 to 1942. Later commissioned as Lieutenant Marie Troup, she had served with the Ninth General Base Hospital Unit in Brisbane, Australia, New Guinea, and other islands in the South Pacific. In 1944, the ANA worked to secure legislation granting commissioned rank to nurses in military service. Flanagan, *One Strong Voice*, 621.

9. "Ninth General Hospital Report for Duty," *The Pulse*, Vol. IV (July 1942), 1; NYW-CMCA.

10. Bessie Parker to Marie Troup, letter, 10 August 1942; box 1, folder 13; Marie Troup Papers: 1927–1982; NYWCMCA.

11. *The Alumnae News*, Vol. 16, No. 1 (January 1943), 10–11; NYWCMCA.

12. Marie Troup to Bessie Parker, letter, 29 April 1946; box 9, folder 6; Records of Office of the Dean, CU-NYHSN: 1923–1963; NYWCMCA.

13. Ibid. In the late 1950s, Muriel Carbery was appointed the second dean of CU-NYHSN and director of nursing service at NYH.

14. Annual Report, NYH, 1942, 15–16; NYWCMCA.

15. Ibid., 16.

16. Minutes, Executive Committee, NYH, 18 December 1941; NYWCMCA.

17. Minutes, Board of Governors, NYH, 9 November 1943; NYWCMCA.

18. Ibid.

19. Annual Report, NYH, 1943, 21; NYWCMCA

20. Minutes, Board of Governors, NYH, 6 October 1941; NYWCMCA.

21. Annual Report, NYH, 1942, 27; NYWCMCA.

22. Minutes, Council, NYH School of Nursing, 9 January 1942; NYWCMCA.

23. Minutes, Board of Governors, NYH, 8 June 1943; NYWCMCA.

24. Minutes, Executive Committee, NYH, 6 May 1941; NYWCMCA.

25. Annual Report, NYH, 1944, 6; NYWCMCA.

26. Minutes, Executive Committee, NYH, 19 December 1944; NYWCMCA. Sister Elizabeth Kenny's title had no religious affiliation, having been bestowed as military rank to nurses in the Australian Medical Corps, in which she served during World War I. Trained as a vocational nurse, she became a controversial figure among some members of the medical community, who rejected her treatment of hot packs and physical therapy for poliomyelitis rather than the traditional practice of immobilization.

27. Annual Report, NYH, 1944, 6; NYWCMCA.

28. Dr. George N. Papanicolaou served on the pathology staff of NYH from 1914 to 1961. He also was on the anatomy faculty of CUMC, director of the Papanicolaou Research Laboratory, and consultant to the Papanicolaou Cytolology Laboratory at the Medical College. Stuart Galishoff, "George Nicolas Papanicolaou," in *Dictionary of Medical Biography*, Vol. II, 576–577.

29. *The Alumnae News*, Vol. 22, No. 4 (Winter 1948), 13–14; NYWCMCA

30. Annual Report, NYH, 1942, 54; NYWCMCA. In 1944, Bessie Parker was appointed acting dean of the School and acting director of nursing service for a term of one year until determining her future status.
31. Minutes, Executive Faculty, CU-NYHSN, 5 August 1942; NYWCMCA.
32. Ibid.
33. Minutes, Executive Faculty, CU-NYHSN, 18 September 1942; NYWCMCA.
34. Annual Report, NYH, 1942, 54; NYWCMCA.
35. Minutes, Executive Committee, NYH, 2 September 1941; NYWCMCA.
36. Minutes, JAB, NYH-CMC, 12 November 1942; NYWCMCA.
37. Minutes, Council, NYH School of Nursing, 19 March 1942; NYWCMCA.
38. Ibid.
39. *Announcements*, CU-NYHSN, Vol. 34, No. 5 (September 1942), 8–9; NYWCMCA.
40. Ibid.
41. Ibid., 10.
42. Ibid., 11.
43. Ibid., 13.
44. Ibid., 16.
45. Ibid., 54.
46. Ibid. See Shirley H. Fondiller, "The Promise and the Reality, 1944–1992," *Healing at Home: Visiting Nurse Service of New York, 1893–1993* (New York: Visiting Nurse Service of New York, 1993), 17. With the advent of World War II, the Henry Street Settlement and the Visiting Nurse Service of New York (VNSNY) evolved in different paths in relation to other aims, administrative concerns, needs, and community focus. In 1944, the VNSNY became a freestanding agency committed to meeting an important community need.
47. Minutes, JAB, NYH-CMC, 18 February 1943; NYWCMCA.
48. Minutes, JAB, NYH-CMC, 13 March 1943; NYWCMCA.
49. Minutes, Board of Governors, NYH, 6 April 1943; NYWCMCA. Lucile Petry had an impressive background at University of Minnesota as associate professor and assistant dean in the school of nursing. Eager to pursue further graduate work, she entered the nursing program at Teachers College at Columbia University, but her studies were interrupted by an appointment in 1941 with the U.S. Public Health Service in Washington, DC, where she had the distinction of being the first woman administrator. Two years later, she accepted the position of dean at CU-NYHSN, but was recalled to the Division of Nursing Education to direct the U.S. Cadet Nurse Corps. In 1965, while attending a meeting of the National League for Nursing in New York, Lucile Petry Leone was a guest of the nursing faculty at the Medical Center's Griffis Faculty Club.
50. Beatrice J. Kalisch and Philip A. Kalisch, "Cadet Nurse, The Girl with a Future," *Nursing Outlook* 21 (July 1973), 445. See Thelma Robinson and Paulie Perry, *Cadet Nurse Stories* (Indianapolis, Indiana: Sigma Theta Tau International, 2001).
51. Lucile Petry, Director of the Division of Nursing Education, U.S. Public Health Service; Report of the U.S. Cadet Nurse Corps; NLNE Board Minutes, 22–26 January 1945, 336; NLNE Archive, microfilm #4.
52. The Honorable Frances Payne Bolton (R-Ohio) was a long time supporter of the nursing profession.
53. Lucile Petry, Director of the Division of Nursing Education, U.S. Public Health Service; Report of the U.S. Cadet Nurse Corps; NLNE Board Minutes, 22–26

January 1945, 336; NLNE Archive, microfilm #4.

54. Annual Report, Department of Measurement and Guidance, National League of Nursing Education, 1951, 3; NLNE Board Minutes, 21–25 January 1952; NLNE Archive, microfilm #5.

55. Annual Report, Acting Dean, CU-NYHSN, in Report of the President, CU, 1943–1944, appendix xxvi; NYWCMCA.

56. *The Alumnae News*, Vol. 17, No. 3 (Fall 1944), 9; NYWCMCA.

57. Annual Report, NYH, 1944, 23; NYWCMCA.

58. *The Alumnae News*, Vol. 17, No. 3 (Fall 1944), 9; NYWCMCA.

59. Bylaws, NYH, chapter XIII, 1944, 12; NYWCMCA.

60. Ibid., 8.

61. Minutes, Board of Governors, NYH, 7 March 1944; NYWCMCA. On 8 June 1944, the Board of Governors announced Parker's official appointment as acting dean with a limited term at the discretion of the Board.

62. Minutes, Executive Committee, NYH, 31 August 1943; NYWCMCA.

63. Transcript of Doris Schwartz interview with Bessie A. R. Parker, 24 July 1970; NYWCMCA.

64. Communication to Bessie Parker, statement, 26 June 1944; folder: 1944–1954; Records of Council, CU-NYHSN: 1931–1970; NYWCMCA.

65. Ibid.

66. Minutes, JAB, NYH-CMC, 21 June 1944; NYWCMCA. The JAB approved two nursing representatives to serve on the Council, which required only one member to be an alumna. The membership was eventually increased to include one individual each from the fields of public health and education, and a layperson. Minutes, JAB, NYH-CMC, 21 June 1946; NYWCMCA.

67. Annual Report, Acting Dean, CU-NYHSN, in Report of the President, CU, 1943–1944, appendix xxvi; NYWCMCA.

68. Ibid.

69. Minutes, Board of Directors, NLNE, 22–26 January 1945, 17; NLNE Archive, microfilm #4.

70. Annual Report, Acting Dean, CU-NYHSN, in Report of the President, CU, 1944–1945, appendix xxv; NYWCMCA.

71. Annual Report, NYH, 1945, 6; NYWCMCA.

72. Ibid.

73. Ibid., 10–11.

74. V-J Day occurred in August, but it was not until 12 September 1945, that the articles of surrender took place.

75. *The Alumnae News*, Vol. 19, No. 3 (Winter 1945), 4; NYWCMCA.

76. Ibid. In April 1943, the Executive Committee had recommended that the seal of the Society and the name of the School be engraved on the medal. At the 28 September 1945 exercises, the graduating class wore a white organdy cap of the School, a white long sleeved uniform, and a shoulder corsage of red rosebuds tied with a silver ribbon. Sitting behind the graduates were the lower classmen, with some wearing the traditional blue plaid and others donning a new look in a blue and white checked uniform.

77. Marie Troup to Bessie Parker, letter, 9 September 1945; box 9, folder 6; Records of Office of the Dean, CU-NYHSN: 1927–1963; NYWCMCA.

78. Ibid. A meritorious service plaque was awarded to the Ninth General Base

Hospital Unit by the commanding general in the Pacific Theatre.

79. "The Nurses' Contribution to American Victory," *American Journal of Nursing* 45, No. 9 (September 1945), 683.
80. S. H. McGuire and D. W. Conrad, "Postwar Plans of Army and Navy Nurses," *American Journal of Nursing* 46, No. 3 (March 1946), 305–306.
81. Ibid.
82. Ibid.
83. Report of the President, CU, 1945–1946, 6; NYWCMCA. The term "Hicksite" refers to the liberal body of Quakers, named after their founder Elias Hicksite, an early American preacher.
84. Ibid.
85. Ibid., 5.
86. Annual Report, NYH, 1945, 5; NYWCMCA.
87. Ibid., 10.
88. Ibid., 23.
89. Minutes, JAB, NYH-CMC, 25 April 1945; NYWCMCA.
90. Alma S. Woolley, "Virginia Matthews Dunbar," in *American Nursing—A Biographical Dictionary*, Vol. 3, Vern L. Bullough and Lillie Senz, edit. (New York: Springer Publishing, 1992), 76. See Minutes, Board of Governors, NYH, 5 February 1948; NYWCMCA.
91. Transcript of Judith Allen interview with Virginia Dunbar, 10 July 1980; NYWCMCA.
92. Minutes, JAB, NYH-CMC, 25 March 1945; NYWCMCA.
93. Transcript of Judith Allen interview with Virginia Dunbar, 10 July 1980; NYWCMCA.
94. Ibid.
95. Hawkins, "Annie Warburton Goodrich," in *Dictionary of American Nursing*, 156.
96. *The Alumnae News*, Vol. 20, No. 2 (Summer 1946), 9; NYWCMCA. On the occasion of Goodrich's 80th birthday, the Yale School of Nursing published an engagement calendar for the year 1946, which showed various stages of her career.
97. Minutes, Board of Governors, NYH, 5 February 1946; NYWCMCA. Transcript of Judith Allen interview with Virginia Dunbar, 10 July 1980; NYWCMCA.
98. Ibid.
99. Ibid.
100. Ibid.
101. Ibid.
102. Woolley, "Virginia Matthews Dunbar," in *American Nursing—A Biographical Dictionary*, 76.
103. Ibid.
104. Helene Jamieson Jordan, "Virginia Dunbar," *The Alumnae News*, Vol. 32, No. 2, (Winter 1958), 6; NYWCMCA.
105. Ibid.
106. Ibid.
107. Ibid. See transcript of Judith Allen interview with Veronica Lyons Roehner, July 1980; NYWCMCA.
108. Transcript of Judith Allen interview with Veronica Lyons Roehner, July 1980; NYWCMCA.
109. Annual Report, Dean, CU-NYHSN in Report of the President, CU, 1945–1946,

appendix xxvi; NYWCMCA.

110. Ibid.

111. Ibid.

112. Ibid.

113. Ibid.

114. Minutes, Board of Governors, NYH, 1 October 1945; NYWCMCA.

115. Ibid.

116. Minutes, Council, CU-NYHSN, 30 October 1946; NYWCMCA.

117. Ibid.

118. Ibid. On 30 April 1948, Dunbar presented a paper on "The Adventure of Thinking Together," at the Boston College School of Nursing, in which she elaborated as follows: "Picking people's brains is a highly respectable occupation. The kind of experience I am referring to gives a sense of being close to people you are working with, of seeing people think. It gives a taste of the excitement of thinking together." Records of Office of the Dean, CU-NYHSN: 1923–1963; box 8, folder 4; NYWCMCA.

119. Annual Report, Dean, CU-NYHSN in Report of the President, CU, 1945–1946, appendix xxvi; NYWCMCA.

120. Report of Public Relations Activities of CU-NYHSN in Minutes, Council, CU-NYHSN, 30 October 1946; NYWCMCA.

121. Ibid.

122. Ibid.

123. Ibid.

124. Ibid.

125. Minutes, Board of Directors, NLNE, 9–10 November 1947; NLNE Archive, microfilm #4.

126. Hospital diploma schools constituted the largest number of basic nursing programs, reaching almost 1200 by 1947.

127. Report of Committee on Statement of Principles, 9–10 November 1947, attached to Minutes, Board of Directors, NLNE, 22–27 January 1947; NLNE Archive, microfilm #4. Anna Wolf had served as chairmen of this important committee.

128. A study of six national nursing organizations was launched in April 1946 under the direction of Raymond Rich Associates, a well-known firm of counselors on public relations, management, and educational promotion. The implications of the Rich Report followed years of arduous debate among the nursing organizations until 1952 when consolidation took place. It produced two major national organizations, the American Nurses Association and the National League for Nursing. See Report of the Joint Coordinating Committee on Structure of the Six National Nursing Organizations in Minutes, Board of Directors, NLNE, 21–25 January 1952; NLNE Archive, microfilm #5.

CHAPTER 8

1. Kalisch and Kalisch, "Cadet Nurse," 445.

2. Annual Report, Dean, CU-NYHSN, in Report of the President, CU, 1946–1947, appendix xxvii; NYWCMCA. The graduating class was admitted to the School in 1943.

3. Ibid.

4. Ibid.
5. Ibid.
6. Minutes, JAB, NYH-CMC, 24 October 1947; NYWCMCA.
7. Transcript of Judith Allen interview with Virginia Dunbar, 10 July 1980; NYWCMCA.
8. "In Memoriam," *The Window* (1999), in Constance Derrell biographical file; NYWCMCA. A native of Trinidad, West Indies, Derrell graduated from Lincoln Hospital School of Nursing, one of only two nursing schools in New York City that admitted black students.
9. Annual Report, Dean, CU-NYHSN, in Report of the President, CU, 1946–1947, appendix xxvii; NYWCMCA.
10. Ibid.
11. Minutes, Council, CU-NYHSN, 17 December 1947; NYWCMCA.
12. Hawkins, "Lydia Elizabeth Anderson," in *Dictionary of American Nursing*, 7–9. On March 4, 1941, the library of NYH School of Nursing was named in honor of Lydia Anderson, a beloved nursing leader and graduate of the class of 1897. At the ceremony, a case was unveiled that contained her nursing insignia, class pin and hospital medal, badge number 3580, and Canadian and U.S flags.
13. Minutes, Council, CU-NYHSN, 17 December 1947; NYWCMCA.
14. Ibid.
15. Annual Report, Dean, CU-NYHSN, in Report of the President, CU, 1948–1949, appendix xxix; NYWCMCA.
16. Minutes, Council, CU-NYHSN, 16 November 1949; NYWCMCA.
17. Transcript of Judith Allen interview with Virginia Dunbar, 10 July 1980; NYWCMCA.
18. Kammen, *Cornell - Glorious to View*, 138, 141. After Dr. Day's departure in 1949, two acting presidents followed him until Malott was appointed.
19. Annual Report, Dean, CU-NYHSN, in Report of the President, CU, 1946–1947, appendix xxvii; NYWCMCA.
20. Helene Jamieson Jordan, "Virginia Dunbar," *The Alumnae News*, Vol. 32, No. 2, (Winter 1958), 7; NYWCMCA.
21. Annual Report, Dean, CU-NYHSN, in Report of the President, CU, 1947–1948; appendix xxvii; NYWCMCA.
22. Virginia Dunbar, " The Adventure of Thinking Together," paper presented at Boston College School of Nursing, 31 April 1948, in Virginia Dunbar biographical file; NYWCMCA.
23. Jordan, *The Alumnae News*, Vol. 32, No. 33 (Winter 1958), 7; NYWCMCA.
24. Annual Report, Dean, CU-NYHSN, in Report of the President, CU, 1946–1947; appendix xxvii; NYWCCA.
25. *The Pulse* (12 April 1947); NYWCMCA.
26. Annual Report, Dean, CU-NYHSN, in Report of the President, CU, 1946–1947; appendix xxvii; NYWCMCA.
27. Ibid. See also Annual Report, NYH, 1947, 36; NYWCMCA.
28. Annual Report, NYH, 1947, 37–38; NYWCMCA.
29. Ibid.
30. Annual Report, NYH, 1948, 45; NYWCMCA.
31. Ibid., 46.
32. Annual Report, NYH, 1949, 12, 37; NYWCMCA.

33. Annual Report, Dean, CU-NYHSN, in Report of the President, CU, 1947–1948; appendix xxvii; NYWCMCA.
34. Supplementary Report to Annual Report of Curriculum Committee, CU-NYHSN, 1946; NYWCMCA. Marjory Overholzer chaired committee.
35. Annual Report, Dean, CU-NYHSN, in Report of the President, CU, 1947–1948; appendix xxvii; NYWCMCA.
36. Annual Report, NYH, 1949, 11; NYWCMCA.
37. Ibid., 26.
38. Ibid., 11.
39. Ibid., 12
40. Ibid. Dr. Stimson was the brother of Julia Stimson, who died on 29 September 1948, at the age of 67.
41. According to CU-NYHSN "Blue Plaid" yearbooks, students who entered the School in 1942 (Class of 1945) were the first to wear the blue check uniform. It remains uncertain, however, as to why students in the Class of February 1947 and the Class of September 1947 continued to wear the blue plaid uniform. Beginning with the Class of 1948 (entered February 1945), the blue check uniform was worn again. By 1951, the students admitted to the School in 1948 were the last group to wear the blue check uniform. Eventually, a manufacturer in the United States was able to replace the blue plaid pattern.
42. Flora Jo Bergstrom, "A Brewery, a Trolley and No Traffic on York Avenue," CUMC Alumni Quarterly, Vol. 45, No. 3/4 (December 1982), 53; NYWCMCA.
43. Louise Lincoln Cady, "The Hated Black Shoes and Stocking," CUMC Alumni Quarterly, Vol. 45, No. 3/4, (December 1982), 52; NYWCMCA.
44. Alma Woolley to Shirley Fondiller, e-mail communication, 30 November 2004; NYWCMCA.
45. Annual Report, Dean, CU-NYHSN, in Report of the President, CU, 1949–1950, appendix xxx; NYWCMCA.
46. Ibid.
47. Ibid.
48. Ibid.
49. Annual Report, Dean, CU-NYHSN, in Report of the President, CU, 1948–1949; appendix xxix; NYWCMCA.
50. Ibid. CU-NYHSN was one of five schools whose graduates qualified for public health nursing.
51. The National Nursing Accrediting Service was established on 11 January 1949, with Helen Nahm as the director. It represented the unification of accrediting activities formerly carried out by the NOPHN, NLNE and the ACSN, and the Council on Nursing Education of the Catholic Hospital Association. In 1952, the new National League for Nursing was officially recognized by the U.S. Department of Education as the accrediting body for all nursing programs. Nahm headed the NLN's Department of Baccalaureate and Higher Degree Programs and later the Division of Nursing Education.
52. Minutes, JAB, NYH-CMC, 12 May 1947; NYWCMCA.
53. Virginia Dunbar to parents of students, letter, 15 September 1948; box 1; Records of Office of the Dean, CU-NYHSN: 1927–1970, NYWCMCA.
54. At the December 1948 event to honor the staff of the newsletter, the speakers shared their thought on the art of self-expression. A representative of *The New*

York Times discussed the techniques of format in publishing.

55. Ibid.
56. Mary Millar to Shirley Fondiller, e-mail communication, 27 February 2004; NYWCMCA.
57. Ibid.
58. Minutes, Board of Governors, NYH, 6 January 1948; NYWCMCA.
59. Ibid.
60. Minutes, Board of Governors, NYH, 1 June 1947; NYWCMCA.
61. Bishop, *History of Cornell*, 518.
62. Stuart Galishoff, "Stanhope Bayne-Jones," in *Dictionary of American Medical Biography*, 146–47.
63. Ibid.
64. Annual Report, Dean, CU-NYHSN, in Report of the President, CU, 1947–1948; appendix xxvii; NYWCMCA.
65. Esther Lucile Brown, *Nursing for the Future: A Report prepared by the National Nursing Council* (New York: Russell Sage Foundation, 1948); NYWCMCA.
66. Ibid.
67. Cited in list of Advisory and Lay Committees in Brown's *Nursing for the Future.*
68. *The Alumnae News*, Vol. 32, No. 2 (1958), 10–11; NYWCMCA.
69. Brown, *Nursing for the Future*, 138.
70. Minutes, Board of Directors, NLNE, 23–24 January 1949, Exhibit II; NLNE Archive, microfilm #4. The Committee for Implementing the Brown Report changed its name to the National Committee for the Improvement of Nursing Services. The chairman was Marion Sheahan, who became the director of nursing service of the newly formed National League for Nursing in 1952.
71. Ibid.
72. Virginia Dunbar to Esther Lucile Brown, letter, 14 April 1949; box 5, folder 4; Records of Office of the Dean, CU-NYHSN: 1923–1963; NYWCMCA.
73. Ibid. The nature of Dr. Brown's illness was not disclosed.
74. Esther Lucile Brown to Laurence G. Payson, letter, 1 March 1950; box 5, folder 4; Records of Office of the Dean, CU-NYHSN: 1923–1963; NYWCMCA.
75. Report of the NLNE President on the National Nursing Planning Conference in Battle Creek, Michigan, 7–10 January 1949, in Minutes, Board of Directors, NLNE, 23–28 January 1949; NLNE Archive, microfilm #4.
76. Authors of the full report of the School Data Analysis were Margaret West and Christy Hawkins. The title was *Nursing Schools at the Mid-Century* (New York: National Committee for the Improvement of Nursing Services, 1950).
77. Minutes, Board of Directors, NLNE, 23–28 January 1949, 51; NLNE Archive, microfilm #4.
78. Fitzpatrick, *National Organization for Public Health Nursing*, 188.
79. Minutes, Council, CU-NYHSN, 16 November 1949; NYWCMCA. A one-page sheet listed the number of schools participating in the school data analysis.
80. Ibid.
81. Ibid.
82. Opdycke, *No One Was Turned Away*, 147.
83. Ibid.
84. Annual Report, NYH, 1947, 7; NYWCMCA.
85. Ibid.

86. Ibid.
87. Ibid.
88. Ibid.
89. Transcript of Judith Allen interview with Virginia Dunbar, 10 July 1980; NYWCM-CA.
90. Annie Goodrich to Lillian Wald, letter, 4 January 1928; box 6, folder 2; Records of Office of the Dean, CU-NYHSN: 1923–1963; NYWCMCA.
91. Annie Goodrich to Lillian Wald, letter, 2 February 1928; box 6, folder 2; Records of Office of the Dean, CU-NYHSN: 1923–1963; NYWCMCA.
92. Lillian Wald to Annie Goodrich, letter, 24 February 1928; box 6, folder 2; Records of Office of the Dean, CU-NYHSN: 1923-1963; NYWCMCA.
93. Virginia Dunbar to Edmund Ezra Day, letter, 26 January 1948; box 6, folder 2; Records of Office of the Dean, CU-NYHSN: 1923–1963; NYWCMCA.
94. Edmund Ezra Day to Virginia Dunbar, letter, 11 February 1948; box 6, folder 2; Records of Office of the Dean, CU-NYHSN: 1923–1963; NYWCMCA.
95. Minutes, Council, CU-NYHSN, 19 November 1949; NYWCMCA.
96. Ibid.
97. Virginia Dunbar to Stanhope Bayne-Jones, memorandum, 3 February 1950; box 6, folder 2; Records of Office of the Dean, CU-NYHSN: 1923–1963; NYWCMCA.
98. Summary of Meeting of Greater Cornell Council in Ithaca, 14 May 1950; box 6, folder 2; Records of Office of the Dean, CU-NYHSN: 1923–1963; NYWCMCA.
99. Laurence Payson to Virginia Dunbar, letter, 7 August 1950; box 6, folder 2; Records of Office of the Dean, CU-NYHSN: 1923–1963; NYWCMCA.
100. Minutes, Board of Governors, NYH, 11 December 1950; NYWCMCA.
101. Stanhope Bayne-Jones to Virginia Dunbar, letter, 15 January 1951; box 6, folder 2; Records of Office of the Dean, CU-NYHSN: 1923–1963; NYWCMCA.
102. Willard Emerson to Stanhope Bayne-Jones, letter, 12 July 1951; box 6, folder 2; Records of Office of the Dean, CU-NYHSN: 1923–1963; NYWCMCA.
103. Minutes, Executive Committee, Board of Governors, NYH, 19 June 1951; NYW-CMCA.
104. Ibid.
105. Virginia Dunbar to Anna Reutinger, letter, 5 July 1951; box 6, folder 2; Records of Office of the Dean, CU-NYHSN: 1923–1963; NYWCMCA.
106. Stanhope Bayne-Jones to Deane Malott, letter, 12 August 1951; box 6, folder 1; Records of Office of the Dean, CU-NYHSN: 1923–1963; NYWCMCA.
107. Bayne-Jones alluded to his meetings with Virginia Dunbar during the year when they explored the need for an endowment for the School of Nursing. See Stanhope Bayne-Jones to Virginia Dunbar, letter, 15 January 1951; box 6, folder 2; Records of Office of the Dean, CY-NYHSN: 1923–1963; NYWCMCA.
108. Stanhope Bayne-Jones to Deane Malott, letter, 12 August 1951, box 6, folder 1; Records of Office of the Dean, CU-NYHSN: 1923–1963; NYWCMCA.
109. Ibid.
110. *The New York Times* (1 November 1951).
111. "Seventy Fifth Anniversary," 12 June 1952; box 6, folder 2; Records of Office of the Dean, CU-NYHSN: 1923–1963; NYWCMCA.
112. Ibid.

CHAPTER 9

1. Lucile Petry Leone, "National Nursing Needs – A Challenge to Education," *Nursing Outlook* 1 (November 1953), 616.
2. Franz Goldman, "Public Policy in Organizing Medical Care," *Annals of American Academy of Political and Social Science* 273 (January 1951), 68.
3. Julien Randell Tatum, "Changing Roles of Professional Personnel in the Field of Medical Care," *Nursing Outlook* 1 (December 1953), 694.
4. John H. Knowles, "The Hospital," *Scientific American* 229 (September 1973), 133.
5. Ibid.
6. Minutes, Board of Governors, 3 April 1951; NYWCMCA.
7. Burton L. Kaufman, *The Korean Conflict* (Westport, Connecticut: Greenwood Press, 1999).
8. Report of the Joint Coordinating Committee on Structure of the Six National Nursing Organizations in Minutes, Board of Directors, NLNE, 21–22 January 1952, Exhibit 2, 2; NLNE Archive, microfilm # 5. See Flanagan, *One Strong Voice*, 158–159.
9. Janet Geister, "One Organization – Why?" *American Association of Industrial Nurses Journal* (March 1959).
10. The three groups included the National Committee for the Improvement of Nursing Services, the Joint Committee on Practical Nurses and Auxiliary Workers in Nursing, and The Joint Committee on Careers in Nursing.
11. Flanagan, *One Strong Voice*, 166–167.
12. Mildred E. Newton, "Nurses Caps and Bachelor Gowns," *American Journal of Nursing* 64 (May 1964), 1787–1789.
13. Margaret Bridgman, *Collegiate Education for Nursing* (New York: Russell Sage Foundation 1953), 113.
14. Ibid.
15. Minutes, Council, CU-NYHSN, 17 October 1951; NYWCMCA.
16. Marion Sheahan, "The Health Needs of the Nation," *Nursing Outlook* 1 (March 1953), 157.
17. Bridgman, *Collegiate Education*, 97.
18. Margaret West and Christy Hawkins, *Nursing Schools at the Mid-Century* (New York: National Committee for the Improvement of Nursing Services, 1950), 71.
19. "Junior College Directory, 1960," *Junior College Journal* 30 (January 1960), 274–306.
20. Mildred L. Montag, *The Education of Nursing Technicians* (New York: G. Putnam's Son, 1961), 3.
21. Ibid., 70, 95.
22. *Report on Associate Degree Programs* (New York, National League for Nursing, 1961), 3.
23. Gwendoline MacDonald, *Development of Standards and Accreditation in Collegiate Nursing Education* (New York: Teachers College Press, Columbia University, 1965), 84.
24. Ibid., 81.
25. Annual Report, Dean, CU-NYHSN, in Report of the President, CU, 1948–1949, appendix xxix; NYWCMCA.
26. R. Louise McManus to Virginia Dunbar, letter, 10 January 1952; box 8, folder 9; Records of Office of the Dean, CU-NYHSN: 1923–1963; NYWCMCA.

27. Helen Bunge to Virginia Dunbar, letter, 10 March 1956; box 8, folder 9; Records of Office of the Dean, CU-NYHSN: 1923–1963; NYWCMCA.

28. Kate Hyden to Virginia Dunbar, letter, 7 October 1952; box 8, folder 9; Records of Office of the Dean, CU-NYHSN: 1923–1963; NYWCMCA.

29. Annual Report, NYH, 1953, 45; NYWCMCA.

30. Ibid.

31. Annual Report, Dean, CU-NYHSN, 1958, 10; NYWCMCA.

32. Student Project Report, 1955; box 8, folder 5; Records of Office of the Dean, CU-NYHSN: 1923–1963; NYWCMCA.

33. Ibid.

34. Annual Report, NYH, 1951, 31; NYWCMCA.

35. Annual Report, NYH, 1950, 22; NYWCMCA.

36. Annual Report, NYH, 1953, 29; NYWCMCA. The nursing program of the Navajo-Cornell Field project explored means of making better care available through the use of trained Navajo day workers called "Health Visitors." The project attempted to determine whether better field and clinic programs would motivate the Navajo to seek the white man's medical care.

37. Annual Report, Dean, CU-NYHSN, 1958, 10–11; NYWCMCA.

38. Annual Report, Dean, CU-NYHSN, 1959, 9–10; NYWCMCA.

39. Annual Report, NYH, 1955, 18; NYWCMCA.

40. Ibid.

41. Ibid.

42. Ibid.

43. Ibid. Thomas Eddy was a Governor of NYH in the 1800s who advocated mental health reform.

44. Annual Report, NYH, 1956, 42; NYWCMCA.

45. Ibid.

46. The Pulse (15 December 1950); NYWCMCA.

47. Muriel Fischer, "Nurses Lose Control of Two B's," New York World Telegram and Sun (8 February 1951). In her later years, Bessie Parker was comfortably located in a new apartment complex near the village of Manville, Rhode Island. She lived there until her death in 1993 at the age of 107.

48. Minutes, Board of Governors, 4 March 1952; NYWCMCA.

49. Ibid. See also transcript of Judith Allen interview with Virginia Dunbar, 10 July 1980; NYWCMCA.

50. Minutes, Board of Governors, NYH, 4 March 1952; NYWCMCA.

51. Ibid.

52. Minutes, Board of Governors, NYH, 15 September 1953; NYWCMCA.

53. Transcript of Judith Allen interview with Virginia Dunbar, 10 July 1980; NYWCMCA.

54. Dr. Hinsey had also served as the faculty representative of CUMC.

55. Minutes, Council, CU-NYHSN, November 1954; NYWCMCA.

56. Minutes, Council, CU-NYHSN, 8 May 1951; NYWCMCA.

57. Minutes Council, CU-NYHSN, 25 March 1954; NYWCMCA.

58. Annual Report, Dean, CU-NYHSN, in Report of the President, CU, 1949–1950, appendix xxx; NYWCMCA.

59. Ibid.

60. Ibid.

61. Minutes, Council, CU-NYHSN, 25 March 1954; NYWCMCA.
62. Ibid.
63. Minutes, Council, CU-NYHSN, 1 October 1956; NYWCMCA.
64. Annual Report, Dean, CU-NYHSN, in Report of the President, CU, 1950–1951, appendix xxx; NYWCMCA.
65. Annual Report, Dean, CU-NYHSN, in Report of the President, CU, 1949–1950, appendix xxix; NYWCMCA.
66. *The Alumnae News*, Vol. 24, No. 2 (Summer 1950) 11; NYWCMCA.
67. Ibid.
68. *The Alumnae News*, Vol. 32, No. 2 (Winter 1958), 5; NYWCMCA.
69. Helene Jamieson Jordan, "Virginia M. Dunbar," *The Alumnae News*, Vol. 32, No. 2 (Winter 1958), 4; NYWCMCA.
70. Annual Report, Committee on Student-Faculty Rounds, CU-NYHSN, October 1955; NYWCMCA.
71. Werminghaus, *Annie W. Goodrich, Her Journey to Yale*.
72. Public Health Traineeships for Professional Health Personnel, Bureau of State Service, U.S. Department of Health, Education, and Welfare, Washington, DC, mimeographed; ANA Archive.
73. Ibid.
74. National League for Nursing, Report of Steering Committee, Division of Nursing Education, *Biennial Reports to the Members*, 1957–1958, 27; NLN Archive.
75. Ibid.
76. Woolley, "Virginia M. Dunbar," in *American Nursing—A Biographical Dictionary*, 76.
77. National League for Nursing, Report of the Department of Baccalaureate and Higher Degree Programs, *Biennial Reports to the Members, 1957–1958*, 54; NLN Archive.
78. Minutes, Board of Governors, NYH, 3 April 1956, 324; NYWCMCA.
79. Minutes, Council, CU-NYHSN, 1 October 1956; NYWCMCA.
80. Ibid.
81. Annual Report, Committee on Student Scholarships, CU-NYHSN, 15 September 1958; NYWCMCA. The name of the Committee on Scholarships was changed in 1958 to the Committee on Financial Aid for Students.
82. Ibid.
83. Eleanor Helm to Virginia Dunbar, letter, 22 April 1954; box 1, folder 12; Records of Office of the Dean, CU-NYHSN, 1923–1963; NYWCMCA.
84. F. Taylor Jones, Commissioner on Institutions of Higher Education, Middle States Association of Colleges and Secondary Schools, to Cooperating Agencies, including National League for Nursing, memorandum, 4 April 1956; box 2, folder 2; Records of Office of the Dean, CU-NYHSN, 1923–1963; NYWCMCA.
85. Virginia Dunbar to Eleanor Helm and Lloyd Elliott, summary report, 1957; box 2, folder 12; Records of Office of the Dean, CU-NYHSN: 1923–1963; NYWCMCA
86. Marie Farrell to Virginia Dunbar, letter, 21 October 1957; box 2, folder 2; Records of Office of the Dean, CU-NYHSN: 1923–1963; NYWCMCA.
87. Report of Visit for Accreditation to CU-NYHSN, NLN, 25 November 1957; box 1, folder 12; Records of Office of the Dean, CU-NYHSN: 1923–1963; NYWCMCA.
88. Eleanor Helm to Virginia Dunbar, letter, 12 December 1957; box 1, folder 2;

Records of Office of the Dean (Addendum): 1927–1970; NYWCMCA.

89. Report of Visit for Accreditation to CU-NYHSN, NLN, 25 November 1957; box 1, folder 12; Records of Office of the Dean, CU-NYHSN: 1923–1963; NYWCMCA.

90. Annual Report, NYH, 1957, 19; NYWCMCA.

91. Annual Report, NYH, 1958, 18; NYWCMCA.

92. Ibid.

93. Ibid.

94. Annual Report, NYH, 1957, 51–52; NYWCMCA.

95. Ibid.

96. Ibid.

97. *The Alumnae News*, Vol. 32, No. 2 (Winter 1958), 5; NYWCMCA.

98. Annual Report, Dean, CU-NYHSN, 1958, 12; NYWCMCA.

99. *The Alumnae News*, Vol. 32, No. 2 (Winter 1958), 5; NYWCMCA.

100. Ibid., 3.

101. Ibid.

102. Transcript of Judith Allen interview with Virginia Dunbar, 10 July 1980; NYWCMCA.

103. Minutes, Board of Governors, NYH, 7 October 1958; NYWCMCA.

104. *The Alumnae News*, Vol. 32, No. 2 (Winter 1958), 9; NYWCMCA.

105. Jean French to members of Alumnae Association, CU-NYHSN, letter, October 1958, in Virginia Dunbar biographical folder; NYWCMCA.

106. Anna Wolf to Alumnae Association, letter, *The Alumnae News*, Vol. 32, No. 2 (Winter 1958), 11–12; NYWCMCA.

107. Annual Report, NYH, 1958, 19; NYWCMCA.

CHAPTER 10

1.   Robert Hamelin, "The Role of Voluntary Agencies in Meeting the Health Needs of Americans," *Annals of American Academy of Political and Social Science* 337, (September 1961), 90.

2.   "Life, Liberty, and the Right to Health Care," *The American Nurse* 8 (15 September 1976), 4.

3.   Henry David, "Manpower Development and Utilization: A Governmental or a Private Responsibility," *Annals of American Academy of Political and Social Science* 325 (September 1959), 72.

4.   William Stewart, "The Changing Challenge of Manpower," paper presented at the Health and Welfare Council of Memphis, 19 September 1966; ANA Archive.

5.   Mary K. Mullane, *The Future of Professional Nurse Education* (New York: American Nurses Association, 1964); ANA Archive.

6.   Report, Department of Baccalaureate and Higher Degree Programs, NLN, Biennial Reports 1963–1964, 28; NLN Archive.

7.   Bernice Anderson, *Nursing Education in Community Junior Colleges* (Philadelphia: J.P. Lippincott, 1966), 15.

8.   Department of Baccalaureate and Higher Degree Programs, NLN, *Biennial Reports 1961–1962*, 8; NLN Archive.

9.   Gwendoline MacDonald, "Baccalaureate Education for Graduates of Diploma and Associate Degree Programs," *Nursing Outlook* (June 1954), 53.

10. Ibid., 52.

11. Ibid., 43–54.
12. *Facts About Nursing, 1970–71* (New York: American Nurses Association, 1971), 173.
13. Annual Report, NYH, 1959, 53; NYWCMCA.
14. Annual Report, NYH, 1959, 20; NYWCMCA.
15. Ibid.
16. Ibid.
17. Annual Report, NYH, 1962, 45; NYWCMCA.
18. Ibid.
19. Ibid., 46.
20. Annual Report, NYH, 1960, 52; NYWCMCA.
21. Ibid.
22. Annual Report, NYH, 1964, 32; NYWCMCA.
23. Annual Report, NYH, 1966, 9; NYWCMCA.
24. Minutes, Board of Governors, NYH, 1 October 1968; NYWCMCA.
25. Annual Report, NYH, 1963, 31; NYWCMCA.
26. Transcript of Judith Allen interview with Mary Klein and Edna Lifgren, 20 July 1980; NYWCMCA.
27. Transcript of Judith Allen interview with Veronica Lyons Roehner, August 1980; NYWCMCA.
28. Ibid.
29. Transcript of Judith Allen interview with Laura Simms, Spring 1981; NYWCMCA.
30. Ibid.
31. Background note, finding aid; Records of Office of the Dean, CU-NYHSN: 1927–1978; NYWCMCA.
32. Ibid.
33. Board of Trustees, CU, to Muriel Carbery, memorandum, 23 January 1960; box 48, folder 1; Records of Office of the Dean, CU-NYHSN: 1927–1978; NYWCMCA.
34. Ibid.
35. Annual Report, Dean, CU-NYHSN, 1962, 9; NYWCMA.
36. Ibid, 2.
37. Transcript of Judith Allen interview with Veronica Lyons Roehner, August 1980; NYWCMCA.
38. Notes of Shirley H. Fondiller interview with Louise Hazeltine, 23 April 2003, at her residence in Trucksville, Pennsylvania; NYWCMCA.
39. Annual Report, Dean, CU-NYHSN, 1959, 3; NYWCMCA.
40. Minutes, Executive Faculty, CU-NYHSN, 20 January 1959; NYWCMCA.
41. Annual Report, Dean, CU-NYHSN, 1959, 2; NYWCMCA.
42. Ibid.
43. Ibid., 1.
44. Minutes, Faculty, CU-NYHSN, 19 June 1959; NYWCMCA.
45. Annual Report, Dean, CU-NYHSN, 1961, 3–4; NYWCMCA.
46. Minutes, Faculty, CU-NYHSN, 15 June 1960. Macgregor's final work was published as *Social Science in Nursing; Applications for the Improvement of Patient Care* (New York: Russell Sage Foundation, 1960).
47. Minutes, Executive Faculty, CU-NYHSN, 16 May 1952; NYWCMCA.
48. Annual Report, NYH, 1964, 5; NYWCMCA. The building was to be named the

Laurence C. Payson House after a prominent member of the Society.

49. Ibid., 24.
50. Annual Report, NYH, 1965, 3; NYWCMCA.
51. Ibid., 4.
52. Annual Report, Curriculum Committee, Faculty, CU-NYHSN, 1961; NYWCMCA.
53. Ibid.
54. Annual Report, Dean, CU-NYHSN, 1962, 7; NYWCMCA.
55. Ibid.
56. Ibid., 8.
57. Minutes, Executive Faculty, CU-NYHSN, 20 January 1962; NYWCMCA.
58. Ibid.
59. Annual Report, Dean, CU-NYHSN, 1962, 7; NYWCMCA.
60. Muriel Carbery to Arthur Jones, letter, 8 May 1961; box 48, folder 3; Records of Office of the Dean, CU-NYHSN: 1927–1978; NYWCMCA.
61. Ibid.
62. Ibid.
63. Minutes, Executive Faculty, CU-NYHSN, 19 September 1962; NYWCMCA.
64. Ibid.
65. Ibid.
66. Transcript of Judith Allen interview with Veronica Lyons Roehner, August 1980; NYWCMCA.
67. Transcript of Judith Allen interview with Laura Simms, Spring 1981; NYWCMCA.
68. Minutes, Medical Board, NYH, 3 January 1963; NYWCMCA.
69. Annual Report, Dean, CU-NYHSN, 1963, 6; NYWCMCA.
70. Ibid., 4.
71. Annual Report, Dean, CU-NYHSN, 1959, 6; NYWCMCA.
72. Ibid.
73. Annual Report, Dean, CU-NYHSN, 1963, 6–7; NYWCMCA.
74. Annual Report, Dean, CU-NYHSN, 1963, 7; NYWCMCA.
75. Ibid.
76. Annual Report, Dean, CU-NYHSN, 1963, 7–8; NYWCMCA. The students who worked in an auxiliary capacity wore a white uniform with a plaid tab on the breast pocket. In contrast, the uniform of the regular student was a plaid dress with a white collar, lapels and cuffs, self-belt, student cap, white shoes, and beige stockings.
77. Ibid. See also Records of Office of the Dean, CU-NYHSN (Addendum): 1927–1970; box 4, folder 1; NYWCMCA.
78. Annual Report, Dean, CU-NYHSN, 1965, 8; NYWCMCA.
79. Ibid., 7.
80. Annual Report, Dean, CU-NYHSN, 1966, 7; NYWCMCA.
81. Minutes, Executive Faculty, CU-NYHSN, 21 March 1962; NYWCMCA.
82. Ibid.
83. Ibid.
84. Minutes, Executive Faculty, CU-NYHSN, 18 September 1968; NYWCMCA.
85. Annual Report, Dean, CU-NYHSN, 1965, 8; NYWCMCA.
86. Ibid.
87. Student Handbook, CU-NYHSN, 1967; NYWCMCA.
88. Ibid.

89. Minutes, Executive Faculty, CU-NYHSN, 20 February 1963; NYWCMCA.

90. Muriel Carbery to Denise Shelly, letter, 5 March 1963; box 2, folder 2; Records of Executive Faculty, CU-NYHSN: 1942–1970; NYWCMCA.

91. Minutes, Executive Faculty, CU-NYHSN, 21 March 1962; NYWCMCA.

92. Minutes, Executive Faculty, CU-NYHSN, 17 June 1964; NYWCMCA. The library also became an excellent resource for students and faculty in the Graduate College of Medical Sciences, established at the Medical Center in 1952.

93. Minutes, Executive Faculty, CU-NYHSN, 19 February 1964; NYWCMCA.

94. Ibid.

95. Muriel Carbery to Dale Corson, letter, 16 July 1964; box 1, folder 2; Records of Office of the Dean: 1942–1983 (addendum); NYWCMCA.

96. Annual Report, Dean, CU-NYHSN, 1965, 6; NYWCMCA.

97. Minutes, Executive Faculty, CU-NYHSN, 20 January 1965; NYWCMCA.

98. Ibid.

99. Ibid.

100. Minutes, Executive Faculty, CU-NYHSN, 19 September 1962; NYWCMCA.

101. Virginia Dericks, "My Role as a Clinical Specialist," paper presented at National Conference on Physician's Assistant, Long Island University, Brooklyn, New York. See Virginia Dericks, "The Role of the Clinical Nursing Specialist," *Centerscope*, Vol. 3 (March 1972), 3; NYWCMCA.

102. Ibid.

103. Ibid.

104. Ibid.

105. Minutes, Executive Faculty, CU-NYHSN, 20 March 1963; NYWCMCA.

106. U.S. Department of Health, Education, and Welfare, *Toward Quality in Nursing— Needs and Goals, Report of the Surgeon General's Consultant Group on Nursing* (Washington, DC: U.S. Government Printing Office, 1963).

107. Ibid.

108. Ibid.

109. Mary K. Mullane to Dr. Luther Terry, letter, 4 December 1963; NLN Archive.

110. Minutes, Coordinating Council, NLN-ANA, 20 January 1964; NLN Archive.

111. Minutes, Executive Faculty, CU-NYHSN, 18 March 1964; NYWCMCA.

112. The Nurse Training Act of 1964 (P.L. 88-581) was the first federal legislation to give comprehensive financial assistance to nursing education. The presidents of the ANA and the NLN stood at President Johnson's side while he signed the historic bill.

113. "NLN Designated as Accrediting Body for the Nurse Training Act," *Nursing Outlook* 12 (December 1964), 8–10.

114. Summary of Provisions of the Nurse Training Act of 1964, 13 October 1964, typescript; ANA Archive.

115. U.S. Commission on Civil Rights, *Civil Rights Under Federal Programs, An Analysis of Title VI* (Washington, DC: U.S. Printing Office, 1965), 15. During the late 1950s and 1960s, the federal government took substantial action in dealing with injustices in civil rights.

116. Minutes, Executive Faculty, CU-NYHSN, 16 September 1964; NYWCMCA.

117. Annual Report, Dean, CU-NYHSN, 1965, 9; NYWCMCA.

118. Ibid.

119. Ibid.

CHAPTER 11

1. U.S. Department of Health, Education, and Welfare, *Toward Quality in Nursing.*
2. National Commission for the Study of Nursing and Nursing Education, *An Abstract for Action* (McGraw-Hill, 1970).
3. Ibid.
4. "National League for Nursing Convention," *Nursing Outlook* 13 (June 1965), 6, 37.
5. Flanagan, *One Strong Voice,* 141–142. See *Educational Preparation for Nurse Practitioners and Assistants to Nurses—A Position Paper* (New York: American Nurses Association, 1965).
6. Ibid., 11.
7. American Nurses Association, *Facts About Nursing,* 1970–71 (New York: American Nurses Association, 1971), 10.
8. *Report of the National Advisory Commission on Health Manpower* (Washington, DC: U.S. Government Printing Office, 1963), 31.
9. Ibid., 24.
10. Ibid.
11. *Healing at Home: Visiting Nurse Service of New York, 1893–1993* (New York: Visiting Nurse Service of New York, 1993), 18–19. See also "Medicare and Medicaid," *Annals of Political and Social Science* 399 (January 1972), 115–124.
12. Minutes, Executive Faculty, CU-NYHSN, 24 February 1966; NYWCMCA.
13. Annual Report, NYH, 1966, 32–33; NYWCMCA.
14. Ibid.
15. Ibid.
16. Ibid., 33–34.
17. Minutes, Board of Governors, NYH, 7 March 1967; NYWCMCA.
18. Ibid.
19. Ibid.
20. Annual Report, NYH, 1968, 11; NYWCMCA.
21. Ibid., 15. See also Minutes, JAB, NYH-CMC, 15 May 1968; NYWCMCA.
22. Annual Report, NYH, 1968, 12; NYWCMCA.
23. Minutes, Board of Governors, NYH, 5 March 1968, 9 September 1969, 7 October 1969; NYWCMCA.
24. Annual Report, NYH, 1961, 52; NYWCMCA.
25. Ibid., 19.
26. Ibid.
27. Brochure, *To the Donors—The New York Hospital-Cornell Medical Center Fund for Medical Progress, 1961–1966*; box 5, folder 5; Records of Development Office, NYH-CMC: 1939–1979; NYWCMCA.
28. Minutes, Steering Committee, Fund for Medical Progress (FMP), 29 June 1961; box 6, folder 9; Records of Development Office, NYH-CMC: 1939–1979; NYW-CMCA.
29. Minutes, Executive Faculty, CU-NYHSN, 20 September 1961; NYWCMCA.
30. Minutes, Board of Governors, NYH, 12 October 1961; NYWCMCA.
31. Annual Report, NYH, 1961, 19; NYWCMCA.
32. Ibid., 50.
33. Ibid.
34. Minutes, Executive Faculty, CU-NYHSN, 17 January 1962; NYWCMCA.

35. Minutes, Executive Faculty, CU-NYHSN, 18 April 1962; NYWCMCA.
36. Minutes, Executive Faculty, CU-NYHSN, 17 January 1962; NYWCMCA.
37. Tozier Brown, "A Special Fund Raising Program—The School of Nursing," preliminary report; box 53, folder 5; Records of Office of the Dean, CU-NYHSN: 1927–1978; NYWCMCA.
38. Ibid.
39. Minutes, Steering Committee, FMP, 8 July 1963; box 6, folder 9; Records of Development Office, NYH-CMC: 1939–1979; NYWCMCA.
40. Minutes, Steering Committee, FMP, 22 July 1963; box 6, folder 9; Records of Development Office, NYH-CMC: 1939–1979; NYWCMCA.
41. Ibid.
42. James Perkins to Emory Morris, letter, 22 October 1963; box 53, folder 5; Records of Office of the Dean, CU-NYHSN: 1927–1978; NYWCMCA.
43. Emory Morris to James Perkins, letter, 10 December 1963; box 53, folder 5; Records of Office of the Dean, CU-NYHSN: 1927–1978; NYWCMCA.
44. Muriel Carbery to Mildred Tuttle, 16 January 1964; box 53, folder 5; Records of Office of the Dean, CU-NYHSN: 1927–1978; NYWCMCA
45. Mildred Tuttle to Muriel Carbery, 16 April 1964; box 53, folder 5; Records of Office of the Dean, CU-NYHSN: 1927–1978; NYWCMCA.
46. Minutes, Steering Committee, FMP, 12 February 1964; box 6, folder 10; Records of Development Office, NYH-CMC: 1939–1979; NYWCMCA.
47. Minutes, Steering Committee, FMP, 23 March 1964; box 6, folder 10; Records of Development Office, NYH-CMC: 1939–1979; NYWCMCA.
48. Report of President Trask's meeting of April 13, 1964, in Washington, DC, with Mrs. Bolton; box 53, folder 5; Records of the Office of the Dean, CU-NYHSN: 1927–1978; NYWCMCA. No further contact ensued with her about prospective donors.
49. Tozier Brown to Muriel Carbery, letter, 4 February 1964; box 53, folder 5; Records of Office of the Dean, CU-NYHSN: 1927–1978; NYWCMCA. Brown described the AHA grant.
50. Ibid.
51. Tozier Brown to Muriel Carbery, letter, 4 March 1964; Tozier Brown to President Trask, letter, 7 April 1964; box 53, folder 5; Records of Office of the Dean, CU-NYHSN: 1927–1978; NYWCMCA.
52. Minutes, Steering Committee, FMP, 11 May 1964; box 6, folder 10; Records of Development Office, NYH-CMC: 1939–1979; NYWCMCA. On May 14, 1964, Tozier Brown wrote to Dean Carbery indicating that he and President Trask were eager to learn of her recommendations after she "digested the material resulting from your conference with Miss Tuttle." See box 53, folder 5; Records of Office of the Dean, CU-NYHSN: 1927–1978; NYWCMCA.
53. Minutes, Executive Committee, Steering Committee, FMP, 9 March 1964; box 6, folder 10; Records of Development Office, NYH-CMC: 1939–1979; NYWCMCA.
54. Minutes, Executive Committee, Steering Committee, FMP, 6 April 1964; box 6, folder 10; Records of Development Office, NYH-CMC: 1939–1979; NYWCMCA. It was not known whether Dean Carbery followed through on a proposal for a professorship since there was no evidence of such an award.
55. Minutes, Executive Committee, Steering Committee, FMP, 15 March 1965; box 6, folder 10; Records of Development Office, NYH-CMC: 1939–1979; NYWCMCA.

56. Minutes, Executive Committee, Steering Committee, FMP, 29 March 1965; box 6, folder 10; Records of Development Office, NYH-CMC: 1939–1979; NYWCMCA.
57. Minutes, Executive Faculty, CU-NYHSN, 20 January 1965; NYWCMCA.
58. Annual Report, Dean, CU-NYHSN, 1964, 11; NYWCMCA.
59. Ibid.
60. Annual Report, NYH, 1966, 3; NYWCMCA.
61. Muriel Carbery to Hamilton Hadley, letter, 4 February 1966; box 53, folder 5; Records of Office of the Dean, CU-NYHSN: 1927–1978; NYWCMCA. Bayne-Jones had enclosed a copy of Mrs. Meyer's letter of 10 January 1966. She was the mother of Katherine Graham, the prominent publisher of the *Washington Post*.
62. Mrs. Eugene Meyer to Stanhope Bayne-Jones, letter, 10 January 1966; box 53, folder 5; Records of Office of the Dean, CU-NYHSN: 1927–1978: NYWCMCA. Apparently, the possibility of funding from Mrs. Meyer did not materialize. There was no record of Carbery communicating with her further.
63. *The Alumnae News*, Vol. 40, No. 3 (February 1966), 2; NYWCMCA.
64. Ibid. Gladys Jones became chairman of the Endowment Fund Committee in 1963. She succeeded Ruth Ernst, also a graduate of the school of nursing.
65. Minutes, JAB, NYH-CMC, October 1966–June 1968; NYWCMCA.
66. Minutes, Executive Faculty, CU-NYHSN, 10 April 1968; NYWCMCA.
67. Minutes, Executive Faculty, CU-NYHSN, 8 May 1968; NYWCMCA
68. Ibid.
69. Minutes, Board of Governors, NYH, 7 October 1969; NYWCMCA.
70. *The Alumnae News*, Vol. 40, No. 3 (February 1966); NYWCMCA. Following her retirement, Veronica Lyons was appointed Professor Emerita.
71. Minutes, Executive Faculty, CU-NYHSN, 1 July 1966–30 June 1968; NYWCMCA.
72. Mary Millar to Shirley H. Fondiller, e-mail communication, 27 February 2004; NYWCMCA.
73. Ibid.
74. Muriel Carbery to Ruth Kelly, memorandum, 4 January 1966, in Minutes, Executive Faculty, CU-NYHSN, 1965-1966; NYWCMCA.
75. Minutes, Executive Faculty, CU-NYHSN, 15 December 1965; NYWCMCA.
76. Ibid.
77. Annual Report, Dean, CU-NYHSN, 1968, 5–6; NYWCMCA.
78. Ibid., 6–8.
79. Annual Report, Dean, CU-NYHSN, 1969, 6; NYWCMCA.
80. Ibid.
81. Annual Report, NYH, 1967, 36; Annual Report, Dean, CU-NYHSN, 1967, 6; NYWCMCA.
82. Minutes, Executive Faculty, CU-NYHSN, 17 March 1965; NYWCMCA.
83. Ibid.
84. Ibid.
85. Minutes, Faculty, CU-NYHSN, 9 March 1965; NYWCMCA.
86. Ibid.
87. Ibid.
88. Ibid.
89. Transcript of Judith Allen interview with Laura Simms, Spring 1981; NYWCMCA.
90. Dorothy Ellison to Muriel Carbery, memorandum, 20 June 1967; box 48, folder 9; Records of Office of the Dean, CU-NYHSN: 1927–1978; NYWCMCA.

91. Dorothy Ellison to Muriel Carbery, memorandum, 19 September 1967; box 48, folder 9: Records of Office of the Dean: 1927–1978: NYWCMCA.
92. Minutes, Executive Faculty, CU-NYHSN, 21 June 1967; NYWCMCA.
93. Minutes, Executive Faculty, CU-NYHSN, 8 May 1968; NYWCMCA. In 1960, the Board of Trustees, CU, dissolved the School's Advisory Council.
94. Minutes, Executive Faculty, CU-NYHSN, 11 June 1968; NYWCMCA.
95. Minutes, Faculty Council, CU-NYHSN, 3 October 1968 and 21 October 1968; NYWCMCA.
96. Ibid.
97. Annual Report, Faculty Council, CU-NYHSN, 1968–1969; NYWCMCA.
98. Minutes, Executive Faculty, CU-NYHSN, 8 May 1968; NYWCMCA.
99. Minutes, Executive Faculty, CU-NYHSN, 17 February 1965; NYWCMCA.
100. Minutes, Executive Faculty, CU-NYHSN, 12 June 1968; NYWCMCA. The title of the Anniversary Program was "The Publick (*sic*) Hospital, 1771–1971."
101. "A Program to Expand the School of Nursing," memorandum, February 1968; box 48, folder 9; Records of Office of the Dean, CU-NYHSN: 1927–1978; NYW-CMCA.
102. Minutes, Executive Faculty, CU-NYHSN, 10 January 1968; NYWCMCA.
103. Annual Report, Dean, CU-NYHSN, 1966, 8; NYWCMCA.
104. Annual Report, Dean, CU-NYHSN, 1969, 4; NYWCMCA.
105. Ibid., 5–6.
106. Ibid., 5. The U.S. Public Health Service had rejected the grant proposal because the design (and not the intent) was unacceptable.
107. Annual Report, Dean, CU-NYHSN, 1969, 4; NYWCMCA. Dean Carbery assigned Ruth Kelly to chair the committee on the experimental program,
108. On 1 June 1970, The New York State Department of Education registered in full the two-year basic baccalaureate program designed for non-nursing graduates of four- year colleges, Registration was extended to September 1973.
109. Annual Report, Dean, CU-NYHSN, 1969, 4; NYWCMCA.
110. Ibid., 2.
111. Minutes, Executive Faculty, CU-NYHSN, 26 February 1968; NYWCMCA.
112. *The Alumnae News*, Vol. 42, No. 3 (April 1968), 9–10; NYWCMCA.
113. Annual Report, Dean, CU-NYHSN, 1968, 8; NYWCMCA.
114. Ibid.
115. Annual Report, Dean, CU-NYHSN, 1969, 9; NYWCMCA.
116. Ibid.
117. Ibid., 8.
118. Ibid., 9.
119. Minutes, Board of Governors, NYH, 9 June 1968; NYWCMCA.
120. R. Palmer Baker, Jr. to Muriel Carbery, letter, 28 August 1968; box 48, folder 10; Records of Office of the Dean, CU-NYHSN: 1927–1978; NYWCMCA.
121. Ibid.
122. Minutes, Board of Governors, NYH, 4 February 1969; NYWCMCA.
123. Muriel Carbery to R. Palmer Baker, Jr., letter, 30 October 1969; box 49, folder 1; Records of Office of the Dean, CU-NYHSN: 1927–1978; NYWCMCA.
124. Ibid.
125. R. Palmer Baker, Jr. to Muriel Carbery, letter, 21 November 1969; box 49, folder 1; Records of Office of the Dean, CU-NYHSN: 1927–1978; NYWCMCA.

126. Minutes, Executive Faculty, CU-NYHSN, 10 December 1969; NYWCMCA.
127. Transcript of Judith Allen interview with Veronica Lyons Roehner, July 1980; NYWCMCA.
128. Transcript of Judith Allen interview with Helen Berg, Summer 1981; NYWCMCA.
129. Transcript of Judith Allen interview with Laura Simms, Spring 1981; NYWCMCA.

CHAPTER 12

1. Minutes, Board of Governors, NYH, 5 May 1970; NYWCMCA.
2. Cornell Newsletter (13 March 1969) in Minutes, Faculty Council, CU-NYHSN: 1968–1969; NYWCMCA.
3. Ibid.
4. Dale Corson to Cornell University community, memorandum, 21 July 1969, in Minutes, Faculty, CU-NYHSN: 1969–1970; NYWCMCA.
5. Ibid.
6. Ibid.
7. Minutes, Faculty Council, CU-NYHSN, 5 June 1970; NYWCMA. The campus protests at Kent State captured the public's attention. Following two days of demonstrations and vandalism, the Mayor of Akron called in the National Guard. A tragic confrontation followed when the guardsmen opened fire on the students, who ignored the order to disperse. Nine students were injured and four killed, including some just passing by.
8. Ibid.
9. Ibid.
10. Minutes, Faculty/Faculty Council, CU-NYHSN, 12 June 1970; NYWCMCA.
11. Annual Report, Dean, CU-NYHSN, 1970, 2; NYWCMCA.
12. Minutes, Executive Faculty, CU-NYHSN, 10 January 1968; NYWCMCA.
13. Minutes, Executive Faculty, CU-NYHSN, 28 February 1968; NYWCMCA.
14. Minutes, Executive Faculty, CU-NYHSN, 8 January 1969; NYWCMCA.
15. Ibid. See Rozella Schlotfeldt and Janette MacPhail, "Experiment in Nursing," American Journal of Nursing 69 (July 1969), 1147–1148.
16. Minutes, Executive Faculty, CU-NYHSN, 8 January 1969; NYWCMCA.
17. Minutes, Faculty Council, CU-NYHSN, 14 February 1969; NYWCMCA.
18. Muriel Carbery, handwritten report, 24 February 1969; Records of Executive Council/Student Senate, CU-NYHSN: 1932–1979; NYWCMCA.
19. Ibid.
20. Minutes, Faculty Council, CU-NYHSN, 28 February 1969; NYWCMCA,
21. "The Cornell University-New York Hospital School of Nursing," AAUP Bulletin (Winter 1970), 388.
22. Muriel Carbery, handwritten report, 24 February 1969; Records of Executive Council/Student Senate, CU-NYHSN: 1932–1979; NYWCMCA.
23. Muriel Carbery to Sister Marcia Hoobler, letter, 27 February 1969; Records of Executive Council/Student Senate, CU-NYHSN: 1932–1979; NYWCMCA
24. Minutes, Student Organization, CU-NYHSN, 3 March 1969; NYWCMCA.
25. Ibid.
26. "The Cornell University-New York Hospital School of Nursing, AAUP Bulletin (Winter 1970), 388.
27. Ibid.

28. Ibid.

29. Ibid.

30. Ibid.

31. Notes of Shirley Fondiller interview with Louise Hazeltine, 23 April 2003; NYW-CMCA.

32. Ibid.

33. "Dedication to Joe Musio," editorial, *The Blue Plaidette*, 1970 yearbook, CU-NYHSN; NYWCMCA.

34. Sister Marcia Hoobler to Muriel Carbery, letter, 1 May 1969; Records of Executive Council/Student Senate, CU-NYHSN: 1932–1979; NYWCMCA.

35. Anne D'Citri to Muriel Carbery, letter, 14 September 1969, Records of Executive Council/Student Senate, CU-NYHSN: 1932–1979; NYWCMCA.

36. Minutes, Board of Governors, NYH, 30 October 1968; NYWCMCA.

37. Hugh Luckey to Faculty, CU-NYHSN, letter, 30 October 1968, in Minutes, Faculty Council, CU-NYHSN: 1968–1969; NYWCMCA.

38. Ibid.

39. Minutes, Joint Administrative Board, NYH-CMC, 15 January 1969; NYWCMCA.

40. Ibid.

41. Minutes, Board of Governors, NYH, 4 February 1969; NYWCMCA.

42. Minutes, Board of Governors, NYH, 1 April 1969; NYWCMCA.

43. Ruth Kelly to Students, memorandum, 6 December 1967; box 1, folder, 6; Records of Academic Standards Committee, CU-NYHSN: 1967–1979; NYWCM-CA.

44. Educational and Administrative Policy Manual, CU-NYHSN; Appendix C: Course Chairmen, October 1967; NYWCMCA.

45. Minutes, Executive Faculty, CU-NYHSN, 21 June 1967; NYWCMCA.

46. Minutes, Executive Faculty, CU-NYHSN, 12 March 1969; NYWCMCA.

47. Minutes, Executive Faculty, CU-NYHSN, 11 February 1970; NYWCMCA.

48. Ibid.

49. Albert Rubin to Eleanor Taggart, letter, 10 October 1969; box 2, folder 14; Records of Alumni Association, CU-NYHSN: 1889–1981; NYWCMCA.

50. Ibid.

51. *The Alumnae News*, Vol. 43, No. 3 (Spring-April 1969), 3; NYWCMCA.

52. Ibid.

53. Ibid.

54. Minutes, Faculty, CU-NYHSN, 16 March 1970; NYWCMCA.

55. Minutes, Board of Governors, NYH, 7 April 1970; NYWCMCA.

56. Ibid.

57. Neal R. Stamp to Muriel Carbery, memorandum, 18 May 1970; box 8, folder 8; Records of Office of the Dean: 1927–1978; NYWCMCA.

58. Notes of Shirley H. Fondiller interview with Louise Hazeltine, 23 April 2003; NYWCMCA.

59. "Nurses for Rockefeller in New York City, 1970," pamphlet, in Eleanor Lambertsen biographical file; NYWCMCA.

60. "NYSNA Board of Directors Endorses Eleanor C. Lambertsen," *The Journal of the New York State Nurses Association*, Vol. l, No. 1 (Spring 1970), 4.

61. Minutes, Faculty/Faculty Council, CU-NYHSN, 5 June 1970; NYWCMCA.

62. Muriel Carbery to Eleanor Lambertsen, letter, 16 April 1970; Muriel Carbery biog-

raphical file; NYWCMCA.

63. John H. Knowles, "The Hospital," *Scientific American* 229 (September 1973), 133.

64. Annual Report, NYH; 1970, 14; NYWCMCA.

65. Ibid.

66. Ibid.

67. Ibid., 6.

68. Ibid.

69. *The American Nurses Association Views the Emerging Physician's Assistant*, official statement of the American Nurses Association, December 1971; ANA Archive.

70. Loretta Ford, "Reaffirmation of the Nurse Practitioner Movement," *The American Nurse* 10 (15 June 1978), 4; ANA Archive.

71. Ibid.

72. U.S. Department of Health, Education, and Welfare, *Extending the Scope of Nursing Practice, Report of the Secretary's Committee to Study the Extended Roles of Nurses* (Washington, DC, U.S Government Printing Office, November 1971).

73. "Community Health Nurses Issue HMO Statement," *American Journal of Nursing* 73 (November 1973), 1925.

74. "Nursing Organizations Meet at Headquarters to Plan Greater Coordination of Activities," *American Journal of Nursing* 73 (January 1973), 7, 9.

75. Shirley H. Fondiller, *The Vision and the Reality—A History of AACN's First 20 Years, 1969–1989* (Washington, DC: American Association of Colleges of Nursing, 1989), 1.

76. Minutes, Executive Faculty, CU-NYHSN, 22 June 1969; NYWCMCA.

77. *The Open Curriculum in Nursing Education*, official statement of the National League for Nursing, February 1970; NLN Archive.

78. Government Relations Department, ANA, to Deans/Directors of Schools of Nursing, ANA Board of Directors, States Nurses Association Executive Directors and Presidents, memorandum, 24 November 1971; ANA Archive.

79. *Washington Report of Medicine and Health* 12 (December 1971).

80. Eleanor Lambertsen to Hugh Luckey, letter, 21 December 1971; Records of Committee on Nursing, Board of Governors, NYH: 1968–1974; NYWCMCA.

81. R. Palmer Baker to the President, Board of Governors, NYH, report, 14 December 1971; Records of Committee on Nursing, Board of Governors, NYH: 1968–1974; NYWCMCA.

82. Annual Report, Dean, CU-NYHSN, 1972, 1; NYWCMCA.

83. Ibid.

84. Ibid., 2.

85. Eleanor Lambertsen, "The Extended Role of the Nurse," convocation address, 2 June 1970, in *The Alumnae News*, Vol. 44, No. 3 (Summer 1970); NYWCMCA.

86. Minutes, Faculty, CU-NYHSN, 2 September 1970; NYWCMCA.

87. Eleanor Lambertsen, "Governance of the School of Nursing," paper, 15 October 1970; box 5, folder 17; Records of Office of the Dean, CU-NYHSN (addendum): 1942–1983; NYWCMCA.

88. Ibid.

89. Ibid. See also Minutes, JAB, NYH-CMC, 18 December 1968; NYWCMCA.

90. Lambertsen, "Governance of the School of Nursing."

91. Ibid.

92. Ibid.

93. Ibid.
94. Ibid.
95. Annual Report, Dean, CU-NYHSN, 1971, 5; NYWCMCA.
96. Ibid.
97. Minutes, Faculty, CU-NYHSN, 23 November 1970; NYWCMCA.
98. "Dedicate Apartment Residence for Cornell Medical and Nursing Students," News Service, NYH-CMC, 31 July 1974; NYWCMCA.
99. Minutes, Capital Gifts Committee, JAB, NYH-CMC, 12 June 1967; NYWCMCA.
100. Ibid.
101. Patricia Long to Jeffrey Hill, letter, 20 April 1970; Records of Residence Committee, Student Organization, CU-NYHSN: 1967–1972; NYWCMCA. Jeffrey Hill was the first male student to enter and graduate from CU-NYHSN. As a result of the increasing number of young men admitted to the School, the name Alumnae Association was changed in 1974 to *Alumni* Association.
102. "Dedicate Apartment Residence for Cornell Medical and Nursing Students," NYWCMCA.
103. Ibid.
104. Ibid.

CHAPTER 13

1. Minutes, Faculty, CU-NYHSN, 18 January 1971; NYWCMCA.
2. The AAUP article was titled, "The Cornell University-New York Hospital School of Nursing: A Report on a Problem of Notice and Academic Freedom," *AAUP Bulletin* (Winter 1970), 387–390.
3. Eleanor Lambertsen to Dorothy Ozimek, letter, 8 April 1971; box 1, folder 3; Records of Office of the Dean, CU-NYHSN (addendum): 1942–1983; NYWCMCA.
4. Ibid.
5. Minutes, Faculty Council, CU-NYHSN, 30 June 1972; NYWCMCA
6. Annual Report, Faculty Council, CU-NYHSN, 1972, 2–3; NYWCMCA.
7. Ibid.
8. Eleanor Lambertsen to Martin Lapidus, letter, 11 April 1975; box 1, folder 7; Records of Office of the Dean, CU-NYHSN (addendum): 1942–1983; NYWCMCA.
9. Ibid.
10. Minutes, Faculty, CU-NYHSN, 3 May 1976; NYWCMCA.
11. Minutes, Faculty, CU-NYHSN, 24 June 1971; NYWCMCA
12. "Primex: Family Nurse Practitioner Program," pamphlet, 1971; box 60, folder 11; Records of Office of the Dean: 1927–1978; NYWCMCA.
13. Ibid.
14. Ibid. The contract was extended 12 months until 23 June 1973.
15. Eleanor Lambertsen to Muriel Carbery, memorandum, 21 December 1971; box 60, folder 11; Records of Office of the Dean, CU-NYHSN: 1927–1978; NYWCMCA.
16. Annual Report, Dean, CU-NYHSN, 1971, 2; NYWCMCA.
17. "Advanced Training Program for Pediatric Nurse Announced," news release, CUMC, 19 April 1972; Eleanor Lambertsen biographical file; NYWCMCA.

18. Annual Report, NYH, 1972, 7; NYWCMCA.
19. Annual Report, Dean, CU-NYHSN, 1971, 8; NYWCMCA.
20. Ibid.
21. Annual Report, Dean, CU-NYHSN, 1971, 10; NYWCMCA.
22. Ibid.
23. Graduate School of Nursing, New York Medical College, catalog, ca. 1963.
24. Minutes, Faculty, CU-NYHSN, 11 May 1970; NYWCMCA.
25. "Long Range Planning Program," CU-NYHSN, 1971, in Agenda, Board of Governors, NYH, 4 May 1971; NYWCMCA.
26. Ibid.
27. Minutes, Faculty, CU-NYHSN, 10 October 1972; NYWCMCA.
28. Ibid.
29. Minutes, Faculty, CU-NYHSN, 8 November 1972; NYWCMCA.
30. Minutes, Faculty, CU-NYHSN, 12 December 1972; NYWCMCA.
31. Annual Report, Dean, CU-NYHSN, 1973, 1; NYWCMCA.
32. Minutes, Faculty, CU-NYHSN, 21 November 1972; NYWCMCA.
33. Louise Hazeltine to Faculty, CU-NYHSN, memorandum, 8 January 1973, in Minutes, Faculty, CU-NYHSN, 1972/73; NYWCMCA.
34. Annual Report, Dean, CU-NYHSN, 1973, 2; NYWCMCA.
35. Annual Report, Dean, CU-NYHSN, 1976, 3; NYWCMCA.
36. Annual Report, Dean, CU-NYHSN, 1973, 2; NYWCMCA.
37. Annual Report, NYH, 1972, 5; NYWCMCA.
38. Annual Report, Dean, CU-NYHSN, 1972, 1; NYWCMCA.
39. David Thompson to Executive Committee, Board of Governors, NYH, memorandum, 20 June 1973, 1–2; NYWCMCA.
40. Ibid.
41. Minutes, Faculty, CU-NYHSN, 22 June 1973; NYWCMCA.
42. Minutes, Board of Governors, NYH, 20 September 1973; NYWCMCA. See 1974 Bylaws of CU-NYHSN, 10; NYWCMCA.
43. Annual Report, NYH, 1974, 10; NYWCMCA. There was speculation among some of the faculty that Lambertsen's appointment in nursing service surprised Muriel Carbery and precipitated an unplanned retirement.
44. "Miss Carbery to be Succeeded by Dr. Lambertsen," *Bulletin and Calendar of Events*, NYH-CMC, Issue 15, No. 35 (May 1974). See *The Alumnae News*, Vol. 48, No. 2 (Summer 1974), 45; NYWCMCA.
45. Annual Report, Dean, CU-NYHSN, 1974, 1; NYWCMCA.
46. Ibid., 2.
47. Annual Report, NYH, 1975, 46; NYWCMCA.
48. List of Faculty Assignments: Spring 1974, in Agenda, Faculty, CU-NYHSN, 10 December 1973; NYWCMCA.
49. Annual Report, Dean, CU-NYHSN, 1973, 2; NYWCMCA.
50. Annual Report, NYH, 1976, 7; NYWCMCA.
51. Annual Report, Dean, CU-NYHSN, 1975, 1–2; NYWCMCA.
52. Administrative Manual, Division of Nursing, NYH, Vol. 1, Section M (2 February 1976); NYWCMCA.
53. Ibid.
54. Ibid.
55. Annual Report, Dean, CU-NYHSN, 1973, 4; 1974, 5; 1975, 7; NYWCMCA.

56. Ibid.

57. Minutes, Faculty, CU-NYHSN, 11 November 1974; NYWCMCA.

58. Eleanor C. Lambertsen to Jeanne B. Dorie, memorandum, 3 September 1976; box 11, folder 10; Records of Office of the Dean, CU-NYHSN: 1942–1983; NYWCMCA.

59. In this flexible, non-traditional program, the student was required to earn a total of 120 semester credits, including 48 nursing credits documented by standardized examinations.

60. Notes of Shirley Fondiller telephone interview with Eleanor Herrmann, 5 August 2004; NYWCMCA.

61. Ibid.

62. Eleanor Herrmann to Colleagues, CU-NYHSN, letter, 9 February 1976; box 11, folder 10; Records of Office of the Dean, CU-NYHSN: 1942–1983; NYWCMCA.

63. Eleanor Lambertsen to Eleanor Herrmann, memorandum, 4 March 1976; box 11, folder 10; Records of Office of the Dean, CU-NYHSN: 1942–1983; NYWCMCA. In August 1976, Eleanor Herrmann resigned from the CU-NYHSN to accept a new position on the faculty of Yale University School of Nursing.

64. Notes of Shirley H. Fondiller interview with Eleanor Herrmann via telephone communication, 5 August 2004; NYWCMCA.

65. Minutes, Board of Governors, NYH, 4 June 1974; NYWCMCA.

66. Minutes, Board of Governors, NYH, 4 March 1975; NYWCMCA.

67. Ibid.

68. Minutes, Faculty, CU-NYHSN, 10 April 1973; NYWCMCA.

69. Minutes, Faculty, CU-NYHSN, 28 August 1973; NYWCMCA.

70. Ibid.

71. Minutes, Faculty, CU-NYHSN, 1 October 1973; NYWCMCA.

72. Annual Report, Dean, CU-NYHSN, 1976, 3; NYWCMCA.

73. Report of National League for Nursing Site Visit, 19–20 November 1974, in Minutes, Faculty, CU-NYHSN, folder: 1975/76; NYWCMCA.

74. Ibid.

75. Ibid.

76. Ibid.

77. Ibid.

78. Ibid.

79. Ibid.

80. Minutes, Faculty, CU-NYHSN, 20 August 1975; NYWCMCA.

81. Ibid.

82. Annual Report, NYH, 1975, 12; NYWCMCA.

83. Minutes, Faculty, CU-NYHSN, 10 February 1975; NYWCMCA.

84. Annual Report, NYH, 1975, 11–12; NYWCMCA.

85. Annual Report, NYH, 1976, 5; NYWCMCA.

86. Ibid.

87. Annual Report, NYH, 1976, 12; NYWCMCA.

88. Ibid., 14.

89. Ibid.

90. Minutes, Board of Governors, NYH, 4 May 1976; NYWCMCA.

91. Ibid.

92. Minutes, Board of Governors, NYH, 10 October 1976; NYWCMCA.

93. Annual Report, Dean, CU-NYHSN, 1976, 4; NYWCMCA.
94. Ibid.
95. Proceedings, Executive Committee, Board of Trustees, CU, 11 May 1976; NYW-CMCA.
96. Ibid.
97. "A Third Century of Progress for The New York Hospital-Cornell Medical Center, A Statement of the Case for Support: 1975–1985," September 1975; box 9, folder 21; Records of Development Office, NYH-CMC: 1939–1979; NYWCMCA.
98. Ibid., 20.
99. "New York Hospital Starts a $200 Million Fund Drive," *The New York Times* (21 May 1976); NYWCMCA.
100. Ibid. Mayor Abraham Beame of New York made the comment.
101. "Summary of the Case for Support, Third Century Program," news release, NYH-CMC, 20 May 1976; NYWCMCA.
102. In 1970, *The Alumnae News* reported the amount of $245,205.20. With the addition of $85,501 from the Fund for Medical Progress and the School's alumnae, the endowment reached the figure of $330,774.29. See *The Alumnae News*, Vol. 39, No 1 (1970); NYWCMCA.

CHAPTER 14

1. Minutes, Board of Governors, NYH, 5 April 1977; NYWCMCA.
2. Proceedings, Board of Trustees, CU, 28–29 January 1977; NYWCMCA.
3. Dale R. Corson, address, 5 May 1977; box 1, folder 10; Centennial Celebration Records, CU-NYHSN: 1975–1978; NYWCMCA.
4. Neil Klein to Eleanor Lambertsen, letter, 5 May 1977; box 2, folder 23; Centennial Celebration Records, CU-NYHSN: 1975–1978; NYWCMCA.
5. Anna Wolf to Reva Rubinstein, letter, 18 April 1977; box 3, folder 4; Records of Office of the Dean, CU-NYHSN: 1942–1983; NYWCMCA.
6. Virginia Dunbar to Jeanne Dorie, letter, 24 March 1977; box 3, folder 4; Records of Office of Dean, CU-NYHSN: 1942–1983; NYWCMCA.
7. *The Alumni News*, Vol., No 3 (Summer 1977), 1; NYWCMCA.
8. Eleanor Lambertsen, "A Century of Excellence," paper, 5 May 1977; box 1, folder 10; Centennial Celebration Records, CU-NYHSN: 1975–1978; NYWCMCA.
9. *The Alumni News*, Vol. 51, No. 3 (Summer 1977); NYWCMCA.
10. Minutes, Faculty, CU-NYHSN, 23 May 1977; NYWCMCA.
11. Ibid.
12. Proceedings, Executive Committee, Board of Trustees, CU, 28 May 1977; Proceedings, Board of Trustees, CU, 29 May 1977; NYWCMCA.
13. Ibid.
14. Ibid.
15. Ibid.
16. Ibid.
17. Minutes, Faculty, CU-NYHSN, 31 May 1977; NYWCMCA.
18. Minutes, Faculty, CU-NYHSN, 7 June 1977; NYWCMCA.
19. Minutes, Faculty, CU-NYHSN, 24 June 1977; NYWCMCA.
20. Minutes, Faculty, CU-NYHSN, 5 July 1977; NYWCMCA
21. Ibid.

22. Eleanor Lambertsen to Alumni, CU-NYHSN, 30 June 1977; box 2, folder 15; Records of Alumni Association, CU-NYHSN: 1889–1981; NYWCMCA.

23. Ibid.

24. Transcript of Judith Allen interview with Helen Berg, Summer 1981; NYWCMCA.

25. Jeanne Dorie to Stanley de Osborne and Robert Purcell, letter, 19 July 1977; box 2, folder 15; Records of Alumni Association, CU-NYHSN: 1889–1981; NYWCMCA.

26. Stanley de Osborne to Jeanne Dorie, letter, 19 July 1977; box 2, folder 14; Records of Alumni Association, CU-NYHSN: 1889–1981; NYWCMCA.

27. Robert Purcell to Jeanne Dorie, letter, 5 August 1977; box 2, folder 14; Records of Alumni Association, CU-NYHSN: 1889–1981; NYWCMCA.

28. Jeanne Dorie to Alumni Members, CU-NYHSN, letter, 7 July 1977; box 2, folder 15; Records of Alumni Association, CU-NYHSN: 1889–1981; NYWCMCA.

29. Eleanor Lambertsen, Progress Report on Termination of Baccalaureate Programs, 15 July 1977; box 2, folder 15; Records of Alumni Association, CU-NYHSN: 1889–1981; NYWCMCA. At the time, the Department of Medicine of the Hospital protested the closing of the School of Nursing.

30. Minutes, Faculty, CU-NYHSN, 30 August 1977; NYWCMCA. See "Little Time to Celebrate," *Cornell Alumni News* (September 1977); NYWCMCA.

31. Minutes, Faculty, CU-NYHSN, 30 August 1977; NYWCMCA.

32. Annual Report, NYH, 1977, 8; NYWCMCA.

33. Eleanor C. Lambertsen to Frank Rhodes, letter, 29 August 1977; box 3, folder 1; Records of Office of the Dean (addendum): 1942–1983; NYWCMCA.

34. Minutes, Faculty, CU-NYHSN, 30 August 1977; NYWCMCA.

35. Ibid.

36. Minutes, Faculty, CU-NYHSN, 6 September 1977; NYWCMCA.

37. Ibid.

38. President's Committee to Evaluate the Possibility of Developing a Master's Level Graduate Program in Nursing, report, 11 October 1977; box 5, folder 14; Records of Office of the Dean, CU-NYHSN (addendum): 1942–1983; NYWCMCA.

39. President's Committee to Review the Possibility of Developing a Master's Level Graduate Program in Nursing, report, 1 May 1978; box 5, folder 14; Records of Office of the Dean, CU-NYHSN (addendum): 1942–1983; NYWCMCA.

40. Eleanor Lambertsen to Dorothy Ozimek, letter, 11 November 1977; box 6, folder 7; Records of Office of the Dean, CU-NYHSN: 1942–1983; NYWCMCA.

41. Ibid.

42. "Statement to the President's Ad Hoc Committee to Examine the Feasibility of a Master's Entry Level Program in Nursing within Cornell University," 15 December 1977, attached to Minutes, Faculty, CU-NYHSN, 16 January 1978; NYWCMCA.

43. Annual Report, NYH, 1977, 5–6; NYWCMCA.

44. Ibid.

45. Ibid.

46. Minutes, Faculty, CU-NYHSN, 13 March 1978; NYWCMCA.

47. Ibid.

48. Minutes, Faculty, CU-NYHSN, 17 April 1978; NYWCMCA.

49. Ibid.

50. Alison Casarett to Eleanor C. Lambertsen, letter, 28 April 1978; box 5, folder 14;

Records of Office of the Dean, CU-NYHSN (addendum): 1942–1983; NYWCM-CA.

51. Statement of Summary Recommendations, April 1978; box 5, folder 14; Records of Office of the Dean, CU-NYHSN (addendum) 1942–1983; NYWCMCA.

52. Ad Hoc Committee to President, CU, report, 1 May 1978; box 5, folder 14; Records of Office of the Dean, CU-NYHSN (addendum): 1942–1983; NYWCM-CA.

53. Ibid.

54. Ibid.

55. Minutes, Faculty, CU-NYHSN, 22 May 1978; NYWCMCA.

56. Minutes, Faculty, CU-NYHSN, 6 June 1978; NYWCMCA.

57. Minutes, Faculty, CU-NYHSN, 20 June 1978, NYWCMCA.

58. Evelyn Gioiella to Frank Rhodes, letter, 4 August 1978; box 1, folder 3; Records of Assistant Executive Director, Nursing Education, NYH: 1932–1985; NYWCM-CA.

59. Frank Rhodes to Evelyn Gioiella, letter, 14 August 1978; box 1, folder 3; Records of Assistant Executive Director, Nursing Education, NYH: 1932–1985; NYWCM-CA.

60. Frank Rhodes to Eleanor C. Lambertsen, letter, 25 October 1978; box 1, folder 3; Records of Assistant Executive Director, Nursing Education, NYH: 1932–1985; NYWCMCA.

61. Minutes of Faculty, CU-NYHSN, 13 November 1978; NYWCMCA.

62. Ibid.

63. Minutes of Faculty, CU-NYHSN, 12 February 1979; NYWCMCA.

64. Special Committee to Consider the Role of College of Human Ecology in the Health Field, CU, report, 2 March 1979; box 5, folder 2; Records of Office of the Dean, CU-NYHSN: 1942–1983; NYWCMCA.

65. Ibid.

66. Ibid.

67. Ibid.

68. Minutes, Executive Committee, Board of Governors, NYH, 3 April 1979; NYW-CMCA.

69. Jerome Ziegler to Frank Rhodes, letter, 16 April 1979; box 5, folder 2; Records of Office of the Dean, CU-NYHSN: 1942–1983; NYWCMCA.

70. Frank Rhodes to Jerome Ziegler, letter, 20 April 1979; box 5, folder 2: Records of Office of the Dean, CU-NYHSN: 1942–1983; NYWCMCA.

71. Jerome Ziegler to Frank Rhodes, letter, 16 April 1979; box 5, folder 2; Records of Office of the Dean, CU-NYHSN: 1942–1983; NYWCMCA.

72. Ibid.

73. Minutes, Council, CU-NYHSN, 6 January 1942; NYWCMCA.

74. Eleanor Lambertsen to William Herbster, memorandum, 6 July 1977; box 3, folder 2; Records of Office of the Dean, CU-NYHSN (addendum): 1942–1983; NYW-CMCA.

75. Ibid.

76. Eleanor Lambertsen to Thomas Martin, memorandum, 27 March 1979; box 10, folder 16; Records of Office of the Dean, CU-NYHSN: 1942–1983; NYWCMCA.

77. Gregory Meredith to Mr. Christaldi, memorandum, 9 April 1979, 10 pp.; box 10, folder 16; Records of Office of the Dean, CU-NYHSN: 1942–1983; NYWCMCA.

78. Ibid., 2.
79. Ibid., 3–5.
80. Ibid., 5–7.
81. Judith Cummings, "Last Class Leaves Cornell Nursing School," *The New York Times* (24 May 1979); NYWCMCA.
82. Ibid.
83. Minutes, Faculty, CU-NYHSN, 14 May 1979; NYWCMCA.
84. Ibid.
85. Judith Cummings, "Last Class Leaves Cornell Nursing School."
86. Ibid.
87. Ibid.
88. Ibid.
89. Frank Rhodes to Eleanor Lambertsen, letter, 30 May 1979; box 1, folder 3; Records of Assistant Executive Director, Nursing Education, NYH: 1932–1985; NYWCMCA.
90. Ibid.
91. Eleanor Lambertsen to Frank Rhodes, memorandum, 31 October 1979; box 5, folder 2; Records of Office of the Dean, CU-NYHSN: 1942–1983; NYWCMCA.
92. Ibid.
93. Ibid.
94. Minutes, Board of Governors, NYH; 8 January 1980; NYWCMCA.
95. Minutes, Alumni Association, CU-NYHSN, 5 May 1984; NYWCMCA.
96. Fran A'Hern Smith, "A Feasibility Study to Assess the Possibility of Establishing a Master's Degree Program in Nursing," April 1980; box 5, folder 15; Records of the Office of the Dean, CU-NYHSN (addendum): 1942–1983; NYWCMCA.
97. Ibid.
98. Ibid., 1.
99. Ibid., 10.
100. Ibid., 13.
101. Ibid., 14.
102. Ibid.
103. Notes of Shirley H. Fondiller telephone interview with Jerome Ziegler, 29 May 2003, and e-mail communication, 7 June 2003; NYWCMCA.
104. Ibid. Professor Ziegler regretted that Cornell's hopes for a master's program in nursing in the College of Human Ecology did not reach fruition, but neither did the proposed master's program in public health. Some reorganization at the University occurred, however, when the program on health administration relocated from the Business College to the College of Human Ecology.
105. The Window, Vol. 2, No. 1 (February–March 1982); NYWCMCA.
106. Ibid.
107. "News of NYH-CMC," *CUMC Alumni Quarterly*, Vol. 46, No. 3 (1983), 27; NYWCMCA.

Bibliography

Special Collections

Archive of the New York Weill Cornell Medical Center, New York, New York. Reports, minutes, official documents, letters and memoranda, proceedings, speeches, newsletters, class records, historical scrapbooks, faculty publications, records of special events and anniversaries, selected documents of Cornell University Medical College and Cornell's Board of Trustees, and histories of The New York Hospital and Cornell University. Also includes individual collections of graduates of the Training School and the Cornell University-New York Hospital School of Nursing, Alumni Association, transcripts of audiotaped interviews, and selected E-mails.

Archive of the American Nurses Association, New York, New York, and Kansas City, Missouri. Reports, minutes, official documents, publications, correspondence, proceedings of ANA Conventions, and assorted memorabilia.

Archive of the National League of Nursing Education, New York, New York. Reports, minutes, letters, proceedings of the conventions of the American Society of Superintendents of Training Schools for Nurses and the NLNE, official statements, and speeches. Microfilm rolls #3–#5.

Archive of the National League for Nursing, New York, New York. Correspondence with the CU-NYHSN, minutes of NLN Board of Directors and committee meetings, policy statements, curriculum conferences, consultations, accreditation reports, and publications.

Barnard College Library, New York, New York. Rare books.

The New York Academy of Medicine, Rare Books Room, New York, New York. Rare books, manuscripts, and historical collections.

Documentary Material

Brown, Esther Lucile. *Nursing for the Future. A Report Prepared for the National Nursing Council.* New York: Russell Sage Foundation, 1948.

Burgess, Mary Ann. *Nurses, Patients and Pocketbooks.* New York: Committee on the Grading of Nursing Schools, 1928.

Committee on the Grading of Nursing Schools. *Nursing Schools Today and Tomorrow.* New York: National League of Nursing Education, 1934.

Cunningham, Elizabeth. *The School Improvement Program of the National League for Nursing, 1951–1961.* New York: National League for Nursing, 1963.

Flexner, Abraham. *Medical Education in the United States and Canada.* Boston: Marymount Press, 1910.

Johns, Ethel and Pfefferkorn, Blanche. *An Activity Analysis of Nursing.* New York: Committee on the Grading of Nursing Schools, 1934.

National League for Nursing. *Proceedings—Open Curriculum Conference—*A project of the NLN study of the open curriculum in nursing education, November 27–29, 1973. New York: NLN, 1973.

_____*Report on Associate Degree Program in Nursing.* New York: NLN, 1961.

National League of Nursing Education. *Curriculum Guide for Schools of Nursing.* New York: NLNE, 1937.

_____*Standard Curriculum for Schools of Nursing.* Baltimore: Waverly Press, 1917.

Nursing and Nursing Education in the United States. Report of the Committee for the Study of Nursing Education. New York: The Macmillan Company, 1923.

West, Margaret and Hawkins, Christy. *Nursing Schools at the Mid-century.* New York: National Committee for the Improvement of Nursing Service, 1950.

Monographs and General Works

Abbott, Edith. *Some American Pioneers in Social Welfare: Selective Documents with Editorial Notes.* Chicago: University of Chicago Press, 1937.

American Nurses Association. *Educational Preparation for Nurse Practitioners and Assistants to Nurses: A Position Paper.* New York: ANA, 1965.

_____*Facts About Nursing, 1970–71.* New York: ANA, 1971.

Anderson, Bernice. Nursing Education in Community Junior Colleges. Philadelphia: J.P. Lippincott Company, 1966.

_____*The Facilitation of the Interstate Movement of Registered Nurses.* Philadelphia: J.P. Lippincott Company, 1959.

Bastable, Susan. "Recruitment of Students into Basic Nursing Education Programs in the United States, 1893–1949: A Historical Survey." EdD Dissertation, Teachers College, Columbia University, 1979. University Microfilms International, catalog number: 8006788.

Beard, Richard Olding. "The University Education of the Nurse." Paper presented at the Fifteenth Annual Convention of the American Society of Training Schools for Nurses, 1909.

Birnbach, Nettie. "The Genesis of the Nurse Registration Movement in the United States, 1893–1903." EdD Dissertation. Teachers College, Columbia University, 1982. University Microfilms International, catalog number: 8313393.

Birnbach, Nettie and Lewenson, Sandra, Editors. *First Words: Selected Addresses from the National League for Nursing.* New York: National League for Nursing Press, 1991.

Birnbach, Nettie and Lewenson, Sandra, Editors. *Legacy of Leadership.* New York: National League for Nursing Press, 1993.

Bishop, Morris. *A History of Cornell University.* Ithaca, New York: Cornell University Press, 1962.

Bridgman, Margaret. *Collegiate Education for Nursing.* New York: Russell Sage Foundation, 1953.

Brown, Raymond Shiland. *The New York Hospital in France: Base Hospital Number Nine AEF. A History of the Work of the New York Hospital Unit During Two Years of Active Service*. New York: Privately Published.

Bullough, Vern L. and Sentz, Lilli, Editors. *American Nursing—A Biographical Dictionary*, Volume 3. New York: Springer Publishing Company, 1992.

Carnegie, M. Elizabeth. *The Path We Tread*. New York: National League for Nursing Press, 1995.

Christy, Teresa E. *Cornerstone for Nursing Education*. New York: Teachers College Press, 1969.

Connors, Helen V. *Laws Regulating the Practice of Nursing*. Lexington, Kentucky: State Governments, 1967.

Conway, Jill K. *The Female Experience in Eighteenth–Nineteenth Century America: A Guide to the History of Women*. New York: Garland Publishing, 1982.

Cumming, Kate. *The Journal of a Confederate Nurse*. Baton Rouge, Louisiana: State Press, 1959.

Fitzpatrick, M. Louise. *The National Organization for Public Health Nursing, 1912–1952: Development of a Practice Field*. New York: National League for Nursing.

Flanagan, Lyndia. *One Strong Voice—The Story of the American Nurses Association*. Kansas City, Missouri: American Nurses Association.

Fondiller, Shirley H. *The Vision and the Reality—A History of AACN's First 20 Years*. Washington, DC: American Association of Colleges of Nursing, 1989.

Harrrar, James A. *Story of the Lying-In Hospital*. New York: The Society of the Lying-In Hospital, 1938.

Healing at Home: Visiting Nurse Service of New York. New York: Visiting Nurse Service of New York, 1993.

Hector, Winifred. *The Work of Mrs. Bedford Fenwick and the Rise of Professional Nursing*. London: The Royal College of Nursing and National Council of Nurses of the United Kingdom, 1970.

Hirsch, Joseph and Doherty, Beka. *The First Hundred Years of the Mount Sinai Hospital of New York*. New York: Random House, 1952.

Jordan, Helene Jamieson. *Cornell University-New York Hospital School of Nursing, 1877–1952*. New York: The Society of The New York Hospital, 1952

Kalisch, Beatrice and Kalisch, Philip. *The Advance of American Nursing*. Boston: Little, Brown and Company, 1978.

Kammen, Carol. *Cornell—Glorious to View*. Ithaca, New York: Cornell University Library, 2003.

Kaufman, Burton L. *The Korean Conflict*. Westport, Connecticut: Greenwood Press, 1999.

Kaufman, Martin, Galishoff, Stuart, and Savitt, Todd L., Editors. *Dictionary of American Medical Biography*. Two volumes. Westport, Connecticut: Greenwood Press, 1984.

Kaufman, Martin, Editor-in-Chief, *Dictionary of American Nursing Biography*. New York: Greenwood Press, 1988.

Larrabee, Eric. *The Benevolent and Necessary Institution—The New York Hospital, 1771–1971*. New York: Doubleday and Company, 1971.

MacDonald, Gwendoline. *Development of Standards and Accreditation in Collegiate Nursing Education*. New York: Teachers College Press, 1965.

Macgregor, Frances. *Social Science in Nursing: Applications for the Improvement of Patient Care*. New York: Russell Sage Foundation, 1960.

Meigs, C. L. *The Invincible Louisa*. Boston: Little, Brown and Company, 1968.

Montag, Mildred, *The Education of the Nursing Technician*. New York: G. Putnam's Sons, 1951.

Mottus, Jane L. "New York Nightingales: The Emergence of the Nursing Profession at Bellevue and New York Hospital, 1850–1920." Ph.D. Dissertation, New York University, 1980. University Microfilms International, catalog number 8017582.

Mullane, Mary K. *The Future of Professional Nurse Education*. New York: American Nurses Association. 1964.

National Commission for the Study of Nursing and Nursing Education. *An Abstract for Action*. New York: McGraw-Hill Book Company, 1970.

Numbers, Ronald. and Leavittt, Judith, Editors. *Readings on the History of Medicine and Public Health*. Madison Wisconsin: QWI Press, 1978.

Opdycke, Sandra. *No One Was Turned Away—The Role of Public Hospitals in New York City Since 1900*. New York: Oxford Press, 1999.

Piemonte, Robert. "A History of the National League of Nursing Education: Great Awakening in Nursing Education 1912–1952" EdD Dissertation, Teachers College, Columbia University, 1976. University Microfilms International, catalog number 7617291.

Poole, Ernest. *Nurses on Horseback*. New York: The Macmillan Company, 1932.

Red, George P. *The Medicine Man in Texas*. Houston, Texas: Standard Printing Company, 1930.

Report of the National Advisory Commission on Manpower. Washington, DC: U.S. Government Printing Office, 1967

Roberts, Mary M. *American Nursing—History and Interpretation*. New York: The Macmillan Company, 1954.

Reverby, Susan and Rosner, David. *Health Care in American Life*. Philadelphia: Temple University Press, 1979.

Robinson, G. Canby. *Adventures in Medical Education*. Boston: Harvard Press, 1957.

Robinson, Thelma M. and Perry, Paulie M. *Cadet Nurse Stories*. Indianapolis, Indiana: Sigma Theta Tau International, 2001.

Siegel, Beatrice. *Lillian Walld of Henry Street*. New York: The Macmillan Company, 1983.

Stewart, William, "The Changing Challenge of Manpower." Paper presented at the Health and Welfare Council of Memphis, September 19, 1966.

Stimson, Julia. *Finding Themselves—The Letters of an American Army Nurse in a British Hospital in France*. New York: The Macmillan Company, 1920.

Thorwald, Jordan. *The Century of the Surgeon*. New York: Pantheon Press, 1956.

U.S. Department of Health, Education, and Welfare. *Extending the Scope of Nursing Practice: Report of the Secretary's Committee to Study the Extended Roles for Nurses*. Washington, DC: U.S. Government Printing Ofice, 1971.

_____*Health Professions Education Assistant Amendments – PL89-290*. Washington, DC: U.S. Government Printing Office, 1965.

_____*Public Health Traineeships for Professional Health Personnel*. Washington, DC: Bureau of State Services, 1956. Mimeographed.

_____*Toward Quality in Nursing—Needs and Goals*. Report of the Surgeon General's Consultant's Group on Nursing. Washington, DC: U.S. Government Printing Office, 1963.

U.S. Public Health Service. *Nursing Education Opportunity Grants*. Arlington, Virginia: Department of Health, Education, and Welfare, 1963

Wald, Lillian. *Windows on Henry Street*. Boston, Little, Brown and Company, 1937.

_____*The House on Henry Street*. New York: Holt, 1915.

Werminghaus, Esther A. *Annie W. Goodrich: Her Journey to Yale.* New York: The Macmillan Company, 1950.

Williamson, Anne. *50 Years in Starch.* Culver City, California: Murray and Gee, 1948.

Articles in the Periodical Literature

Anonymous. "Hospital Life in New York," *Harper's New Monthly Magazine* (July 1878).

Beard, Richard Olding. "Hospital Economics of the Nursing Situation," *Modern Hospital* 21 (October 1923): 394.

"Community Health Nurses Issue HMO Statement," *American Journal of Nursing* 73 (November 1973): 1925.

Cummings, Judith. "Last Class Leaves Cornell Nursing School," *The New York Times* (24 May 1979).

Fischer, Muriel. "Nurses Lose Control of Two B's," *New York World Telegram and Sun* (8 February 1951).

Ford, Loretta. "Reaffirmation of the Nurse Practitioner Movement," *The American Nurse* 10 (15 June 1978): 4

Geister, Janet. "One Organization—Why?" *American Association of Industrial Nurses Journal* (March 1959).

Hamelin, Robert. "The Role of Voluntary Agencies in Meeting the Health Needs of Americans," *Annals of American Academy of Political and Social Science* 337 (September 1961): 93–102.

"Junior College Directory, 1960," *Junior College Journal* (January 1960): 274–306.

Kalisch, Beatrice and Kalisch, Philip. "Cadet Nurse: The Girl with a Future," *Nursing Outlook* 21 (July 1973): 444–449.

Kalisch, Philip. "Heroes of '98: Female Army Nurses in the Spanish American War," *Nursing Research* 24 (November–December 1975): 410–425.

Keyes, Jessie M. "Present Day Opportunities," *American Journal of Nursing* 11 (February 1911): 46.

Knowles, John H. "The Hospital," *Scientific American* 229 (September 1973): 128–137.

Leone, Lucile Petry. "National Nursing Needs—A Challenge to Education," *Nursing Outlook* 1 (November 1953): 616–619.

"Life, Liberty and the Right to Health Care," *The American Nurse* 8 (15 September 1976): 4.

MacDonald, Gwendoline. "Baccalaureate Education for Graduates of Diploma and Associate Degree Programs," *Nursing Outlook* 23 (June 1964): 52–56.

McGuire, S. H. and Conrad, D. W. "Postwar Plans of Army and Navy Nurses," *American Journal of Nursing* 45 (September 1945): 683.

"NLN Designated as Accrediting Body for the Nurse Training Act," *Nursing Outlook* 12 (December 1964): 8–10.

Newton, Mildred E. "Nurses Caps and Bachelor Gowns, " *American Journal of Nursing* 64 (May 1964): 73–77.

"New York Hospital Starts a $200 Million Fund Drive," *The New York Times* (21 May 1976).

"NYSNA Board of Directors Endorse Eleanor C. Lambertsen," *The Journal of the New York State Nurses Association*, Volume I (Spring 1970): 4.

"Oliver H. Payne Gives $1,500,000 to Form a Medical College," *The New York Herald* (September 1898).

Roberts, Mary. "The Social Security Act and the Nurse," *American Journal of Nursing* 36 (December 1936): 155.

Schlotfeldt, Rozella and MacPhail, Janetta. "Experiment in Nursing," *American Journal of Nursing* 69 (July 1969): 1475–1480.

Shannon, M. L. "Our First Four Licensure Laws," *American Journal of Nursing* 75 (August 1975): 1329.

Sheahan, Marion. "The Health Needs of the Nation," *Nursing Outlook* 1 (March 1953): 156–157.

"The Cornell University-New York Hospital School of Nursing: A Report on a Problem of Notice and Academic Freedom," *AAUP Bulletin* (Winter 1970): 387–390.

Tatum, Julien Rundell. "Changing Roles of Professional Personnel in the Field of Medical Care," *Nursing Outlook* 1 (December 1953): 694–696.

Subject Index

Name Index

Adams, Polly, 144
Addams, Jane, 33
Alcott, Louisa May, 4
Allen, Lucile, 108
Anderson, Lydia E., 61, 65
Anthony, Susan B., 3
Argondizzo, Nina, 191, 197
Aufhauser, Trude, 165

Baker, George F., 37, 64
Baker Jr., R. Palmer, 170
Barr, David P., 112, 128
Barton, Clara, 4, 17, 39
Bayne-Jones, Stanhope, 115, 119–121,
    129–130, 162
Beard, Mary, 18, 45, 60–61, 65, 67, 69,
    81, 87, 108–109
Belcher, Helen, 144
Belmont, Mrs. August, 115
Berg, Helen, 159, 171, 180
Bergstrom, Flora Jo, 113
Bird, Alice, 17
Bolton, Frances, 160
Bower, Ralph F., 93
Bradshaw, Fannie, 78
Breckinridge, Mary, 57–58
Brennan, Agnes, 29
Brewster, Mary, 16, 32
Bridgman, Margaret, 125
Brinker, Dorothy, 150
Brown, Eliza W., 10–11
Brown, Esther Lucile, 115–117, 136
Brown, Raymond, 52
Brown, Tozier, 159, 161

Buchanan, Robert, 185
Bundy, MacGeorge, 180
Bunge, Helen, 127
Burgess, May, 116

Cady, Louise Lincoln, 113
Carbery, Muriel, 93, 109, 129, 137,
    141–149, 153, 158–162, 164–165,
    167–171, 174–176, 178–181, 190–191,
    195, 204, 227, 230, 232
Casarett, Alison, 208, 210–211
Cooper, Theodore, 214
Cornell, Ezra, 5–6, 75
Cornell III, Ezra, 204
Corson, Dale, 173–174, 193, 199, 201,
    203, 205, 218
Curtis, James, 208

Danielson, Edna, 196
Davis, Carolyn, 208
Day, Edmund Ezra, 75, 80–81, 83–84,
    87–88, 91, 96, 98, 100–102, 109,
    118–119
de Roulet, Mrs. Vincent, 202
Dericks, Virginia, 151–152
Derrell, Constance, 108
Dines, Alta E., 93
Dix, Dorothea Lynde, 3–4
Doane, Marion, 221
DonDero, Alice, 191
Dorie, Jeanne, 197, 206
Dubois, Eugene, 69, 84
Dunbar, Virginia Matthews, 101–105,
    107–108, 110, 112–120, 125–134, 136,